A Handbook for the Sheep Clinician

8th Edition

Dedication

To the memory of Michael Clarkson and Bill Faull who started it all in 1983, and to the many sheep keepers and veterinary surgeons who have generously shared their time and knowledge over the last 40 years.

A Handbook for the Sheep Clinician

8th Edition

Agnes C. Winter and Dai Grove-White

School of Veterinary Science,
University of Liverpool,
UK

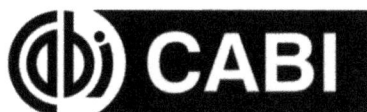

CABI

CABI is a trading name of CAB International

CABI
Nosworthy Way
Wallingford
Oxfordshire OX10 8DE
UK

CABI
200 Portland Street
Boston
MA 02114
USA

Tel: +44 (0)1491 832111
E-mail: info@cabi.org
Website: www.cabi.org

Tel: +1 (617)682-9015
E-mail: cabi-nao@cabi.org

The views expressed in this publication are those of the author(s) and do not necessarily represent those of, and should not be attributed to, CAB International (CABI). Any images, figures and tables not otherwise attributed are the author(s)' own. References to internet websites (URLs) were accurate at the time of writing.

CAB International and, where different, the copyright owner shall not be liable for technical or other errors or omissions contained herein. The information is supplied without obligation and on the understanding that any person who acts upon it, or otherwise changes their position in reliance thereon, does so entirely at their own risk. Information supplied is neither intended nor implied to be a substitute for professional advice. The reader/user accepts all risks and responsibility for losses, damages, costs and other consequences resulting directly or indirectly from using this information.

CABI's Terms and Conditions, including its full disclaimer, may be found at https://www.cabi.org/terms-and-conditions/.

A catalogue record for this book is available from the British Library, London, UK.

ISBN-13: 9781800626331 (paperback)
        9781800626348 (ePDF)
        9781800626355 (ePub)

DOI: 10.1079/9781800626355.0000

Commissioning Editor: Alexandra Lainsbury
Editorial Assistant: Helen Elliott
Production Editor: Shankari Wilford

Typeset by Straive, Pondicherry, India

Contents

About the Editors

Agnes Winter grew up on a small family farm in the Yorkshire Dales. After graduating from the University of Liverpool Veterinary School in 1965 she worked in mixed practice in north Wales concentrating on farm animal work. With her Welsh farmer husband she kept a flock of sheep, further developing her interest, skills and knowledge of the species. After some years she returned to Liverpool Veterinary School to undertake a PhD supervised by the late Professor Michael Clarkson, with whom she co-authored several previous editions of this book. Along the way she obtained several specialist qualifications in sheep health and disease. The rest of her career was spent at this vet school where she finished her academic career as Head of the Department of Veterinary Clinical Science, becoming an Honorary Professor on retirement. She is a past President of the Sheep Veterinary Society and has received several prestigious awards for her contributions to the sheep industry.

Agnes C. Winter BVSc, PHD, DSHP, DipECSRHM, FRAgS, FRCVS
Honorary Professor, School of Veterinary Science, University of Liverpool
Email: a.winter@liverpool.ac.uk

Dai Grove-White graduated from the University of Liverpool in 1975. Following a period of working overseas in the Middle East and Africa, he worked in Bala, North Wales in primarily beef and sheep practice. Whilst in practice he carried out research on acid base balance and fluid therapy in calves for which he was awarded FRCVS in 1997. In 2000 he returned to the University of Liverpool as a member of academic staff. He gained an MSc in Veterinary Epidemiology in 2005 and was awarded a PhD in 2008 for work on the molecular epidemiology of *Campylobacter* spp in ruminants. In addition to undergraduate and postgraduate teaching, he was active in research in the fields of dairy calf nutrition, equine obesity and sheep lameness. From 2012 until his retirement in 2019, he was Head of the Department of Livestock Health and Welfare. In his retirement, he keeps a small flock of sheep and is an Associate Editor for a well established veterinary journal in addition to carrying out peer review for a number of journals.

Dai Grove-White BVSc MSc(epi) DBR DipECBHM PhD FRCVS
Department of Livestock and One Health, Institute of Infection, Veterinary and Ecological Sciences, University of Liverpool, Leahurst Campus, Neston, Wirral, CH64 7TE
Email: daigw@liverpool.ac.uk

Contributors

All contributors to the 8th edition are from the Department of Livestock and One Health, Institute of Infection, Veterinary and Ecological Sciences, University Liverpool.

Dr Joseph Angell BVSc MSc DipLSHTM PhD MRCVS
(also of Wern Vets CYF, North Wales)
Email: joseph@wernvets.co.uk
ORCID ID: 0000-0002-3684-0277

Niall Connolly BSc BVSc Cert AVP FHEA MRCVS
Email: conno11y@liverpool.ac.uk
ORCID ID: 0009-0007-1019-7811

Dr Peers Davies MA VetMB PhD MRCVS
Email: Peers.Davies@liverpool.ac.uk
ORCID ID: 0000-0001-6085-9763

Professor Jennifer Duncan BVM&S, BSc. Hons, Dip. ECSRHM, Dip.VEPH, PhD, SFHEA, MRCVS
Email: jsduncan@liverpool.ac.uk
ORCID ID: 0000-0002-1370-3085

Dr Emma Fishbourne BSc (Hons), BVSc, PhD, DBR, FHEA, MRCVS
Email: emma.fishbourne@liverpool.ac.uk

Dr John Graham-Brown BVSc MSc PhD FHEA MRCVS
Email: J.Graham-Brown@liverpool.ac.uk
ORCID ID: 0000-0001-7305-5262

Dr Dai Grove-White BVSc MSc(epi) DBR DipECBHM PhD FRCVS
Email: daigw@liverpool.ac.uk
ORCID ID: 0000-0002-5969-5535

Jo Oultram BVSc CertCHP DBR SFHEA ARSM DipABRSM MRCVS
Email: joultram@liverpool.ac.uk
ORCID ID: 0000-0003-3169-1361

Professor Robert Smith BSc BVSc PhD DipECAR DipECBHM FRCVS
Email: robsmith@liverpool.ac.uk
ORCID ID: 0000-0003-0944-310X

Helen Williams BVSc CertCHP DipECBHM FHEA MRCVS
Email: he1enw@liverpool.ac.uk
ORCID ID: 0000-0003-0846-7329

Professor Agnes Winter BVSc PhD DSHP DipECSRHM FRAgS FRCVS
Email: a.winter@liverpool.ac.uk

Abbreviations

µg	micrograms
1-BZ	benzimidazoles
2-LV	levamisole
3-ML	macrocyclic lactones
4-AD	amino-acetonitrile derivatives
5-SI	spiroindoles
AFBI	Agri-Food and BioSciences Institute
AGID	agar gel immunodiffusion
AHDB	Agriculture and Horticulture Development Board
AI	artificial insemination
APHA	Animal and Plant Health Agency
BCS	Body condition score
BDV	Border Disease virus
BOHB	Beta-hydroxybutyrate
BSE	Bovine spongiform encephalopathy
BT	Bluetongue
BTV	Bluetongue virus
BVDv	Bovine Virus Diarrhoea virus
BW	Bodyweight
CAE	Caprine arthritis and encephalitis
CAP	Common Agricultural Policy
CCN	Cerebro-cortical necrosis
CK	creatine kinase
CL	corpus luteum
CLA	Caseous lymphadenitis
CNS	Central nervous system
CODD	Contagious ovine digital dermatitis
CP	Crude Protein
CPD	Continuing Professional Development
CS	Condition score [BCS]
CSF	Cerebro-spinal fluid
CT	Computed tomography scan
D value	Digestibility value
DEFRA	Department for the Environment, Food and Rural Affairs
DM	Dry matter
DMI	Dry Matter Intake
DNA	Deoxy-ribonucleic acid
DOMD	Digestible organic matter in the dry matter
EAE	Enzootic Abortion of Ewes
EBV	Estimated Breeding Value
eCG	equine chorionic gonadotrophin
EID	electronic identification
ELISA	Enzyme-linked Immunosorbent Assay

EM	electron microscopy
epg	eggs per gram
EU	European Union
FECRT	faecal egg count reduction test
FMD	foot and mouth disease
FMDV	foot and mouth disease virus
FR	Footrot
FSH	follicle stimulating hormone
FSS	Food Standards Scotland
FWEC	faecal worm egg count
GGT	Gamma glutamyl transferase
GI	gastro-intestinal
GSHPx	Glutathione Peroxidase
ID	interdigital dermatitis
IgA	Immunoglobulin A
IgG	Immunoglobulin G
IgM	Immunoglobulin M
IM	intra-muscular
iu	international units
IV	intravenous
KOH	Potassium hydroxide
LA	long-acting
LH	luteinising hormone
LPS	lipo-polysaccharide
LWG	Liveweight Gain
Ma	*Mycoplasma agalactia*
MAP	*Mycobacterium avium* subspecies *paratuberculosis*
Mcc	*M. capricolum* subsp. *capricolum*
ME	Metabolizable Energy
MJ	Megajoule
MMc	*M. mycoides* subsp. *capri*
MOET	multiple ovulation embryo transfer
Mp	*M. putrefaciens*
MRI	Magnetic resonance imaging
mRNA	messenger RNA [Ribonucleic acid]
MSD	Merck Sharp & Dohme
MV	Maedi Visna
NADIS	National Animal Disease Information Service
NOAH	National Office of Animal Health
NSA	National Sheep Association
NSAID	Non-steroidal anti-inflamatory drug
NSD	Nairobi sheep disease
OIE	Office International des Epizooties
OJD	Ovine Johne's disease
OMAGOD	Ovine mouth and gum obscure disease/idiopathic oral ulceration
OP	organophosphate
OPA	Ovine pulmonary adenocarcinoma
p.o.	*per os*
PCR	Polymerase chain reaction
PCV	Packed cell volume
PGE	parasitic gastroenteritis

PI3	Parainfluenza 3 virus
PII	Plasma Inorganic Iodine
PME	Post mortem examination
PMSG	pregnant mare serum gonadotrophin
PNA	peanut agglutinin
PPE	Personal Protective Equipment
PPR	Peste de petits ruminants
PrP	Prion protein
PT	Pregnancy toxaemia
RAMA	registered animal medicines advisors
RVF	Rift Valley fever
SBV	Schmallenberg virus
SCOPS	Sustainable Control of Parasites in Sheep
SFP	Single farm Payment
SMCO	S-methylcysteine sulfoxide
SP	synthetic pyrethroid
SPA	Sheep pulmonary adenomatosis
SRUC	Scotland's Rural University College
SVS	Sheep Veterinary Society
TB	Tuberculosis
TBD	tick-borne disease
TBF	tick-borne fever
TSE	transmissible spongiform encephalopathy
TST	Targeted selective treatment
UreaN	Urea Nitrogen
UV	Ultra-violet
VIO	Veterinary Investigation Officer
VMD	Veterinary Medicines Directorate
WAHIS	World Animal Health Information System
WOAH	World Organisation for Animal Health

Preface

It is now over 40 years since the booklet 'Notes for the Sheep Clinician', the ancestor of this book, was first produced by Professor Michael Clarkson and Mr W. B. (Bill) Faull for students in their clinical years at the University of Liverpool Veterinary School. After I returned to the Vet School in 1986, I also contributed to new editions, becoming joint author with Michael after Bill retired.

In the early 1980s Michael and Bill were developing the concept of teaching flock health, encouraging a year-round holistic veterinary input into care of sheep flocks, rather than the more common 'fire brigade' work often practised previously. Veterinary surgeons and sheep farmers soon indicated that they found the notes helpful and, because it had a green cover, it became known as the 'Liverpool Green Book'. Anecdotally, we were told of ancient copies turning up in various obscure and far-flung parts of the world. Originally published by the Liverpool University Press until 1997, it was then regularly updated internally until CABI published the 7th edition in 2012. The content of that edition was considerably expanded both in information and geographical range covered in the hope that it would be of interest in other important sheep-keeping countries.

When CABI suggested a new edition was again due I was the only surviving author. Now retired, I felt I could not undertake this task alone. I felt strongly that the book should retain its Liverpool heritage, so recruited members of the Department of Livestock and One Health to assist in updating the content; thus it is now a multi-author book. I am most grateful to my colleague Professor Jennifer Duncan for recruiting contributors as well as contributing chapters herself; to the university staff who have updated various chapters; and most of all to Dr Dai Grove-White for much help in contributing to and editing the new edition. Although parts have again been expanded in the light of new information and practices (particularly with regard to parasite control, mitigating anthelmintic and parasiticide resistance and antimicrobial resistance), we have tried to keep to the practical clinical aspects of sheep medicine without attempting to cover more unusual or uncommon conditions, or sheep kept for milk production, or details on pathology or micro-organisms which can be obtained elsewhere. One major difference now is the abundance of information on the internet, so throughout, web addresses are given for the many useful resources available on-line.

Many veterinary surgeons and farmers have contributed to the knowledge condensed into this book. Alun Davies must be acknowledged for his contribution to early editions on feeding sheep, much of which survives in this edition. The Sheep Veterinary Society has contributed enormously to the sum of knowledge on sheep keeping and diseases over the past 50 years and membership is essential for anyone with an interest in sheep and their diseases.

My sincere thanks go to my veterinary friends Judith Charnley, Fiona Lovatt and Heidi Svensgaard who have all helped with various aspects of the book and to my friend Dianna Bowles who allowed me to use the lovely photo of her Herdwicks for the cover.

Thanks to the staff of CABI, especially Alex Lainsbury (Commissioning Editor), Ali Thompson (Managing Editor), Shankari Wilford (Production Editor) and Helen Elliott (Editorial Assistant) for their help and encouragement.

Agnes Winter
March 2024

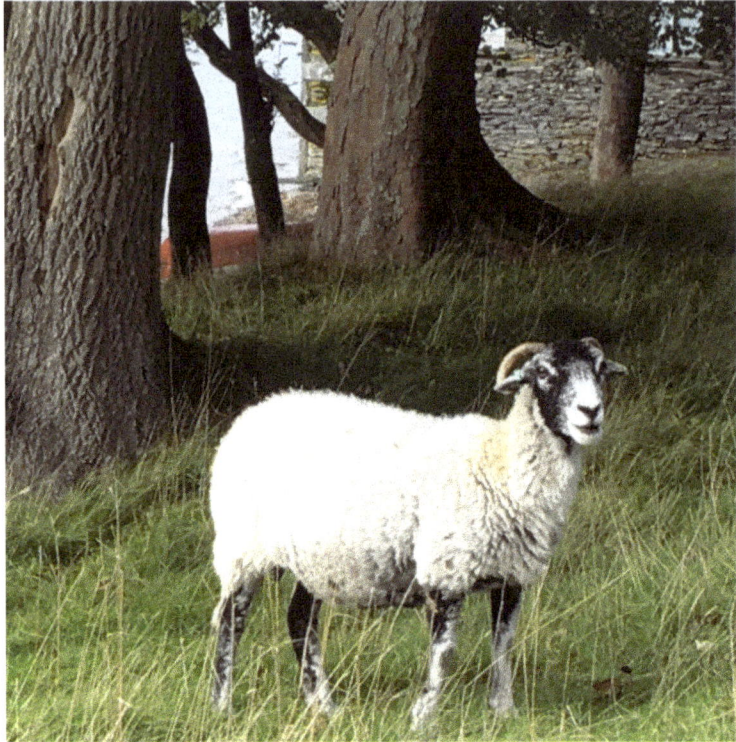

1 Production

DAI GROVE-WHITE*

Department of Livestock and One Health, Institute of Infection, Veterinary and Ecological Sciences, University of Liverpool, UK

Abstract

This first chapter covers the way in which the sheep industry is organized, particularly in the UK, with reference to those in some other countries, important breeds, and assessment of financial and physical performance of flocks including government support, if any. It also covers feeding throughout the production cycle in order to maximize performance. It mentions the effect that future policies on environmental and sustainable concerns may have on sheep-keeping and always being aware of effects on sheep welfare.

Structure of the Sheep Industry and Economics

Sheep are found in almost every country in the world and due to breeding and selection are able to live in environmental extremes, from dusty deserts and snowy peaks, with their exact management being dependent on both environmental and social factors. In many pastoral societies, their role is crucial for human survival as a source of protein and shelter. It has been estimated that there are over one billion sheep and lambs in the world with the greatest number in China, with 128 million, followed by Australia with 73 million, India with 65 million, Iran with 54 million, Sudan with 52 million and Nigeria with 35 million. New Zealand and the UK have a similar number of around 33 million. The USA has six million and Canada less than one million sheep and lambs. Considerable numbers of sheep are found in South America, especially in Argentina, Uruguay, Peru and Chile.

In the countries of the European Union (EU), Spain has a breeding flock of approximately 14 million ewes, with Greece, Italy and France having around seven million breeding ewes each. In total, the EU has about 35 million breeding ewes whilst the UK breeding ewe population is approximately 15 million.

It is important that veterinary surgeons involved in sheep work should have a working knowledge of the structure and economics of the sheep industry in their own country (Fig.1.1). This should include an appreciation of the often relatively low value of individual sheep such that individual animal-based interventions may have a minimal, neutral or even negative impact on flock profitability. This is in contrast to the way flock profitability can be improved considerably by structured veterinary advice and involvement. It is increasingly recognized that, as in other livestock enterprises, a population-based ('whole flock') approach will help maximize productivity, profitability and animal welfare. Furthermore, improving productivity by minimizing the impacts of disease will have a positive benefit in terms of reducing the carbon footprint of the enterprise, which will be of increasing importance in the future. However, there is a dilemma, with veterinary surgeons saying that farmers are not willing to pay for advice and, on the other hand, many farmers complaining that their veterinary surgeon is not willing (or possibly not able!) to provide an overall flock-based service for sheep. This service should involve more than the occasional visit to investigate an abortion outbreak, for example, or to carry out a caesarean operation on a ewe which has been brought to the surgery. The development of subscription-funded Flock Health Clubs (https://www.flockhealth.co.uk/flock-health-

*Email: daigw@liverpool.ac.uk

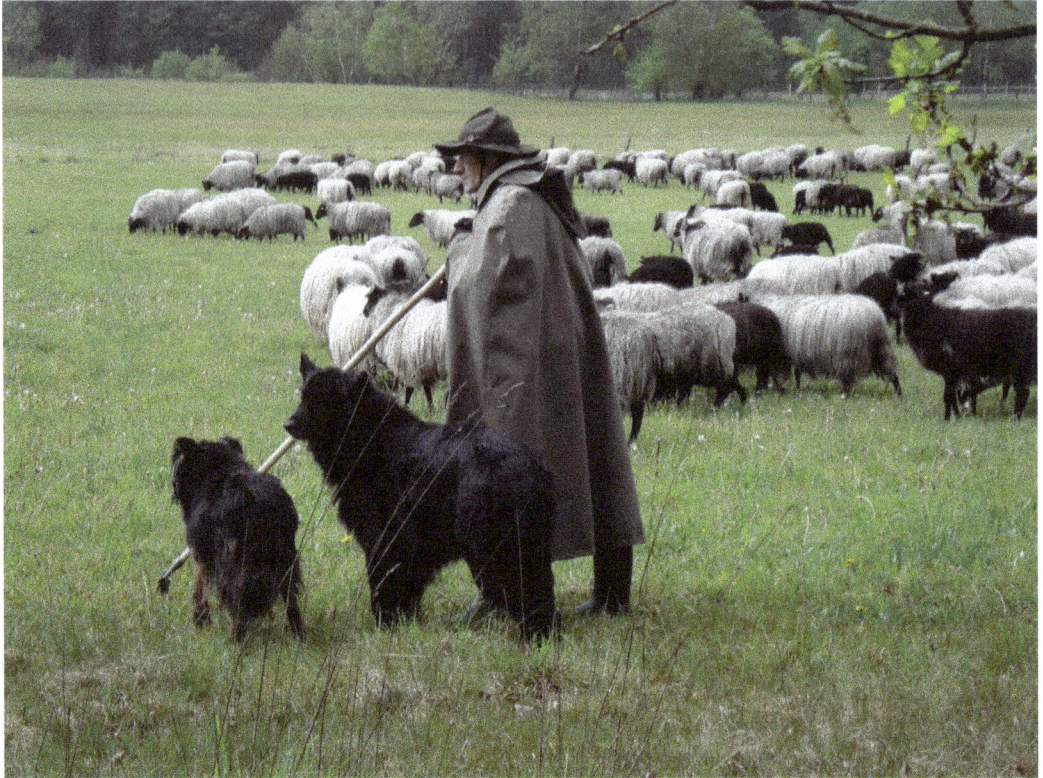

Fig. 1.1. Sheep-keeping systems vary throughout the world; this flock on German heathland is still kept in a traditional way with the shepherd staying with the sheep as they move around the grazing (photo Agnes Winter).

clubs - accessed 28/10/24) by veterinary practices offers a route whereby population-based services can be offered economically by practices to their more enthusiastic sheep clients. Flock Health Clubs offer both the farmer and veterinarian the opportunities to learn from each other and from other farmers as well as facilitation of farmer education via regular group meetings where specific topics can be discussed with invited experts where appropriate.

However, flock-based medicine requires the development of specific skills by the veterinarian and these are best learnt both by experience, and by attendance and participation at continuing professional development (CPD) meetings. Membership of organizations like the Sheep Veterinary Society (SVS, https://sheepvetsoc.org.uk - accessed 28/10/24) and the National Sheep Association (NSA, https://www.nationalsheep.org.uk - accessed 28/10/24) is essential for the successful sheep clinician who wishes to practise flock-based medicine.

Sheep are kept under a wide variety of systems which need to be understood for the clinician's own country. For example, in the UK the stratification system of hill or mountain, upland and lowland farms should be understood (see Fig. 1.2) and the physical and financial performance of a client's farm should always be considered in the context of these three strata.

Many sheep clinicians have learnt and gained 'street credibility' by keeping some sheep of their own as there is nothing that sheep farmers like talking about more than sheep! This personal involvement, even on a small scale, gives experience the production, marketing disease problems and financial constraints, which are similar on large commercial flocks.

It is also invaluable to know the main breeds of sheep and particularly those that are likely to be encountered in the area in which you work. It would be an expert who was able to identify the more than 60 breeds in the UK, but finding information about examples of the main breeds in the different layers of the stratification system is relatively easy with the aid of the internet and the excellent charts which are available from many sources such as British Wool (https://www.britishwool.org.uk - accessed 28/10/24), for example. The main hill breeds are Scottish Blackface, Welsh Mountain and Swaledale (Fig. 1.3), all of which are now bred in large numbers and can be found a long distance from their area of origin. These breeds are bred pure on the mountains for three or four lamb crops, then moved to upland farms as draft ewes where they are crossed with a ram of a long-wool breed, especially the Border or Bluefaced Leicester (Fig. 1.4.), to give the Mule or the Halfbred, which forms the breeding ewes of the lowland farms. These are then crossed with a terminal sire such as the Texel or Charollais to produce the prime lamb for slaughter. Other terminal sire breeds include Down-type breeds and the Suffolk.

The sheep industry has traditionally lagged behind the cattle industries in adoption of strategies for genetic improvement of sheep breeds. However, that is changing with the advent of commercial breeding companies such as Innovis and the uptake of recording schemes for key health and production parameters allowing the generation of estimated breeding values (EBV) to guide producers in selection of breeding stock (https://signetdata.com/technical/sheep-recording/-accessed 28/10/24).

Figures for physical and financial performance are obtainable for many sheep systems in many parts of the world, by internet searches, from flocks involved in recording schemes. These flocks are likely to be above average in their production so may act as targets to improve production by veterinary advice. In England, for example, the Agriculture and Horticulture Development Board (AHDB) produces information from its recorded flocks and divides this into the average of a particular sector and the performance of the top-third farms in that sector. In addition, they provide a 'benchmarking tool' (https://ahdb.org.uk/farmbench - accessed 28/10/24) allowing easy comparison of individual farm performance with industry standards, thereby identifying areas for possible improvement. Such tools can be invaluable for the keen sheep clinician in motivating change on their clients' farms. The main factors which distinguish the flocks in the top third of the sector

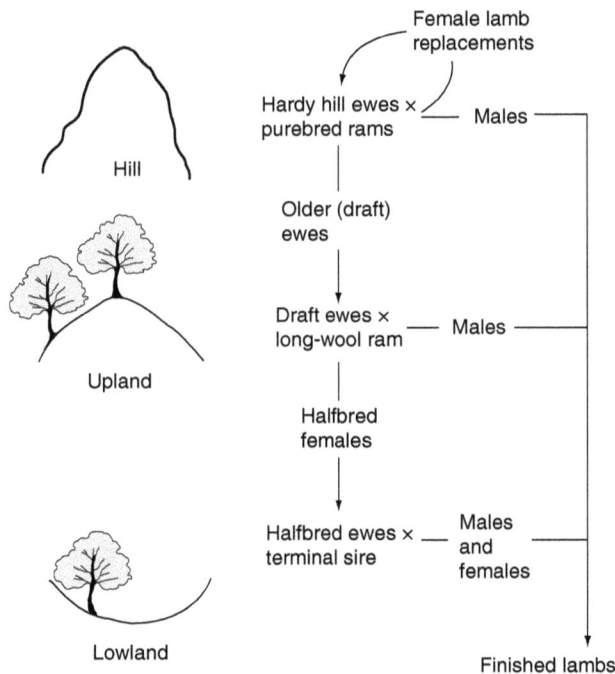

Fig. 1.2. Stratification of sheep in the UK.

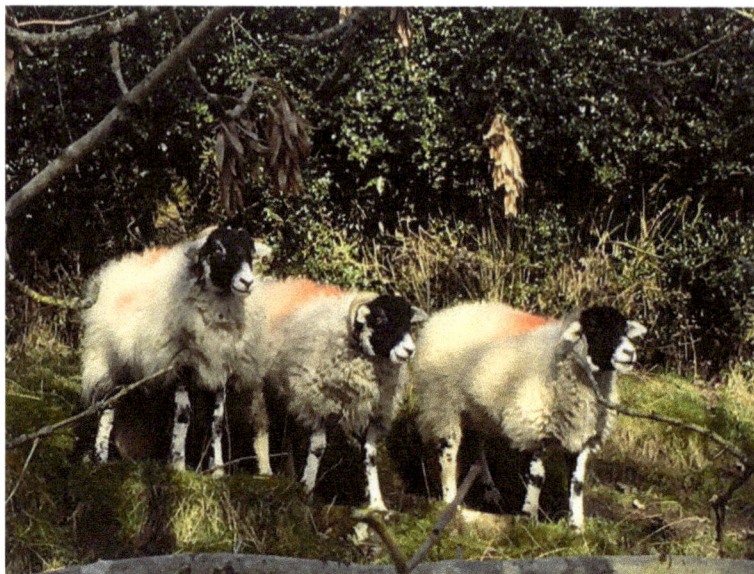

Fig 1.3. Swaledale sheep, a common hill breed (photo Agnes Winter).

are number of lambs reared and stocking density, suggesting several areas where veterinary input and the production of farm health programmes can contribute significantly to farm economics. Similar data are available for Scotland and Wales and for many other countries. Production figures are usually expressed as a quantity per 100 ewes which are put to the ram (tupped). Representative figures of lamb performance in the UK are 110 lambs per 100 ewes tupped for mountain farms, 140 for upland farms and 170 for lowland farms, with an average of 10% lamb mortality across all three systems.

While the physical performance figures have differed little over recent years, the financial information may show marked variation due to fluctuating market conditions, but up-to-date figures for the cost of cull ewes and prime lambs can be obtained online. The sheep clinician will find this information invaluable in discussions with farmers.

In many countries, including New Zealand, Australia and the USA, there are currently no government-funded support schemes for the sheep industry, but this is not the case in Europe. In the EU there is a complex and massive support mechanism for many agricultural systems, including sheep, dating back to the post-war period. The Common Agricultural Policy (CAP) of the EU originally made payments based on ewe numbers or lamb production but since 2005,

this payment, known as the Single Farm Payment (SFP) has been independent of production. However, it is likely that emphasis of funding will change with increased importance being placed on social and environmental factors. The UK left the EU in 2021 and thus left the CAP. Currently (2024), payments equivalent to the SFP are continuing but these will reduce considerably over the next few years with future monies being paid for specific environmental improvements and climate change mitigation measures. In the past, different methods have been used to calculate the SFP for England, Scotland and Wales and producers have indicated that without such support, sheep farms will be unable to continue to exist. Some estimates would suggest that removal of SFP may reduce farm income by 40–80% in some hill areas of Wales with devastating social consequences in such areas. It is likely that within all the countries of the UK, payments will continue, albeit at a lower rate, but targeted specifically at environmental management and animal welfare rather than production *per se*. It is important for the sheep clinician to understand the main features of the schemes in their local area as these may allow or demand a greater input from clinicians into flock health schemes, which may become mandatory for receipt of specific payments in the future.

Feeding Management

(This section provides general advice on feeding sheep. AHDB produces excellent guides to sheep nutrition which may be downloaded at https://ahdb.org.uk/knowledge-library - accessed 30/10/24. See Appendix 4 for a practical exercise on the specific common problem of how to assess a diet which is being fed to sheep for adequacy.)

Grass, either fresh or conserved as hay or silage, is the main and cheapest food for sheep in the UK. However, because of seasonality of grass growth coupled with its effect on quality and quantity of the crop and the varying requirements of ewes throughout the production cycle, alternative foods may be used to replace and/or supplement grass, either grazed or conserved. Supplements include simple or complex rations of cereals and protein sources and mineral supplements used when copper, cobalt and selenium concentrations are deficient in grass grown on certain soil types.

Feeding the Ram

Many rams are purchased by sheep farmers each year. These, almost invariably, will be in body condition score (BCS) 3.5–4.5 having been well fed with concentrates in preparation for sale. It is important that this concentrate feeding is continued up to mating, at no more than 400 g/day. This should minimize the effects of diet change from mainly concentrates to grass only, and at the same time prepare the rams for the mating period during which concentrate feeding of the rams only can be difficult.

Rams already on the farm should have a BCS of 3.5 (i.e. be fit not fat) 6–8 weeks prior to the beginning of mating. Overfat rams usually have reduced reproductive performance. Most rams will be in correct condition provided reasonable grazing has been available during the summer months.

If there is insufficient grass and/or rams are in poor condition, concentrates and hay will need to be provided during the premating period and possibly during the mating period itself. The amount of concentrates required will vary depending on BCS, but up to 600 g/day of a concentrate containing 160 g/kg (16%) crude protein (CP) can be provided. Proprietary ewe concentrates should be avoided, especially if large amounts are being fed, because of the high concentrations of magnesium and phosphorus which they contain, predisposing to urinary calculi. Coarse mixes of cereals, sugarbeet pulp and vegetable protein sources with a minimum addition of minerals are recommended.

Feeding the Ewe

Condition scoring is an essential guide to feeding management (see Chapter 4).

Pre-mating

The production cycle can be considered to end and start at the time of weaning. At this time, the BCS of ewes will depend not only on the amount of food which has been available but also on within-flock factors such as previous suckling load. The period from weaning to mating provides an opportunity to adjust the feeding so that ewes are in optimum condition at mating.

In lowland conditions, where high lambing percentages are expected, the BCS at mating should be 3 or 3.5 but in hill flocks, where much lower lambing percentages are required, the optimum score will normally be 2.5.

Increasing the nutrition in the 2–3 weeks pre-mating so that ewes gain 0.5 of a BCS (flushing effect) will increase ovulation rate and reproductive performance if ewes are below BCS 3. However, if ewes are in good condition, flushing has little advantage over simply maintaining ewes in condition, and there is a risk that flushing ewes already in good condition will lead to ewes becoming overfat, which may result in reduced reproductive performance.

Grass, provided it is in good supply, should meet the requirements of the ewe for maintenance and some increase in body condition. However, in late-lambing flocks in which mating takes place in late November and December, grass will need to be supplemented with concentrates and probably conserved forage also. Feed blocks and liquid molasses diets can be an alternative to concentrates and do not require to be replenished daily. The aim in these circumstances should be to have ewes in good condition 3 weeks pre-mating and then to provide a maintenance ration for them over the mating period. If conditions are very wet, windy cold, maintenance needs will increase.

Post-mating

MATING TO 42 DAYS During pregnancy, 20–25% of embryos/fetuses die and some of these deaths are caused by a combination of incorrect nutrition and handling and climatic stress, the latter especially in late-mating flocks. The aim should be to feed ewes at maintenance level or just below. Both overfeeding, with ewes gaining in weight, or significant underfeeding will increase embryo and fetal losses. Above-average losses may also be attributable to grazing low-selenium content herbage and to grazing pasture containing large amounts of red clover, although recent work casts doubt regarding the role of red clover in embryonic loss. Alternative forage crops, such as kale and rape, should also be avoided.

Low-cobalt-content herbage has also been found to have an important longer-term effect by reducing the vigour of the lamb at birth and its resistance to disease.

Grass will meet the needs of the ewes for nutrients in the post-mating period during the early part of the mating season, but in areas where cobalt and selenium are known to be deficient in herbage, providing a small amount of concentrates containing enhanced amounts of these minerals may be beneficial. It should be noted that cobalt and selenium concentrations of herbage are usually at their lowest in late summer and autumn and are most likely to be below requirements in wet seasons.

PERIOD 42–90 DAYS The fetus grows slowly throughout this period but growth of fetal membranes and the placenta is considerable, especially during the later weeks. This results in an extra energy requirement above maintenance of approximately 2 MJ/day at 90 days. However, 1 kg of loss will provide 20 MJ of metabolizable energy (ME), so the extra needs can easily be met by a small loss in ewe condition. Only severe underfeeding will reduce placental growth and hence lamb birthweight. Virtually no placental growth occurs after 90 days.

The aim should be to maintain CS in the 3–3.5 range for lowland ewes. Ewes which have been scanned to have three or more lambs should be carefully managed so that their CS does not decrease below 3–3.5, but in lowland ewes with twins and singles and in hill ewes carrying singles, some loss of condition (up to 0.5 CS) can be tolerated and will be desirable in ewes in CS 4 or above. In contrast, thin ewes and ewe lambs and shearling ewes which are still growing will need an above-maintenance ration; the ME required for 1 kg liveweight gain = 24 MJ. Grass will often not be abundant throughout the period and will have to be supplemented with conserved forage and, in some cases, concentrates or feed blocks. Medium- to good-quality hay or silage should easily meet the nutrient requirements of the ewe, so, provided these forages are available, concentrate supplementation is unnecessary.

PERIOD 90 DAYS TO LAMBING During this period, fetal growth accelerates rapidly with the fetus doubling its size in the last 4 weeks of pregnancy (Fig. 1.5). Mammary growth also occurs, especially in the final 2 weeks before lambing, when udder weight increases by more than 100%.

The net result of the above is an increasing requirement for nutrients for fetal and mammary tissue growth and development.

The appetite limitations of the ewe during this period impose considerable restrictions on ration formulation. The dry-matter intake (DMI) of an adult ewe is estimated to be 2–2.25% of bodyweight, equating to a daily DM intake of 1.5–1.8 kg for an adult ewe weighing 65–80 kg, although it declines during the last 2–3 weeks of pregnancy.

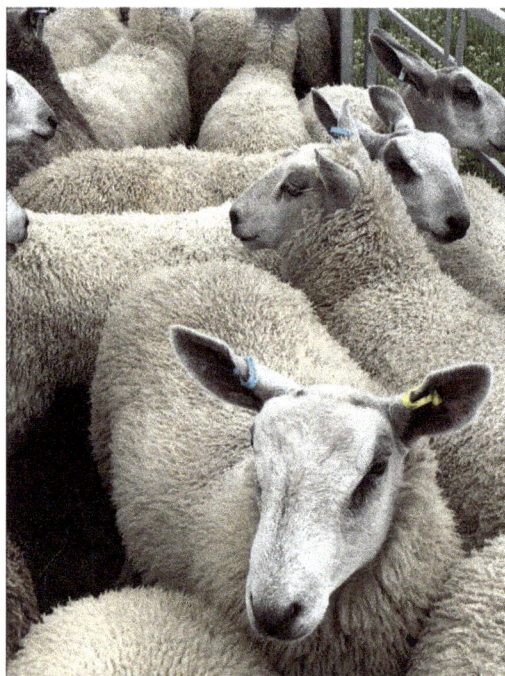

Fig 1.4. Young Bluefaced Leicester ram lambs, commonly crossed with Swaledales to create the Mule (photo Agnes Winter)

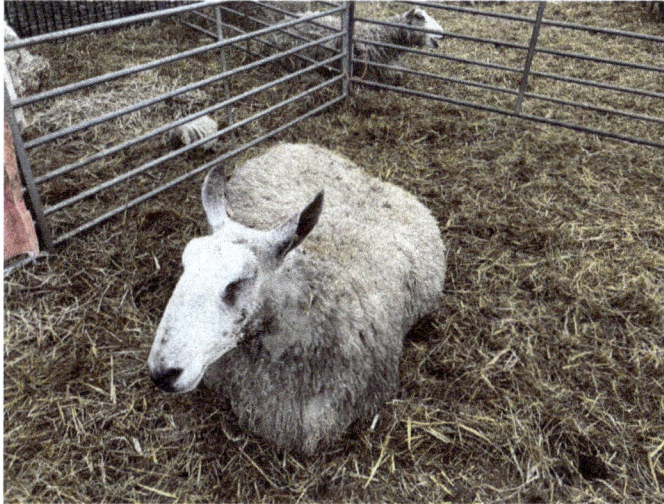

Fig. 1.5. Most of this heavily pregnant ewe's abdomen is taken up with the uterus and its contents, reducing rumen capacity (photo Agnes Winter).

This decline will depend in part on diet fed but may be up to 30%, i.e. down to 1.0–1.2 kg. The digestibility of the forage(s) and concentrates fed will also impact on appetite with higher intakes occurring with higher forage digestibilities (due to faster rumen outflow allowing more food to be consumed), thus high-quality fodder production is key to successful nutrition of the pregnant ewe. Although not widely practised, shearing of housed ewes, results in a 25% increase in DMI. It is increasingly recognized that the physical presentation of foodstuffs is critical in housed ewes thus attention should be paid to both adequacy of fodder presentation and concentrate feed barrier space (0.45 cm per ewe) together with ensuring adequate pen space (1.0–1.4 sq. m/ewe) for all ewes.

Quality of forage not only indicates feeding value but is also indicative of the likely daily intake. Hay is very variable in quality and a chemical analysis of a representative sample is recommended.

Silage usually has higher ME and CP values than hay but DM intakes are lower (approximately 90%) than those of equivalent ME value of hay. However, as a general rule, well-made silage results in better intakes than hay due to the likely higher digestibility (DOMD), and thus ME, of silage compared to hay. The intake of long material in a big bale will be 85% of precision-chopped material. Furthermore, precision-chopped silages are likely to have a better fermentation profile and consequent digestibility compared to bagged long-fibre silages.

Straws may also be used as forage. Spring barley varieties are most suitable but all cereal straws can be used.

Chemical analysis of the whole straw is not a suitable means of assessing feeding quality because in most cases the ewes only eat the 25% of the straw which is most readily consumable and has the highest feeding value. The remainder should be discarded and used as bedding. Fresh straw should be provided daily either in a rack or on the floor. In the former system, uneaten straw should be removed from the rack daily. Straw feeding value may be enhanced by treatment with a strong alkali or urea.

The body tissue of the ewe may be considered as a reservoir of nutrients which can be built up and depleted to a certain extent without adverse effects provided the depletion occurs slowly. An alternate 'flat-rate' feeding system has been devised which utilizes this fact. It is first necessary to calculate the total concentrate needs of the ewe over the period and then to provide the same daily amount throughout the period. Ewes gain weight at first and then, as lambing approaches, lose condition. Practically, this is an easy-to-operate system and it also avoids the risk of metabolic acidosis occurring when ewes are fed large amounts of concentrates in late pregnancy. Lamb birthweights are similar to those obtained when ewes are fed on the traditional increasing plane of nutrition, but, especially in young ewes, colostrum production may be somewhat reduced and there is increased possibility of hypocalcaemia. A single-step system therefore may be more appropriate with ewes fed at a first flat rate up to approximately 3 weeks pre-partum when the quality of the concentrate can be increased and then fed at a second increased flat rate until the end of pregnancy.

WATER REQUIREMENTS   Housed pregnant ewes require a daily intake of 2.5 kg water in mid-pregnancy and up to 5 kg in late pregnancy.

Lactation

Colostrum production and consumption by the lamb is crucial. Sufficient colostrum should be available to meet the passive immunity requirements and also the energy demand in the first day of life. Output to 24 h post-partum will vary from 1.5 to 3.5 kg.

In early lactation, ewes suckling singles are likely to be producing a daily average milk yield of 2 kg or more, those suckling twins 3 kg or more and those suckling triplets 4 kg or more, provided they are well fed. Maximum daily yields occur at approximately 4 weeks post-partum and will vary from 2 to 5 kg. After 4 weeks, there is a slow, steady decline in yield but ewes will still be producing 1.5–2 kg at 10 weeks after lambing.

Nutrient requirements largely reflect the milk production of the ewe. The production of 1 kg of milk requires 7.1 MJ ME and 72 g of metabolizable protein. Formulation of rations to meet these requirements is modified by a number of factors including: (i) stage of lactation; (ii) BCS of the ewe; and (iii) foods which are available.

In the immediate post-partum period, ewes are hungry and careful rationing of concentrates to avoid gorging and consequent digestive upsets is necessary. Post-lambing DM intake increases steadily up to 5–7 weeks of lactation. Despite this increase in appetite, lactation demands usually outstrip the intake and ewes usually lose condition in the first month of lactation. A loss of one CS is not uncommon and is frequently a reflection of high milk yields. Growth rate(s) of the lamb(s) are a good indicator of milk yield in the early stages of lactation. Yields may be calculated from live-weight gain by assuming the DM content of ewes' milk is 200 g/kg and the conversion ratio of milk solids to live-weight gain is 1:1.

In practice, many ewes will be at grass throughout the lactation period. It is quite likely that grass will be limited at the beginning, which results in a considerable loss in body condition. Limitation is indicated by a sward length below 4 cm and ewes spending more than 9 h/day grazing. When sward length is below 2 cm, supplementation should be given to provide almost all nutrient needs (i.e. forage and concentrates). When the sward length is 2–3 cm, concentrates can provide approximately half of nutrient needs.

Concentrate feeding is also a vehicle by which magnesium can be made available to the ewe. An intake of 6 g/day of calcined magnesite, equivalent to 4 g of magnesium, should prevent hypomagnesaemia, which can be a problem in early spring when young grass high in protein is being grazed. High intakes of non-protein nitrogen and a rapid rate of passage through the gut both reduce magnesium absorption. Feeding of a high-energy concentrate food such as sugarbeet pulp should be a considered option to minimize the problem. Providing ewes with shelter to reduce environmental stress is also beneficial.

Feeding the Lamb

Providing the lamb with a supply of colostrum is essential. Ideally, the lamb will receive this from its dam within a few hours of birth and will continue to suck its dam and receive further amounts in the following 48 h.

Ewes vary widely in production. In the first 24 h, the mean yield should be 3.0 l but some ewes will produce 500 ml and others more than 4 l.

For details of substitute colostrum preparations, see section on lamb survival (Chapter 7).

Most post-lambing mortality occurs in the first few days of life and the major cause is starvation. Insufficient colostrum or milk may be causative but the ewe not allowing the lamb to suck and lack of sucking drive and udder problems, such as blocked teats, may also be responsible. Starvation after the first few days is usually the result of poor feeding of the ewe in lactation, sore teats, mastitis or mismothering.

The lamb is dependent almost entirely on the ewe's milk until 4 or 5 weeks of age. Solid food consumption will begin at 3–4 weeks of age when the lamb starts to consume measurable amounts of grass and/or, if available, concentrate creep feed. The timing of the onset of grazing is important as it is obviously when lambs commence to ingest significant numbers of parasite infective larvae.

Feeding the naturally reared lamb post-weaning

Most lambs will be weaned between 14 and 22 weeks of age. Some of these, especially single lambs, will be ready for slaughter at the time of weaning and will be finished off on grass or grass with a minimum concentrate supplementation in the autumn. The system depends on having available good-quality grass such as aftermaths (the fresh grass growth after a crop of hay or silage has been taken off) and cow grazing. If such pastures are not available, performance figures will be disappointing, partly because of low intakes. Intakes and performance will also be depressed if the grass is deficient in trace minerals such as cobalt. The post-weaning period is particularly problematic, especially if the grass is lush. In areas of cobalt deficiency, providing concentrates which contain minerals could, paradoxically, be more beneficial when there is lots of grass following a good rainfall in the late summer and early autumn than in drier conditions when less grass is available.

Many of the lambs, especially wether lambs from hill and uplands, will be managed so that they reach the required slaughter weight between Christmas and Easter. During the winter period, these lambs may graze green forage crops, turnips or sugarbeet tops. However, increasingly, they are being fed on silage with some concentrate supplementation. Growth rates of between <50 g/day and >200 g/day may be obtained, depending on the quantity and quality of the supplement provided. Farmers who rear store lambs have the option of finishing these store lambs early or late.

Grass silage, if fed solely, even if of high DM and digestibility (D) values, will be unlikely to give growth rates in excess of 80 g/day. Part of the problem is that of low intakes which become more apparent: (i) if the DM is below 220 g/kg; (ii) if the pH is <4.0; and (iii) if the material is big bale rather than precision chopped. Maize silage has also been fed successfully.

Supplementing silages with 200 g concentrates/day will increase total intake and give growth rates between 120 and 150 g/day and 400 g concentrates will give growth rates of 175–225 g/day.

Shearing lambs in late summer and autumn usually results in higher food intakes and improved growth and carcass weight performance. Shearing may be particularly useful if the final finishing period is indoors because of nutritional and non-nutritional factors such as reduced space allowance and cleaner sheep being sent for market.

It is increasingly recognized that pre-lambing ewe nutrition is key to successful lamb production via its impacts on twinning (nutrition at mating) and lamb survival, with the latter being mediated via lamb birthweight and adequacy of colostrum production. Assessment of adequacy of nutrition is a key management practice and revolves around regular body condition scoring, observation of the animals, correct diet formulation and presentation. When troubleshooting nutritional problems it is worth remembering the old '4 diet' adage: 'There are four diets fed to animals and the aim should be for all four to be the same!'

1. The diet formulated by the nutritionist
2. The diet prepared by the farmer
3. The diet placed in front of the animals by the farmer
4. The diet actually consumed by the animals

As can be seen, this encompasses all aspects of ewe nutrition from forage production through to diet presentation and building adequacy if animals are housed.

Targeted blood sampling of ewes in late pregnancy is increasingly being performed routinely together with BCS measurement to 'ask the ewe herself' as to the adequacy of the diet she is receiving. Blood constituents and metabolites measured include Beta Hydroxy Butyrate (BOHB), blood Urea, Albumen, Total Protein, Ca, Mg, Plasma Inorganic Iodine (PII) and indicators of trace element status. In most cases, BOHB, Urea and Albumen are sufficient to assess dietary energy and protein status. Usually, 10–20 animals is recommended for sampling and care must be taken in selection of ewes, i.e. a random sample, representative of the group, should be aimed for.

Future Trends

With the increasing focus on care for the environment and sustainability within agriculture, there is increasing interest in management and nutritional practices that are considered to have less of a negative environmental impact and may rather have a positive effect, e.g. improving soil health and biodiversity and reducing the need for synthetic inputs such as anthelmintics, insecticides etc. Many of these practices fall under the broad banner of 'regenerative agriculture' where farming practices are utilized that improve soil health and biodiversity, e.g. no-till arable farming, crop rotation, utilization of grazing livestock as a source of nitrogen for arable crops, mixed farming rather than monoculture etc. In the context of sheep-keeping, the following practices are all worthy of consideration. In many cases they may be practised in conjunction with each other:

- Mob grazing
- Mixed grazing
- The use of herbal leys
- Integration of sheep into arable farming as a source of nitrogen.

Mob Grazing

This is increasingly popular and is based on the observation of the grazing behaviour of free-roaming herds of ungulates in the African Savannah where vast numbers of animals will graze a small area for a short period before moving to fresh grazing. The theory is that the upper third of the plant will be consumed by the grazing animal with the remainder being trampled underfoot into the soil along with fresh animal faeces, thereby improving soil structure and biodiversity long term, since grazing will not select for particular grass species. There is also evidence that it may increase soil sequestration of carbon. Key to the practice are very high stocking densities for very short periods of time with a large lag period before animals return to graze, e.g. one acre could be grazed by approximately 100 cattle or 400 sheep for one day with a grazing interval of 30–60 days. For successful mob grazing, the pasture must be diverse, with modern single-species leys being unsuitable. Thus, the use of herbal ley mixtures containing a diversity of plant species is a popular adjunct to mob grazing. Cattle, with their unselective grazing behaviour, are considered by many to be more suitable than sheep for mob grazing due to their selective grazing behaviour.

Mixed Grazing

This is usually carried out with cattle, although horses may occasionally be utilized in mixed-grazing strategies. Mixed grazing, with, e.g., cattle and sheep, may be simultaneous or sequential. Benefits include better pasture-usage efficiency and reducing parasite challenge, thereby increasing ruminant production for no increase in inputs. Furthermore, it can have a positive effect on pasture quality and plant biodiversity.

Herbal Leys

Herbal leys or multi-species pastures are defined as pastures containing up to 15–40 different grass, legume and herb species in contrast to the more usual pasture sward that may contain less than five different species. Their use is associated with an increase in animal productivity associated with both an enhanced nutritional quality and direct anthelmintic properties of some of the constituent plant species, e.g. birdsfoot trefoil and chicory. This property is of particular importance today with the looming spectre of anthelmintic resistance.

2 Reproduction

ROBERT SMITH*

Department of Livestock and One Health, Institute of Infection, Veterinary and Ecological Sciences, University of Liverpool, UK

Abstract

Managing reproduction in a sheep flock is a key aspect of the production cycle so that lambing takes place over a relatively short period when all necessary resources can be available to care for the ewes and to maximize lamb survival. This chapter covers the hormonal control of natural breeding and how this can be manipulated. It also covers checking rams for fertility, artificial insemination and some diseases affecting rams.

Control of Breeding

Most breeds in the UK are seasonally anoestrus, although the Dorset Horn or Polled Dorset and its crosses and some continental breeds will breed most of the year (Box 2.1). The Merino, which is a very important breed in countries such as Australia and South Africa, is not strongly seasonal so can be stimulated to breed at most times of the year. In seasonal breeders, the breeding cycle is controlled by decreasing daylight length (short-day breeders) and so ewes and rams (tups) both show peak reproductive activity in the autumn. This is controlled by melatonin from the pineal gland, with light blocking its production.

Biologically, mating was controlled by seasonal anoestrus to synchronize birth of offspring with feed resources, particularly spring grass growth. However, farmers may also target specific finished lamb markets or ram sales which require out-of-season lambing to maximize lamb growth. There are a range of complementary and additive methods to advance the breeding season or synchronize mating (tupping) and lambing. These interventions have a greater effect as the normal breeding season approaches compared to when the ewes are in deep anoestrus. In general, breeds native to higher latitudes are more seasonal than those native to lower latitudes and the seasonality of less seasonal breeds is easier to overcome with treatments.

Once out of seasonal anoestrus, ewes typically display oestrus every 16–18 days with 3–4 follicular waves stimulated by follicle stimulating hormone (FSH) during each oestrus cycle. Luteinizing hormone (LH) pulses grow the dominant follicles in each wave but these regress whilst progesterone production is high from the corpus luteum (CL) formed from the previous ovulation. When the CL regresses, a LH surge takes place and ovulation occurs accompanied by behavioural oestrus during which the ewe will actively seek out and be receptive to the ram. Rams should remain with the ewes (1 ram / ~30 ewes) for at least 35 days (1 ram/120 ewes quoted for the Romney breed) to allows ewes which did not conceive when first mated to be bred again at the subsequent oestrus. Harnesses with coloured chalk or wax blocks (raddle) can be used on rams to mark ewes mated and the colours changed to indicate those served at different time points.

Genetics

The ideal number of lambs per ewe varies between hill vs. lowland farming systems and the level of farmer supervision. Several breeds have been developed with high fecundity and the underlying genetics have been elucidated. The number of oocytes that develop on the ovary is controlled by a signaling system associated with a range of bone

*Email: robsmith@liverpool.ac.uk

morphometric proteins (named after the first tissue they were identified in). Mutations in different molecules, or their receptors, are associated with increased fecundity in different breeds (Booroola, Inverdale, Lleyn, Belclare and Cambridge). Usually, having a single copy of the mutation (heterozygosity) is associated with increased fertility but two copies (homozygosity) is associated with reduced fertility or infertility. Thus, careful breeding is needed to maximize benefit without the downside.

The ram effect

Introduction of a novel male or reintroduction of males after at least 2 weeks' absence (Fig. 2.1) can stimulate luteinizing hormone (LH) pulsatility and follicular development 1–2 months early in the season. This can be mimicked by male odour alone.

Introduced rams can be vasectomized so they cannot mate or be intact rams placed in the field in a pen or trailer to prevent mating. Some ewes will ovulate quickly after ram introduction, have a short cycle, ovulate again and then have a normal cycle returning to oestrus about 21–26 days after ram introduction whilst most ovulate immediately, start a normal-length cycle and come into oestrus at 16–19 days after ram introduction. To maximize fertility and synchronization, fertile rams should be introduced 14 days after initial ram contact. Ewes that conceive to the first round of mating will lamb 163–176 days after initial ram introduction. As rams may also be out of season and several ewes come into oestrus per day, one ram to ten ewes is recommended to achieve the best conception rate. A vasectomized ram may also be used to withdraw individual ewes as they are raddled so they can be served by a fertile ram or for artificial insemination. This is also a cheap method of inducing a degree of oestrous synchronization but requires careful management.

Nutrition – 'flushing'

Flushing by suddenly increasing nutritional inputs is a very old technique, first scientifically reported

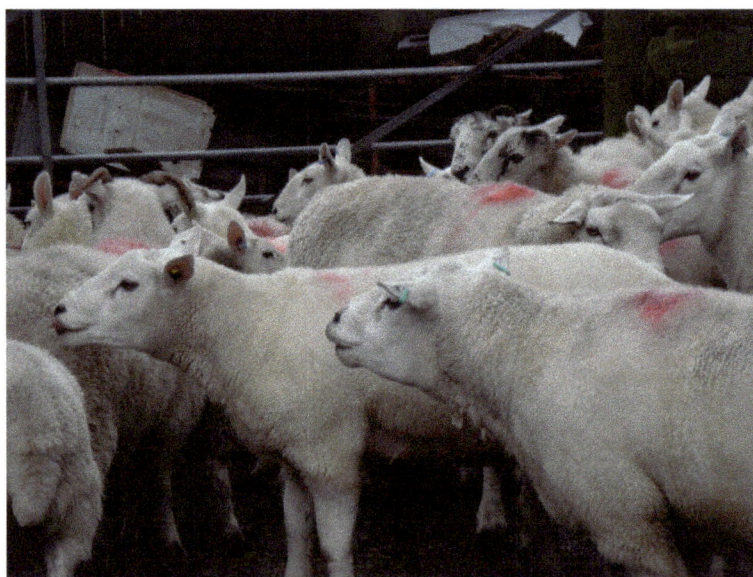

Fig. 2.1. These Texel rams (foreground) with a group of ewes are showing the Flehman response (curling the upper lip) which helps detect ewes in oestrus (photo Agnes Winter).

in 1837. There is a short-term effect of acutely increasing feeding or energy or protein for 3–7 days before an increased ovulation rate occurs and also a longer-term benefit of an increased plane of nutrition for 6 to 8 weeks before breeding. There is a 'static effect' whereby ewes in better body condition score (BCS) have higher ovulation rates but also a 'dynamic effect' whereby a shorter-term increase in bodyweight in thin animals gives a higher ovulation rate than in animals already in good condition. So regardless of the starting body condition of ewes, both short-term and long-term feeding strategies can increase percentage pregnant, ovulation rate and thus number of lambs born per ewe. This is in addition to any genetic effect in prolific breeds of sheep.

Day length

Seasonality can be manipulated by exposure to either shortening days or long days, although animals will become refractory to the day length signal (stop responding) if they are kept in that environment for a long period, for example 16 hours per day for 2 months. Housing and exposing a flock of ewes to light can be difficult and expensive. Exposing a smaller number of rams to shorter day length to bring them into season early and then use the ram effect to bring the females into season is more practical. It is probably more practical to choose a less seasonal breed of sheep to obtain tupping at the required date.

Melatonin ear implant

Melatonin is a hormone produced by the pineal gland in the brain. Exposure to light blocks production so it is the body's internal signal of day length. Treating with melatonin simulates the longer nights coming into winter, stimulating both ewes and rams to enter oestrous. The UK- and EU-authorized product (Regulin, Ceva Animal Health) contains 18 mg of melatonin and is injected subcutaneously at the base of the ear. The ability to bring forward mating depends on the underlying seasonality of the sheep treated. In less seasonal breeds, such as Suffolk and their crosses, implants can be used in the UK from mid-May to late June for ram introduction in late June and July. In more seasonal animals, such as the Mule and Halfbreds, they can only successfully be used from early June to late

July for ram introduction from mid-July to late August.

A suggested protocol is:
Day 1 – (30 weeks before wanting to lamb) move ewes from sight, sound and smell of ram.
Day 7 – Implant ewes at the base of the ear.
Day 42 – (30–40 days after implantation) introduce rams.
Peaking mating will occur at 25–35 days after ram introduction. Use vasectomized rams for the first 14 days to stimulate ewes but not impregnate them to obtain a compact lambing period. Thus, practical use is also incorporating the ram effect.

The exact timing of all the protocols described above will depend on the latitude, genetics of the sheep and nutrition. Treating a small number of animals with a protocol based on studies published in your geographical region, with sheep of similar genetics, and monitoring the effect is suggested before large-scale use in a subsequent year.

Manipulating the timing of oestrus and ovulation with progestogen devices

Breeding may be advanced by up to 6 weeks by the use of progestogen intravaginal devices with or without injection of pregnant mare's serum gonadotrophin (PMSG), also known as equine chorionic gonadotropin (eCG), that has predominantly FSH activity in the sheep but with a longer duration of action than endogenous FSH (Table 2.1). The authorized product in the UK is PMSG Intervet 5000IU (MSD Animal Health).

Sponges impregnated with flugestone acetate, a synthetic progesterone-like compound, have been available around the world for decades (Chronogest, MSD Animal Health). Medroxyprogesterone acetate is another synthetic progesterone-like compound that has also previously been used but is no longer available in the UK. Progesterone itself embedded in silicone around a plastic T (CIDR-OVIS in UK (Zoetis), CIDR-G in many other countries) has become available more recently and has a similar effect. They are basically a corpus luteum on a stick! When in the vagina–the progestogen is absorbed into the circulation and prevents ovulation until removal 12 days later. This timing ensures that any endogenous CL has regressed so on removal of the device the ewe comes into oestrus. If a shorter regime is needed, after 6 days a prostaglandin analogue (Dinoprost or Cloprostenol) can be injected to cause luteolysis of any endogenous CL and then the device removed. Injection of PMSG (300–750 IU using the higher dose in July, reducing in August) at sponge removal will stimulate follicle development and lead to improved twinning and conception rate, particularly near seasonal anoestrus. The farmer should be warned that individual ewes react differently to the same dose of PMSG and the results are unpredictable so unwanted multiple pregnancies are a risk. Its effect may also reduce over repeated use in an individual.

A mild vaginitis does occur during use of intravaginal devices but this does not seem to compromise conception rate. We have seen chronic vaginitis in animals where the strings of Chronogest sponges have disappeared intravaginally and owners have assumed they have fallen out but, they have been left in. Farmers should be cautioned to check carefully and not assume they have fallen out if the strings are not visible.

An unlicensed alternative to progestagen intravaginal devices to time the fall in progesterone and timing of oestrus is to give two injections of prostaglandin analogue ((Dinoprost or Cloprostenol) either 7, 9 or 11 days apart to synchronize the fall in progesterone. All three timings give similar results.

Ewes and rams should be in good condition (CS 3) and fit. Put the rams near the ewes at device withdrawal then put them with the ewes 48 h after withdrawal, for 48 h. If possible, remove ewes from the ram when they have been marked (raddled) convincingly, to avoid repeated serving of favourites. Introducing rams at sponge withdrawal reduces the pregnancy rate drastically (68–40% in one trial). Two weeks after first oestrus, put rams, with a different raddle crayon, with the ewes for 1 week and then remove. The usual advice is to allow one ram for ten ewes, though it is possible with some individual rams to achieve good fertility with more ewes. There are considerable differences between breeds and individuals in the ability of rams to breed outside the usual season.

Table 2.1 provides an example of a schedule for early lambing with progestogen sponges (for normal conditions in the UK, although a similar schedule can be used at any time during the breeding season by substituting appropriate dates).

Roughly 70% of the ewes should lamb to the induced oestrus and most have twins. Results vary widely, according to: (i) breed; (ii) feeding; (iii) time of year; and (iv) weather. Test a batch of ewes and record the results in order to find out whether the procedure is worthwhile on a particular farm.

Only well-managed farms can benefit from early, concentrated lambing. Housing and labour for lambing must be planned well or welfare is compromised and lamb mortality may be high.

Induction of parturition

Induction can be used routinely after synchronization of tupping to allow close lambing supervision over a short period of time, such as for smallholders with full-time jobs. Inducing lambing to reduce metabolic load on ewes with pregnancy toxaemia can also be a useful treatment.

Initially, pregnancy is maintained by progesterone from the corpus luteum formed on the ovary after ovulation. After approximately 60 days of gestation pregnancy is also maintained by placental progesterone so cannot be terminated reliably by exogenous prostaglandin alone acting to cause luteolysis. Normal parturition is triggered by corticosteroids secreted by the fetal adrenal glands. This also stimulates final maturation of the lungs. This can be mimicked by injection of dexamethasone or

Table 2.1. Example of devising a schedule for early lambing (15–23 December), working backwards from desired lambing date.

Calculate	Activity	Date
Longest gestation 150 days[a]	Last lambing required	23 December
Shortest gestation 144 days[b]	First lambing anticipated	15 December
Last mating date	Remove rams	26 July
First mating date[c]	Introduce rams	24 July
Sponges in for 14 days	Remove sponges	22 July
	Insert sponges	8 July

[a]Counting 150 days back from 23 December the last mating date can be calculated (26 July).
[b]Counting 144 days back from 15 December the first mating date can be calculated (24 July).
[c]The sponges need to be removed 2 days before the rams are introduced (i.e. 22 July).

Robert Smith

other synthetic corticosteroids. Dexamethasone is authorized in the UK for other food-producing animals so can be used under the cascade for induction of lambing in ewes. Two types of product are available, dexamethasone sodium phosphate alone (e.g. Dexadreson) and a mixture dexamethasone sodium phosphate and dexamethasone phenylpropionate (e.g. Dexafort). Dexamethasone sodium phosphate is absorbed rapidly from the injection site, whilst dexamethasone phenylpropionate is absorbed more slowly, thus altering the duration of action from approximately one day to four days. There are no data comparing use of these two formulations and many studies do not differentiate but generically state 'dexamethasone'. Studies have demonstrated that 16 mg (8 ml of 2 mg/ml) dexamethasone is required to provide reliable induction. If the typical gestation length of the ewes on a holding is known, then inducing just before they are likely to start naturally will provide the best lamb viability. This may be 140–147 days depending on the gestation length typical on the farm. Injection on the evening on day 1 will result in most lambing in the daytime of day 3. So injecting at 8 p.m. on Thursday evening 144 days since the ram went in will result in most ewes lambing 8 a.m. – 8 p.m. on the following Saturday, ideal for smallholders who work during the week. Occasionally, some lambs will be born on the Sunday. If rams are left in for more than one cycle, personal experience is that ewes served in the second cycle will not respond and they will lamb 2–3 weeks later. It is best to have the ram in only for 7 days or less or use coloured raddles and induce in batches.

Theoretically, if dates are not accurately known, a longer-acting version of dexamethasone may better induce lung maturation but no studies have directly compared the two versions available.

Ram Examination

This is best done 3 months before tupping time as part of a flock health visit as sperm takes about 60 days to develop and any problems detected need time to resolve and unaffected sperm produced. About 10% of rams have poor fertility. Many of these can be detected by palpation of testicles without the need for electroejaculation but there are some conditions which are missed if examination of fresh semen is not carried out.

Examination of a ram lamb before use, or of a newly bought ram, is a wise investment (Fig. 2.2). An infertile ram which is not detected can lead to ewes lambing 2 months late. If several rams of the

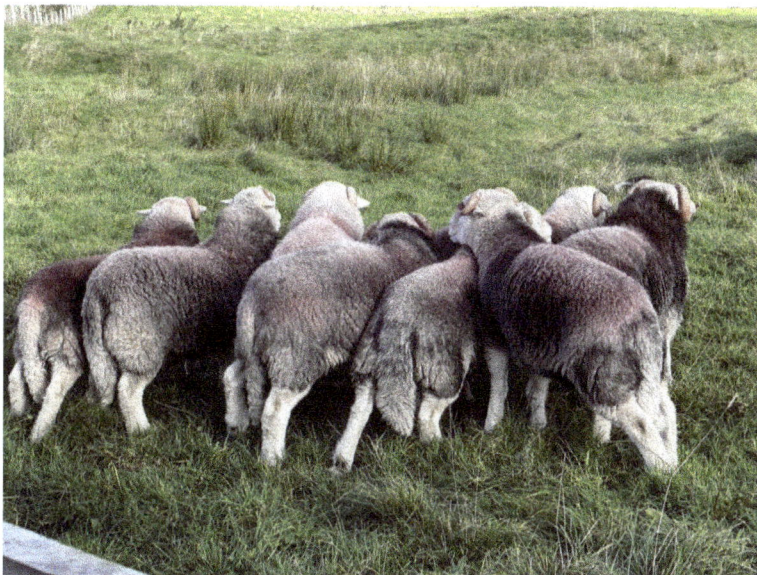

Fig. 2.2. Group of Herdwick rams. These rams should be checked 6–8 weeks before putting in with the ewes (photo Agnes Winter).

same breed work together, an individual infertile ram may never be detected but may result in a reduction in overall fertility of the flock.

Any history based on good breeding records is valuable. Illness, however brief, can lead to temporary infertility up to and beyond 2 months later. If the ram is examined before entry to the flock, its conformation and any inherited condition should be checked. Teeth should make contact with the dental pad. Orf should be looked for around the lips. The CS should be 3 to 3.5. Feet should be checked for foot rot and CODD, brisket for abscesses and lymph nodes for Caseous Lymphadenitis.

Before the breeding season (before July in the UK), the size of testicles and numbers of spermatozoa are lower, especially in more seasonal breeds.

The testicles should be of similar size, very resilient (turgid) and move freely in the scrotum (compare with others of the same age and similar breed). The scrotal circumference ranges from 30 to 44 cm in mature lowland rams and from 30 to 40 cm in hill breeds. The scrotal circumference of ram lambs at 9 months old should be at least 28 cm in lowland and 26 cm in hill breeds. Testicular hypoplasia is incurable; no spermatozoa are produced, though libido may be normal. The head and tail of the epididymis should be palpated for evidence of pain, lumps or adhesions since epididymitis is a common cause of reduced fertility in rams.

A variety of organisms may be associated with epididymitis but *Brucella ovis* infection is of great importance in southern European countries, Australia, New Zealand, South Africa and North and South America. Control schemes have been described where rams are tested and culled. This infection is not present in the UK where it is a notifiable disease but other bacteria have been found in epididymitis cases including *Mannheimia* and *Histophilus*. Even prolonged antimicrobial treatment is usually unrewarding.

Epididymitis may occur in outbreaks in groups of intensively reared, trough-fed rams that spend more time lying than grazing. This risk may be reduced by keeping growing rams in small groups at grazing and rotating to clean paddocks.

Ultrasound examination of the testicles is not a standard part of ram examination but can be useful to further differentiate the cause of any asymmetry or abnormalities noticed on palpation. Recent research suggests blood flow, testicular volume and pixel heterogeneity are correlated with testosterone production and sperm morphology so this may become more commonly performed in future once predictability of fertility from findings becomes clearer.

The penis can be extended with care, with the ram in the sitting position, to check for rare defects, by holding the prepuce and pushing forwards with the other hand at the sigmoid flexure, which is found at the base of the testicles. (Have a bit of practice so you can do it well!.) The vermiform appendage should be free from a persistent frenulum and approximately 10 mm long. Although not needed for successful mating, if it is short or absent this may suggest that the ram has had urolithiasis and there is a risk that residual uroliths could be present in the bladder and cause further urolithiasis episodes.

There are a number of battery-operated electro-ejaculators which can be used to obtain semen samples from rams when placed per rectum at the level of the pubic brim. Older 'on/off' types allowed little control of intensity of stimulation. Recently, the Lane pulsator ejaculators (www.lane-mfg.com) have become the predominant product used in the UK for both bull and ram electroejaculation. Each probe has three longitudinal electrodes arranged along the ventral surface. They allow either programmed or manually increasing electrical stimulation in a wave with current between the electrodes rather than from the probe to earth via the legs. They allow a subtle stimulation that can be adapted to the response of the individual and appear to be better tolerated than the old-fashioned equipment. The semen can be collected in a warm beaker or in a small transparent plastic bag. Between 0.5 and 2 ml of dense creamy semen is normally collected from a fertile ram. Semen obtained by electroejaculation is not necessarily typical of a natural ejaculate. An alternative is collection by artificial vagina, which needs training for the ram, or semen can be recovered from the vagina of a ewe just served by the suspect ram.

Semen examined immediately on a warm slide in a warm room should show good wave motion (as if being vigorously stirred). If a poor sample is obtained, a second sample should be taken. After mixing one drop of semen on a warm slide with five drops of nigrosin-eosin (1.67 g eosin, 10.0 g nigrosin, 100 ml water) for 3 minutes, a smear can be made. Further evidence of the likely fertility is provided by: (i) the total number of spermatozoa; (ii) the number of live (unstained) spermatozoa; and (iii) the number of spermatozoa free of morphological abnormalities.

Smears can be stained by Romanowsky or Diff-Quick methods as used for blood smears to detect the presence of polymorphs, suggesting an inflammatory response.

If the history and examination of the ram and semen show reduced fertility, treatment is not normally possible. A potentially valuable ram may be tested again 2–3 months later, as infertility is occasionally temporary. A report should always remind the client that the only final evidence of fertility is the production of lambs.

Rams should be permanently marked for identification and reports should be made on the special certificates designed by the British Veterinary Association (BVA) 'Certificate of Veterinary Examination of a Ram Intended for Breeding', which can be downloaded by BVA members or found on the SVS website (www.sheepvetsoc.org.uk - accessed 1/11/24). This certificate also contains guidelines for semen collection by electroejaculation.

Libido can be tested by observing mounting ability with ewes in oestrus, mating dexterity by viewing intromission (which is aided by shearing the rear of the ewe) and serving capacity by counting the number of ewes served over a set time. These tend to be used as a secondary investigation as ewes need to be in the breeding season and synchronized to be in oestrus so they cannot easily be performed ahead of the breeding season as a check.

Artificial Insemination (AI) and Multiple Ovulation Embryo Transfer (MOET)

The vast majority of sheep are bred by natural service. AI is not widely used due to the difficulty of transcervical insemination because of the anatomy of the sheep cervix. Most AI is performed on high genetic value animals by specialist companies using laparoscopy. Throughout the UK, a wide range of breeding services including AI and MOET are available from Innovis (www.innovis.org.uk) and have been responsible for advances in flock performance. Similar organizations exist in most sheep-producing countries.

AI with fresh semen

Synchronization of ewes with a progestogen device and injection of PMSG at withdrawal is used, with AI 56 h after device withdrawal. Fresh semen can be placed in the vagina but better results are obtained by placing semen by pipette just into the cervix. One ejaculate will inseminate 20 ewes with a conception rate of around 70%. This procedure has been used for many years in large flocks in eastern Europe and Scandinavia.

AI with frozen semen

Conception rates with frozen ram semen given into the cervix are low (30%)

Intrauterine insemination by laparoscopy, under local analgesia, with diluted frozen ram semen, allows one ejaculate to be used to inseminate 100 ewes with a conception rate of 60–70%.

A pilot study under UK conditions inseminated 20 ewes with frozen-thawed sperm using 2 straws of $\leq 200 \times 10^6$ spermatozoa into the vagina 12–24 hours after standing oestrus and obtained a 50% pregnancy rate. This equates to 20 ewes served per ram ejaculate compared to 250–500 for cattle AI. It remains to be seen if AI becomes more common in the UK.

Breed and Flock Improvement

Breed improvement has always been a feature of sheep farming from its earliest days in the development of different breeds suited to particular areas of the world. The naming of breeds of sheep according to the geographical area of origin such as Suffolk, Clun Forest and Swaledale indicates the selection which has taken place over centuries. The selection of rams and ewes according to breed standards was also an attempt to improve flocks though physical features were not necessarily associated with production criteria. In the past 60 years, recording of data on production, the recognition that much of this data is genetically inherited and the introduction of breeding techniques such as AI and MOET have given sheep breeders objective measurements to guide improvements and have made marked advances in flock performance.

Ram evaluation run by Signet Breeding Services (https://signetdata.com - accessed 1/1//24.) in the UK identifies superior rams for a number of criteria and the production of estimated breeding values (EBV) for each criterion including for ewes and lambs in pedigree flocks. The pedigree and performance data are analyzed to estimate how much of a sheep's performance is due to its genetic make-up and how much to the flock environment. An EBV is measured in the same units as the trait (e.g. 8-week weight in kg) and expressed as a positive or negative value compared with the average for the trait.

A ram having a value of +5 kg for 8-week lamb weight, for example, means that, on average, its progeny will be 2.5 kg better than those from a ram with a zero value, since only half its genes are transmitted. A recorded ram will have a value for each trait and, in addition, different individual EBVs are combined to give breeding indexes to identify superior rams for the different stratifications in the UK sheep industry.

Similar schemes are used in other countries and many breed societies use Sire Referencing Schemes and EBV values to increase the rapidity with which genetic improvement can be made across flocks by identifying superior rams from the whole breed. Genomic selection is also starting to gain traction in the sheep industry with the first genomic evaluations being launched in the UK by Signet in 2023.

Diseases Affecting Ram Lambs, Rams and Wethers

Pizzle Rot (Balanoposthitis)

This is seen in both rams and wethers (castration effects development of the area so they urinate inside the prepuce). Signs range from small ulcers and discharge at the prepuce to scabbing causing blockage of the prepuce and also fly strike on the affected area. The causative organism is usually *Corynebacterium renale*. This organism produces ammonia from urea in urine. High protein concentrates and lush grass are risk factors. Access to water, salt or ammonium chloride to increase drinking and acidify urine are preventative. Affected animals should be isolated to reduce environmental contamination, with unaffected rams moved to a clean paddock or housing. Wool around the prepuce should be clipped away and the area cleaned. Systemic antibiotics, such as amoxicillin, should be administered and fly treatment to avoid fly strike.

Scrotal Mange

This is caused by a sheep-adapted strain of *Chorioptes bovis* and characterized by crusty scabs on the lower third of the scrotum. These may crack and expose a sore, weeping dermis. Rams may nibble their teeth when the area is touched in a 'gratification reflex'. It can also affect the lower legs and poll of the head. If lesions are extensive then the raised blood flow and testes temperature can lead to testicular degeneration and reduced sperm quality. Diagnosis can be confirmed by tape strip from several locations as there is a low number of mites

in the tissue debris. Long-acting avermectins such as doramectin may be effective but a single shorter acting treatment with ivermectin is not. Diazinon sheep dips are effective and as these are used less often this condition may become more of a problem.

Urolithiasis

This is mainly a hazard for the housed 2–4-month-old castrated male lamb or in ram lambs being fed a lot of concentrate in preparation for sales, although it does occasionally occur in adult males, particularly heavily fed pedigree rams. We have also seen outbreaks when ram lambs have had access to ewe nuts with high mineral content instead of lamb creep feed, or if compounding errors have left out ammonium or calcium chloride included in the feed to acidify the urine and avoid crystal formation. The fine sand-like calculi, usually consisting of magnesium ammonium phosphate, obstruct the penis most commonly at the vermiform appendage or at the sigmoid flexure. Other types of urolith do occur in other countries depending in geology and plant species consumed.

Clinical signs

- The affected animals show discomfort with straining ('hiccups'), kicking at the abdomen, twitching of the tail and general restlessness.
- A precipitate of crystals may be found on the preputial hairs which may feel sticky or be dry and sometimes bloodstained.
- 'Water belly' may occur, with urine leaking subcutaneously from a ruptured urethra leading to 'pitting oedema', or into the abdominal cavity from a ruptured bladder so a fluid thrill can be felt on the opposite side of the abdomen in one side is balloted.

Treatment (not easy, but urgent)

Assess the state of the animal as treatment differs depending on whether salvage or retention of breeding potential is the aim. Check whether the bladder is intact by ultrasonography and/or abdominocentesis and consider decompressing the bladder with a long needle through the abdominal wall. For valuable breeding animals, take blood for haematocrit, urea, creatinine and potassium, sodium and chloride concentrations. Ultrasonographic assessment of the cortex to medulla ratio of the kidneys is useful (1:1 is expected) to determine if back pressure and hydronephrosis have led to kidney damage, worsening the prognosis.

Possibilities then are:

- Examine the vermiform appendage. If this is obstructed, cut it off at the base with a pair of clean scissors. If you are lucky and this is the only obstruction, urine will flow, but keep a close check as blockage may recur. Obtain client consent as this will be detected at pre-purchase ram examination. In animals castrated early in life, the penis may not have developed sufficiently to be exteriorized and a pair of Metzenbaum scissors can be placed inside the prepuce under sedation and local anaesthetic to indicate the lumen of the prepuce and a scalpel used to cut down onto the prepuce two-thrids along its length. The glans of the penis can then be located within the lumen and examined. The wound can be left open to heal by secondary intention. This is probably only cost-effective in castrated pet animals.
- Give a spasmolytic and analgesic injection. Xylazine, detomidine and Buscopan (butylscopolamine and metamizole) are authorized in food-producing animals so can be used under the cascade. Acepromazine and diazepam are not authorized. The efficacy of spasmolytics and analgesics is not well determined and if urination is not observed within 30 minutes after administration, further action must be taken; the animal should not be left 'to see what happens'.
- If the obstruction is higher, there are no calculi palpable in the pelvic urethra using a finger into the rectum and the animal is not required for breeding purposes, do a perineal urethrostomy under caudal epidural anaesthesia and sedation. If urine still does not flow, you can attempt retrograde flushing into the bladder, but catheterization is difficult because of the urethral diverticulum. The urethrostomy is completed by transection of the penis and exteriorizing the stump through the skin incision below the anus. The distal portion of the penis is left *in situ*. This is probably the best method where urethral rupture has occurred at the sigmoid flexure.

- For breeding animals, either:
  - do a laparotomy, open the bladder and attempt to flush down the urethra. This is also an option if the bladder has already ruptured (usually on the dorsal aspect) and repair is to be attempted; or
  - insert a Foley catheter into the bladder percutaneously or via the laparotomy and exteriorize the tube next to the incision. The bladder can be flushed daily with Walpole's solution in an attempt to dissolve the stones. The catheter can be closed off for increasing time daily to apply some pressure onto the blockage. Recanalization can occur in 7–14 days.
- For all cases, correct the fluid deficit and electrolyte balance with intravenous fluids, if required.
- For all cases, drench twice daily with 5 g ammonium chloride or other urine acidifier, but not until metabolic acidosis has been corrected.

These cases can be complex and the prognosis is always guarded.

Control when cases are occurring

- Check the type and amount of concentrate being fed. Make sure it is formulated for feeding to breeding rams or fattening lambs and is not being fed in excessive amounts.
- Ensure plenty of fresh water is available.
- Supply salt (NaCl) as licks, or in the ration to encourage drinking.
- Add 2% ammonium chloride to the ration.
- Contact the feed supplier to alert them to a possible problem, particularly if feeding instructions have been correctly followed.

Control in future

- Ensure no magnesium is added to concentrates; do not exceed 200 g MgO/t.
- Ensure calcium:phosphorus ratio is at least 1.2:1 up to 2:1; include 1.5% ground limestone in the diet if necessary.
- Ensure there is a minimum of 1% salt in the concentrate.
- Ensure there is plenty of fresh water available.
- Avoid castration.

3 Vaccination

DAI GROVE-WHITE* AND JO OULTRAM

Department of Livestock and One Health, Institute of Infection, Veterinary and Ecological Sciences, University of Liverpool, UK

Abstract

Vaccination is a key tool in the management of disease in the sheep flock. The relatively low individual animal value together with the trends for increasing flock size and reduced labour availability on farms often precludes individual animal treatment. Prevention of disease is thus paramount for farm viability. Biosecurity measures such as testing and quarantine can reduce the likelihood of novel diseases entering into a flock and biocontainment measures can limit spread within the flock, but they will have little effect on the occurrence of endemic diseases such as due to *Clostridia* spp. and *Pasteurella* spp which are ovine commensals present in all flocks. Vaccination is a key tool in control of such diseases. This chapter discusses the key vaccines used in the sheep industry and briefly describes the types of vaccines available and likely future trends in development.

Vaccination Background

Vaccination as a tool in disease control is receiving renewed interest at the time of writing (2024). This is in part due to the recognition that control of infectious disease via vaccination can result not only in improved flock health and profitability with a concurrent reduction in the carbon footprint of a sheep enterprise but also in a reduction in the use of antimicrobials. There have been massive strides made in vaccinology resultant on the COVID-19 pandemic and this acquired knowledge and expertise will undoubtedly spill over into the animal health sectorz e.g. development of novel viral vectored vaccines for diseases such as louping-ill. There is considerable research interest in the development of vaccines against both ectoparasites such as sheep scab and endoparasites including *Fasciola hepatica* (liver fluke) and *Teladorsagia circumcincta* and it is likely that such vaccines will be commercially available in the next few years. This follows on from the development of Barbervax by the Moredun Institute as an aid to reducing *Haemonchus contortus* faecal egg shedding. It is currently licensed in Australia and South Africa but not in the UK.

Traditionally, veterinary vaccines have been categorised into two groups (Table 3.1) – live and killed vaccines, each with their advantages and disadvantages, although with the advent of new technologies these classic distinctions become less clear, e.g. viral vector, DNA and mRNA vaccines.

In the UK, flock health planning has become a standard practice for many sheep enterprises and, as such, a vaccination schedule should be in place as part of each flock health plan, based upon the particular disease risks within the flock. In the UK, the National Organization of Animal Health (NOAH, https://www.noah.co.uk) has produced detailed guidelines for vaccine usage in sheep (https://www.noah.co.uk/wp-content/uploads/2022/05/NOAH-Livestock-Vaccination-Guideline-August-2022.pdf#page=32; accessed 17/11/24) and broadly places vaccines into one of two categories (Table 3.2).

All licensed vaccines in the UK are supported by efficacy data suggesting their use is beneficial, although this may not be the case in all countries. However, for a vaccine to produce the desired level of protection, it must be stored and administered correctly, as recommended by the manufacturers in their data sheets. It has been shown that this is often not the case with UK sheep, with incorrect storage and administration being commonplace. In terms of storage, maintenance of a 'cold chain' is

*Email: daigw@liverpool.ac.uk

Table 3.1. Types of vaccines used in animal health.

Vaccine Type	
Modified live vaccine	Inactivated (killed) vaccines
Advantages	**Advantages**
• Rapid response	• Usually, safer
• Usually, single primary dose	• No risk of contamination with other live pathogens
• Usually, no adjuvant required	• More stable in handling and storage
• Better induction of cell mediated immunity (CMI) so get:	
○ CMI & antibody responses	
• Better able to stimulate IgA production	
Disadvantages	**Disadvantages**
• Potential for undesirable effects due to live antigen, e.g. abortion	• Usually, slower response
• Potential for reversion to virulence	• Two primary doses required
• Potential for contamination by other live pathogens	• Adjuvant* required for maximal response
• Sensitive to environmental factors (light, temperature)	• Usually, do not stimulate cellular immunity (CMI) so get:
• Must be used quickly after reconstitution	○ Antibody response only
	• More frequent vaccinations required, compared with live vaccines
	• More expensive to produce

Adjuvant = chemical(s) added to vaccine to improve immune response, e.g. aluminium hydroxide, Quill A, mycobacterial cell wall fractions

Table 3.2. Sheep vaccines used in the UK (NOAH, 2022, modified)

UK sheep diseases and vaccination categories

Category 1	**Category 2**
(consider use for all flocks)	**(Consider use in specific disease circumstances)**
• **Clostridia**	• **Orf – parapox virus**
Clostridium **spp.**	• **Louping-ill virus*****
• **Pasteurellosis**	• **Johne's disease***
Mannheimia haemolytica	*Mycobacterium avium* **var** *paratuberculosis*
Bibersteinia trehalosi	• **Mastitis**
• **Footrot**	*Staphylococcus aureus*
Dichelobacter nodosus	• **Erysipelas****
• **Abortion**	*Erysipelothrix rhusiopathiae*
Chlamydia abortus (EAE)	• **Caseous lymphadenitis***
Toxoplasma gondii	*Corynebacterium pseudotuberculosis*
	• **Arboviruses**
	Bluetongue***
	Schmallenberg***

* can be imported into UK under specific import licence
** used under cascade
*** if vaccine available

key, with the optimal temperature range being from 2°–4° centigrade. Administration should be as per the manufacturer's instructions, usually by the subcutaneous route. Whilst true sterility is not achievable with the use of multi-dose syringes, cleanliness can be maximized by frequent needle changes and the use of devices such as the Sterimatic system (https://www.sterimatic.co.uk - accessed 2/11/24) whereby the needle is automatically disinfected between animals (Fig. 3.1). Finally, consideration should be given to the physiological state of the target animals to be vaccinated in order to both protect the health of the animal and maximize the vaccinial response. Poor nutritional status, presence of concurrent disease or stressors (recent or current) are all likely to have a negative impact. Always read the data sheet before using vaccines as instructions and protocols sometimes change.

At the time of writing, vaccines are available in the UK and many other sheep-producing countries for control of the following:

- clostridial diseases;
- pasteurellosis;
- combined clostridial diseases and pasteurellosis;
- enzootic abortion of ewes (EAE);

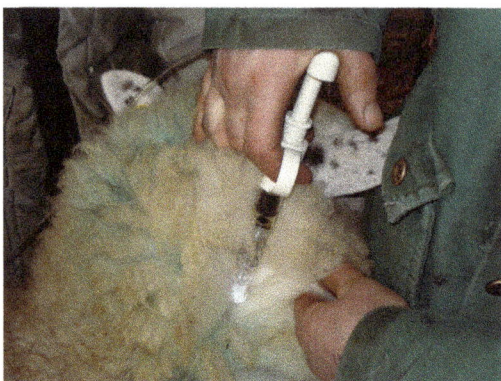

Fig. 3.1. Vaccination should be carried out carefully and cleanly (photo Agnes Winter).

- toxoplasmosis;
- footrot (FR);
- orf;
- Schmallenberg virus; not available in UK currently (March 2024);
- Louping-ill. There is currently no vaccine available but it is likely that a new viral vectored recombinant vaccine will become available in the near future.

Other diseases for which vaccines can be used in special circumstances in the UK are caseous lymphadenitis, botulism, Johne's disease, mastitis, erysipelas and specific arboviruses such as Bluetongue. In some countries and circumstances, diseases such as Q fever (*Coxiella burnetti*), foot and mouth disease (FMD), Peste de petits ruminants (PPR), Anthrax (*Bacillus anthracis*), Sheep pox and *Brucella melitensis* may be controlled by vaccination.

Bluetongue vaccine was used in the UK while the threat of disease existed in 2007 but is not available currently for the 2023–4 outbreak (see below for more information). See also under specific diseases in relevant chapters.

Clostridial Diseases

Clostridial diseases (see Table 3.3), other than tetanus and botulism, generally cause rapid collapse and death; therefore diagnosis and control are key issues. The diseases are an ever-present risk in virtually all flocks and

Table 3.3. Clostridial infections and associated diseases.

Disease	*Clostridium* sp.	Age affected	Season	Trigger factors
Enterotoxaemias				
Lamb dysentery[a]	*perfringens* type B	<2 weeks	Spring	Flush of milk
Struck[a]	*perfringens* type C	Growing lambs and adults	Spring	Flush of milk or grass
Pulpy kidney[a]	*perfringens* type D	>2 weeks	Any	Flush of milk, grass or concentrates
Braxy[a]	*septicum*	4–8 months	Autumn	Frosted food
Black disease[a]	*novyi* type B	Adults	Winter	Liver fluke
Bacilliary haemoglobinuria[a]	*novyi* type D	Adults	Winter	Liver fluke
Acute abomasitis[b]	*Paeniclostridium sordellii*	Growing lambs and adults	Spring	Intensive feeding
Gas gangrenes				
Blackleg[a]	*chauvoei*	Any	Any	Injury, wounds
Big head	*novyi* type A	Adults	Any	Fighting, wounds
Neurotropic				
Tetanus[a]	*tetani*	2 weeks–4 months	Spring	Docking, castrating
Botulism[c]	*botulinum*	Adults	Any	Toxin in food

[a] Included in 8-in-1 vaccines.

[b] *P. (formerly Clostridium) sordellii* is increasingly being implicated by laboratories as a cause of death; included in 10-in-1 vaccine.

[c] *C. botulinum* is rare in sheep and usually associated with chicken litter but is included for the sake of completeness.

should be controlled by vaccination. It is common for mistakes to be made in timing of vaccine administration or accidentally missing individuals or groups. It is also quite common to find farmers who do not routinely use these vaccines either on the grounds of cost (questionable as they are not expensive) or the mistaken belief that their farm is not subject to this group of diseases. Clostridial organisms are commonly found in the intestinal tract, are widespread in soil and form resistant, long-lasting spores, so it is never safe to assume freedom from these diseases.

Vaccination against clostridial diseases

There are several vaccines available ranging from comprehensive '8- or 10-in-1' to single component for blackleg. *Mannheimia* (*Pasteurella*) *haemolytica* and *Pasteurella trehalosi* antigens are also combined with clostridial in one of the commonly used vaccines. Clostridial vaccines are defines as killed formalized toxoid and bacterin-toxoid vaccines. By using a multicomponent vaccine and efficient primary and secondary doses, it is possible to maintain a protective level of immunity throughout the year in both ewes and lambs, against all the common clostridial diseases. Vaccines containing fewer antigens may be cheaper and are sometimes used for growing lambs, but it is arguably better to have a fully comprehensive insurance policy for these killing diseases.

Two doses of vaccine at a 4–6-week interval produce sufficient antibodies to protect a ewe for the first year with sufficient spare, via colostrum, to protect its lamb(s) for up to about 16 weeks, providing the secondary or booster dose is given approximately one month before lambing (Fig. 3.2). In subsequent years, only one pre-lambing booster injection is required to protect both ewe and lamb(s).

Assuming a flock to have no initial protection, one effective vaccination schedule is as follows.

Ewes

- Primary as soon as possible
- Secondary – 4–6 weeks later
- Booster – 4–6 weeks before lambing
- Repeat booster annually

Lambs (ewe and ram)

Those to be kept over 16 weeks (for slaughter or breeding):

- Primary – at 10–12 weeks
- Secondary – at 14–16 weeks

- Booster (for breeding lambs only) with the adult ewes and rams pre-lambing time.

Bought-in ewes (for breeding) and store lambs (for slaughter)

Unless there is reliable vaccination information, it is best to assume that these have not been vaccinated, or at least that their immunity has waned, and to give them the full course of primary and secondary injections, starting as soon as possible after purchase. A short cut is often taken with the bought-in ewes (with some justification if there are no obvious winter clostridial risks, e.g. black disease) and that is to vaccinate them on arrival but delay the secondary injection until 4–6 weeks before lambing, but this strategy can be risky.

Bought-in rams

If their vaccination status is in doubt, give two doses at a 4–6-week interval, followed by an annual booster.

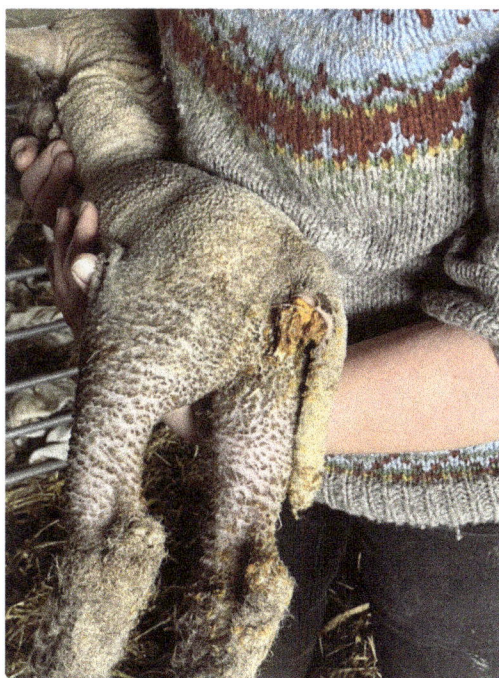

Fig. 3.2. This day-old lamb has passed sticky orange meconium, a sign that it has had a good feed of colostrum providing antibodies providing its mother was correctly vaccinated (photo Agnes Winter).

Lambs out of unvaccinated or inadequately vaccinated ewes

These lambs should either be vaccinated (primary in first week, secondary at 6 weeks) or rely on 200 ml of colostrum (fresh or frozen) taken from a vaccinated ewe and given at birth.

In an outbreak

Control measures in the rest of the flock consist of:

- Remove sheep from the predisposing source (where possible), for example take off the lush grass or reduce the concentrates.
- Give an antibiotic injection (e.g. penicillin) for those with local infection, for example 'gas gangrene' and tetanus.
- Give antitoxin, if available, to all at risk, but in the UK this is now only available for tetanus. As the protection provided by antitoxin persists for only approximately 2 weeks, it is appropriate to inject a primary dose of vaccine at the same time (but at a different site), followed by the secondary dose of vaccine 4 weeks later, thus providing both immediate and long-term cover; the potency of the antigen overcomes any significant interference by circulating antibody.

Pasteurellosis

Vaccines targeting *Pasteurella* and *Mannheimia* spp. are killed vaccines which produce high levels of specific antibodies targeting the so-called iron-regulated proteins, which are produced when the bacteria are grown in iron-depleted cultures. In flocks experiencing pasteurellosis, a combined vaccine containing clostridial and *Pasteurella* antigens is often used on the same schedule as for clostridial vaccination. A specific vaccine for pasteurellosis is available if, for any reason, the combined vaccine is not suitable. Note that passive antibodies to *Pasteurella/Mannheimia* spp. obtained by lambs from colostrum only protect for 2–4 weeks compared with up to 16 weeks for clostridial protection. If pneumonia is a problem in young lambs, they can be vaccinated with a single vaccine from 3 weeks of age with a booster after 4 weeks.

Abortion

Effective vaccines are available to protect against the two major causes of abortion in the UK namely EAE (caused by *Chlamydia (Chlamydophila) abortus*) and toxoplasmosis (*Toxoplasma gondii*).

Although there has been an effective dead vaccine to protect against EAE, this is not available at the time of writing (March 2024). It had the advantage of being able to be administered to already pregnant ewes. There are currently two live vaccines available (Enzovax: MSD, and CEVAC Chlamydia). Both these contain a live, temperature-attenuated vaccine strain 1B of *Chlamydia abortus* and must be given at least 4 weeks before mating. Boosters are recommended a few years after the initial dose, but, in practice, most sheep are only vaccinated once. Outbreaks of vaccine-associated abortion have been reported from which the vaccine strain 1B of *Chlamydia abortus* has been isolated. Genomic analysis suggests that the vaccine strain is not, in fact, attenuated and that occurrence of abortion in inoculated animals is associated with administration of low doses of *Chlamydia abortus* insufficient to produce immunity. This would suggest that it is important to ensure vaccinated ewes receive a full dose as per the manufacturer's recommendations. Given the potential for serious economic losses, it is advisable that all flocks that purchase replacement animals, irrespective of vendor's EAE status, vaccinate these animals as a matter of routine. Vaccination may not be required in the minority of flocks that do not purchase any replacements or do not have other sheep flocks as direct neighbours, providing they practise strict biosecurity and investigate all abortions.

The vaccine against toxoplasmosis is a live vaccine and should only be given to non-pregnant sheep at least 3 weeks before tupping. The EAE vaccine and that for toxoplasmosis can be given at the same time but from different syringes at different sites (e.g. on each side of the neck).

The third most common cause of abortion in sheep is uterine infection with *Campylobacter* spp. commonly *C. fetus fetus* or *C. jejuni*. Outbreaks are usually self-limiting but killed vaccines may be imported into the UK under special licence if desired.

Footrot (FR)

Lameness in sheep remains a major health and welfare issue in the UK sheep industry and, furthermore, is a major driver of antibiotic usage. Control revolves around the 'Five Point Plan' which includes vaccination as a key component. One vaccine (Footvax: MSD) is available and should be used as part of a package of control measures when dealing with an infected flock. It is a killed vaccine containing ten strains of *Dichelobacter nodosus*. It is prepared in an oily adjuvant, which can lead to lumps developing at the injection site. The vaccine can be curative as well preventative, with a response usually noticed after a single dose. Boosters are needed, the frequency and timing depending on individual flock circumstances and identification of particular high-risk times for disease spread. Whilst it is licensed for control of footrot caused by *D. nodosus*, it also has an impact on the incidence of Contagious Ovine Digital Dermatitis (CODD) associated with infection by *Treponema* spp. This is likely due to the role that *D. nodosus* plays in the aetio-pathogenesis of CODD.

Monovalent vaccines have been used in some places where only a single strain of *D. nodosus* has been implicated, for example in Nepal. Research is ongoing looking at candidate antigens in order to develop a better vaccine for the future.

Erysipelas

In flocks experiencing problems of chronic arthritis of lambs shown to be caused by *Erysipelothrix rhusiopathiae*, or where post-dipping lameness is a recurrent problem, vaccination with an erysipelas vaccine is usually highly effective in preventing future problems. The vaccine used is licensed for pigs and can be used under the cascade. It is a dead one and requires two injections 3 weeks apart to produce immunity. Young lambs are protected through colostral antibodies so vaccination should be carried out on a similar schedule to clostridial vaccines, with pre-lambing boosters in succeeding years.

Louping-ill

Louping-ill is a flavivirus transmitted by the *Ixodes ricinus* tick which appears to be increasing its geographical range. It infects a number of species both domesticated, e.g. sheep, cattle, and wild, e.g. mountain hares. It can also cause high mortality in red grouse on affected moorlands. A killed vaccine for sheep was developed in the 1930s and was available until 2017 when it was discontinued. However, a novel recombinant vaccine is currently under development at the Moredun Research Institute in Scotland and should be available commercially in the near future. It is expected that the novel vaccine will provide passive protection to

lambs via colostral antibodies. This vaccine will only be necessary in tick-infested areas where louping-ill is a known or potential problem in sheep or red grouse.

Orf

Orf (syn: ovine ecythma, scabby mouth, contagious pustular dermatitis) caused by a parapox virus, is highly contagious and widespread in the UK national flock. Orf vaccine may be employed as a control measure in infected flocks. It consists of a live, fully virulent virus, capable of causing clinical disease and should NOT be used in flocks which have no previous history of the disease. Care is needed in handling the vaccine, which can cause infection in people. It is administered by scarification of the skin in the inner thigh or shoulder region. A scab forms at the vaccination site and this contains live virus and may be shed into the environment for up to 7 weeks where it may persist for many months under suitable environmental conditions, as may occur in farm buildings. It is therefore important that contamination of lambing pens and fields is avoided by not putting recently vaccinated sheep into them. Ewes should not be vaccinated within 7 weeks of lambing. It can be used in lambs but risks transmitting infection to ewes' teats. Similarly, it may be transmitted from vaccinated lactating ewes to their lambs by the lamb becoming exposed to infected scabs as it seeks the teats. Thus, it is generally considered advisable to vaccinate both ewes and lambs on infected farms, ensuring ewes are vaccinated at least 8 weeks prior to lambing. Lambs may be vaccinated from a few days of age. As with all vaccines, read the data sheet thoroughly before recommending vaccination.

Ovine Johne's disease (paratuberculosis)

Ovine Johne's disease (OJD), caused by infection with *Mycobacterium avium* var. *paratuberculosis* (MAP), is being increasingly recognized as a major 'iceberg disease' and an important cause of economic losses in the UK sheep industry. Its prevalence in the UK is unknown although a recent study found 64% of 50 flocks to have evidence of infection. By analogy with cattle, it is believed that infection is acquired via the oro-faecal route from contaminated environments with adult sheep representing the primary source of infection. A killed oil-based adjuvant vaccine (Gudair) would appear to offer effective control of clinical and subclinical disease. It has been shown to reduce markedly MAP excretion into the environment thereby reducing the probability of lambs becoming infected. The vaccine is usually administered to lambs, destined to be replacements, at between 4 weeks to 6 months of age (usually 3–6 months). The vaccine is not licensed in the UK but may be imported under special licence.

Bluetongue

Bluetongue is an arbovirus with at least 24 different strains or serotypes. Until recently it has been considered to be a disease of tropical and subtropical climes. However, in 2006, Bluetongue appeared in northern Europe and continued in 2007 causing devastating losses in some sheep flocks. Cases appeared in the east of England in 2007. A novel serotype A killed vaccine against the specific serotype (BTV-8) was developed and was widely used in 2008 and 2009. This resulted in no further disease in the UK and a huge reduction involving this serotype elsewhere. However, the disease remains active in countries around the Mediterranean involving other serotypes, namely BTV-1, 3, 4 & 8. At the time of writing (November 2024) there has been a large outbreak of BTV-3 in northern Europe, with heavy losses of animals, which has since spread to the East of England. A general licence to use an inactivated vaccine is currently in place in England (see https://www.gov.uk/government/publications/general-licence-for-bluetongue-serotype-3-btv-3-vaccine, accessed 13/11/24). Live, multivalent vaccines are manufactured and used outside Europe, e.g. South Africa, but there is a risk of reversion to virulence with such vaccines and their use is not allowed in Europe or the UK (see Chapter 17 for more information).

Schmallenberg disease

This is another disease spread by infected midges which first appeared in the UK in 2012–13 with another outbreak in 2017 and currently (2023–24). In sheep, its major effect is deformity of fetuses leading to abortion or lambing difficulties. A vaccine has been available but is not at the time of writing (March 2024).

Dai Grove-White and Jo Oultram

4 Thin Sheep

PEERS DAVIES* AND JOHN GRAHAM-BROWN

Department of Livestock and One Health, Institute of Infection, Veterinary and Ecological Sciences, University of Liverpool, UK

Abstract

Thinness in sheep is extremely common and is a cause of welfare issues and loss of productivity. Where many animals are involved, incorrect or inadequate feeding is a common cause and should always be investigated. A number of common chronic diseases may also be responsible, which often require laboratory tests and post-mortem examination on which to make a correct diagnosis.

Thin ewes are interesting and important for the following reasons:

- They are common, which should encourage us to do something about them.
- They are economically important, as thin ewes are less productive in terms of fertility, fecundity, milk yield and even mothering ability.
- They are likely experiencing poor welfare in one form or another depending on the cause.
- The causes are not infinite; in fact, for most cases, the list is short:
  - lack of food (quality and/or quantity)
  - inadequate teeth – particularly the cheek teeth
  - chronic disease, for example chronic lameness (e.g. joints or severe feet lesions, e.g. CODD), chronic parasitism, chronic pneumonias, Johne's disease.

This should encourage us to diagnose them accurately.

First, consider:

- What is thin? To an extent, this is a subjective decision and the 'normal' range of body condition is not universal across all breeds at all times of the year. However, in the authors' opinion, we can consider sheep below BCS 2.0 to be 'thin' regardless of breed or stage in the production cycle. Lowland ewes would typically be expected to carry more condition during the year so a BCS less than 3.0 represents a likely problem and reduced productivity.
- How many are thin? The prevalence of the problem will influence the relative likelihood of specific differential diagnoses and will also influence the economic rationale for different types of intervention. To establish the extent of the problem you need to sample the BCS of a representative number of the flock. In an ideal situation you may wish 100% of the ewes to be at the target BCS at any given time of year but this is unrealistic given the normal biological variation between individuals. Instead, it may be more appropriate to consider a normal distribution (bell curve) of body condition scores centred around the target score, with 95% within half a score thinner or fatter. That would mean you should have no more than 2.5% of the flock thinner than half a score below the target. Calculating the prevalence of the problem will not only help you identify the cause from your differential list but also give you a benchmark from which you can judge the success of your intervention. Malnutrition and parasitism are far more likely to be the cause of a large proportion of thin ewes than tooth loss or chronic lameness, for example.

*Email: Peers.Davies@liverpool.ac.uk

- Who is thin? Understanding which groups of animals within a flock are thin can be very helpful in identifying a cause. Age and litter size are arguably the two most important group variables to consider, but others such as management group and flock of origin (if they are purchased replacements) can both be important, especially in the case of infectious causes.
- Thinness may be reversible or irreversible (i.e. they may not get better); indeed, the ability of a ewe to regain condition after weaning is considered an important trait in some selection programmes as is the ability to maintain body condition through the production cycle. Both traits can be used in combination with other production metrics.
- Thin ewes are not 'worth' much, especially if they are thin due to irreversible causes, but deserve a lot because they represent a serious welfare problem. Their real value may be in the opportunity to diagnose underlying disease management issues in the flock which impact on the rest of the population.
- With respect to parasitic diseases, chronically infected animals may be an important source of pasture contamination for other high-risk stock (e.g. grazing lambs) through persistent egg shedding.
- Thin ewes are generally unprofitable for the following reasons:
  - If thin at tupping, their ovulation rates are reduced and therefore they produce fewer lambs (peak ovulation rate happens at BCS 3.5 for most breeds).
  - If thin in late pregnancy, they produce smaller lambs and risk pregnancy toxaemia.
  - If thin at lambing, they produce less colostrum, of lower quality and show less interest in their lambs, which in turn are more susceptible to disease.
  - If thin in early lactation, they produce less milk leading to poor growth rate in their lambs.

Condition Scoring

One of the reasons for the number of thin ewes being underestimated in sheep compared to other species is that visual assessment of body condition is not reliable as the fleece masks their condition. It is only when the ewe is shorn or handled that the thinness is revealed leading to a delay in taking the necessary remedial action. Condition scoring was introduced to overcome this problem and is now an essential tool in good flock management as well as in the clinical examination of individual sick sheep. In some countries (e.g. New Zealand, Australia) bodyweight is an essential monitoring tool, but cannot be generally applied in the UK because of the large number of breeds and wide variation in mature bodyweight, whereas a more standard breed type is found in these other countries. Condition scoring does not suffer from breed differences though it will be necessary to use different ideal target scores for different breeds, particularly between hill and lowland sheep.

The crucial element in the technique is to decide, by feeling the mid-lumbar region, whether the ewe is 'too thin' or 'too fat' or just about right (Fig. 4.1), so that action follows, for example, by separating and supplying extra, or occasionally less, food (see Fig. 4.2).

A number score (1 to 5, where 1 is emaciated and 5 is so fat you can't feel anything else) is given and it needs practice across the full range of scores and standardizing with other scorers from time to time. Each condition scoring session usually requires

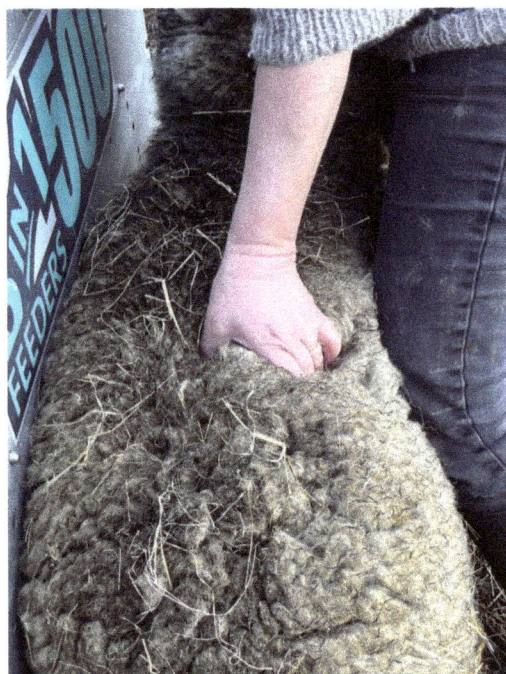

Fig. 4.1. Condition scoring by feeling muscle and fat cover over the loin is a vital technique (photo: Agnes Winter).

Peers Davies and John Graham-Brown

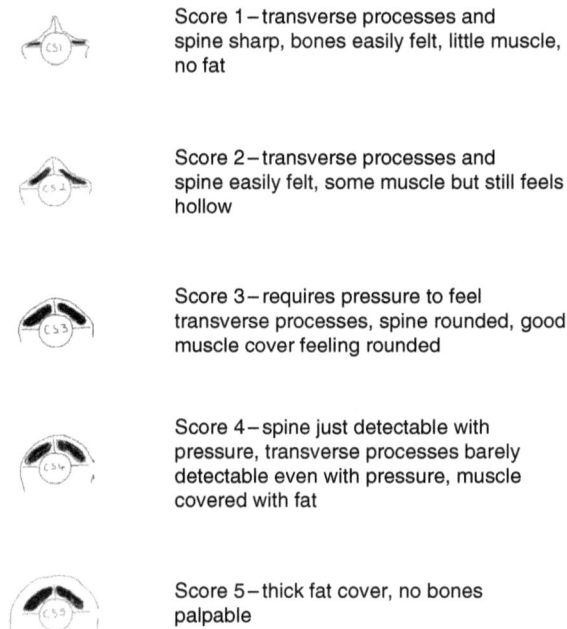

Score 1 – transverse processes and spine sharp, bones easily felt, little muscle, no fat

Score 2 – transverse processes and spine easily felt, some muscle but still feels hollow

Score 3 – requires pressure to feel transverse processes, spine rounded, good muscle cover feeling rounded

Score 4 – spine just detectable with pressure, transverse processes barely detectable even with pressure, muscle covered with fat

Score 5 – thick fat cover, no bones palpable

Fig. 4.2. Condition scoring: descriptions of the mid-lumbar region denoting condition score (CS) 1–5.

doing a few 'to get your hand in', but it is a technique that is learnt quickly and needs no kit, only one sensitive hand. Half-scores are useful as most people find the distinction between full scores too large for decisiveness. It is usually possible to teach the technique rapidly with agreement within half a score.

Two vital times when farmers should condition score their flock are 6–8 weeks pre-tupping and 6–8 weeks pre-lambing (see Table 4.1), because then there is time to intervene by reallocating resources such as food, housing and shepherding (N.B. It will take 1 month to gain 0.5 BCS on a high plane of nutrition). Repeat scoring in about 4 weeks is advisable to assess progress, although it may be too late by then to alter some of the events, particularly late in pregnancy when the demands by the fetuses are high. Lowland ewes with a BCS of less than 3 (hill 2.5) should be separated and clinically checked. Most will require

more, perhaps better, food while some will require treatment or even culling.

Feeding

An adequate diet throughout the year is fundamental to the productivity of a flock. See Chapter 1 for details of feeding throughout the production cycle. Further information is also available at https://ahdb.org.uk/knowledge-library/feeding-the-ewe - accessed 2/11/24.

Assessing the Suitability of a Diet

This is an essential part of any investigation into the cause of excessive thinness in a group of sheep (particularly pregnant ewes) or whether a specific disease is involved. See Appendix 4 for an example of how to carry out such an assessment on farm. As well as the composition of the diet, do not forget to check that all sheep in the group have equal access.

Metabolic Profiling

Blood biochemistry can be a very useful diagnostic tool for the thin ewe where parameters such as

Table 4.1. Target condition scores at crucial stages in production cycle.

	Tupping	Mid-pregnancy	Lambing
Hill breeds	2.5	2.5	2.0–2.5
Upland breeds	3.0–3.5	2.5–3.0	2.5
Lowland breeds	3.5	3.0	3.0

beta-hydroxybutyrate (BHB or B-OHB), albumin and urea nitrogen (UreaN) are most informative. BHB is a particularly useful marker of energy status as it is produced as a by-product of fat metabolism when energy supply is too low. In contrast, UreaN is a marker of current protein intake and should be considered alongside BHB, whereas albumin can be depleted by long-term underfeeding of protein but also by other factors such as chronic parasitism, due to liver fluke or *Haemonchus*, for example, and these differentials may be explored with other tests such as packed cell volume (PCV) and liver enzyme levels to look for evidence of blood loss or hepatic damage, respectively.

Teeth

It is very important to be able to examine sheep teeth properly, not only for ageing (see Fig. 4.3, Fig.4.4. and Table 4.1) but also because faulty teeth are one of the most common causes for adult sheep to be thin (Fig. 4.5).

With regards to teeth, the following points are worth noting as there is a lot of variation within and between flocks, and some confusing features:

- Eight worn permanent incisors can look like eight temporaries and *vice versa*, especially in mountain breeds such as Welsh Mountain. Generally, the temporaries are smaller, more triangular and without a table (i.e. a flat surface). However, since this means that a yearling is being compared with an old ewe, it is usually possible to tell the difference by general observation, so common sense is needed rather than unthinking application of the data shown in Table 4.1 and Fig. 4.3.
- The permanent corner incisor is usually less obvious than the other permanent incisors (it sometimes never erupts). It can look like a temporary tooth, making the sheep appear like a 3-year-old (six teeth).
- In rapidly growing lowland breeds, eruption of incisors can take place earlier than indicated in Table 4.1. The first set of permanent incisors can be present by 15 months, the second set by 21 months, the third set by 2 years 3 months and a full mouth by less than 3 years.
- Age the sheep in relation to the time of year and the normal time of lambing (e.g. in the autumn in the UK, most sheep will be X years

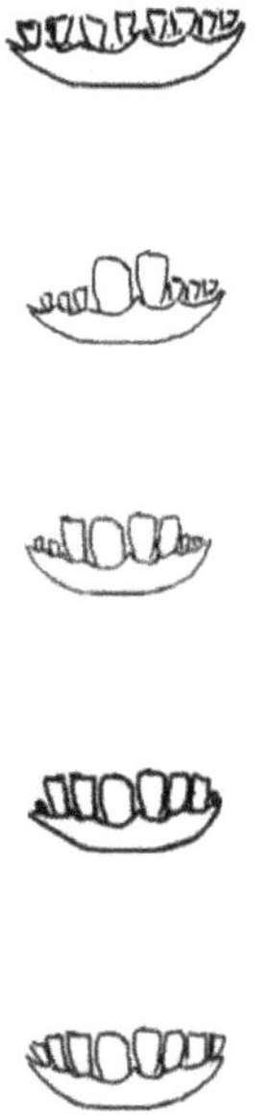

Eight temporary teeth – the animal is less than about 1 year 3 months old

One pair of permanent teeth – about 1.5 years old

Two pairs of permanent teeth – about 2 years old

Three pairs of permanent teeth – 2.5 to 3 years old

Full mouth – more than 3 years old

Remember that a full set of small permanent teeth can look like temporaries – look at the animal to gauge if it is old or young.

Fig. 4.3. Teeth and ageing.

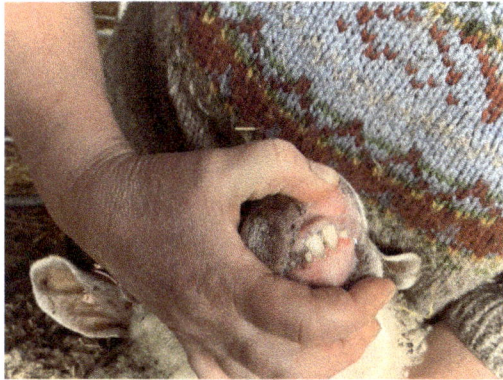

Fig. 4.4. This sheep has its second pair of permanent incisors just erupting, therefore it is about 2 years old (photo Agnes Winter).

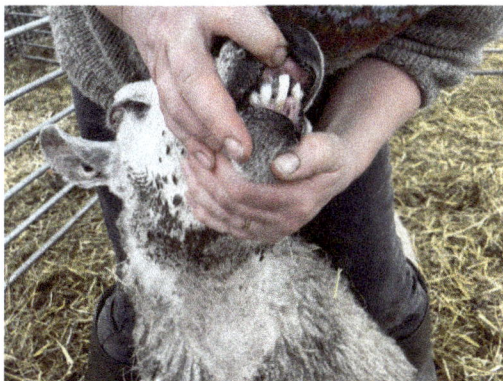

Fig. 4.5. This ewe has long, loose and missing incisors – a poor mouth in a 5-year-old (photo Agnes Winter).

plus or minus 6 months, while in the spring they will be just X years, since most ewes are born in March).

- Periodontal disease causes premature incisor and molar tooth loss and sheep then look older than they really are.
- The first and second molars (fourth and fifth cheek teeth) are present early in the lamb's life and a year or more before the temporary premolars are shed and the permanent premolars erupt. The region between the third premolar and the first molar is, therefore, a very susceptible site for food impaction and progressive disease, starting in the first year or so of life. It is almost certainly the reason why the mid-ramus is the area most

prominently affected (lump and sinus) in periodontal disease of the cheek teeth so this area should always be carefully examined.

Teeth problems

Incisors

Very occasionally, faulty eruption occurs and a dentigerous cyst may result which ultimately causes considerable bony deformity and may cause premature culling, though it is surprising how efficiently such sheep maintain condition. Malposition in relation to the dental pad (over- or undershot) is quite common but it is probably not significant, unless extreme. It has low heritability, and the selection for good apposition (bite or occlusion) is unreliable before 3 years old. Premature loss of incisors (broken mouth) is extremely common and is connected with periodontal disease.

To some extent, tooth eruption always causes a local 'itis', but in many sheep there is a serious progressive gingivitis leading to gum recession early in life and subsequent loosening of teeth following subgingival plaque formation and periodontitis. Osteomyelitis, abscessation and sinus formation are natural consequences of the initial gum pathology. The reason for such serious progression is uncertain; the role of some oral bacteria has been investigated and there is a strong suspicion that gritty food may be involved, which may help to explain why the prevalence of the disease is much higher on some farms than others, where the soil types and grazing environments differ. Feeding blocks or molasses may also have an adverse effect on teeth. Sometimes, there is a family or breed prevalence within a flock, suggesting a genetic component.

Premature loss of incisors in hill and upland sheep reduces the ability of ewes to maintain body condition and to feed their lambs well, and so often results in premature culling. Its effect on lowland sheep is not so serious providing the cheek teeth are not involved, and therein lies the problem. Broken-mouthed sheep should always have their cheek teeth checked, because incisor loss often means molar loss, although occasionally the incisors may appear healthy while the cheek teeth are not (and *vice versa*). The customary reliance on incisor examination alone (ageing) can be very misleading and all thin sheep need their cheek teeth examining

Table 4.2. Ageing – a rough-and-ready guide (see points worth noting in text).

Age (years)	Incisors	Cheek teeth (one side)
Up to 1 (lamb, hogg)	Four pairs (eight teeth) temporary	Three premolars – temporary, two molars – permanent
1–2 (yearling, shearling)	One pair permanent (two teeth), three pairs temporary	Three premolars – permanent, three molars – permanent
2–3	Two pairs permanent (four teeth), two pairs temporary	As above
3–4	Three pairs permanent (six teeth), one pair temporary	As above
Rising 4 and over (sometimes to a grand old age)	Four pairs permanent (full mouth)	As above
Old sheep	Less than four pairs permanent (broken mouth)	May lose some premolars and/or molars

by external palpation of the jaws. Studies have shown a poor correlation between incisor loss and body condition but a good correlation between molar tooth disease and condition.

Cheek teeth

First examine from outside (most problems can be detected by this method, but a more detailed examination can be done if considered necessary – see below).

- Note CS, dribbling, staining of lips and mouth, mouthing (when trying to eat) and quidding (swelling of cheeks with wads of food and spilt quids and cuds on the ground). Observe sheep chewing the cud and regularity of movement of lower jaw.
- Feel along the outside of the cheek for evidence of pain (flinching on pressure) and for irregularity of teeth (shear mouth and wave mouth).
- Feel with finger and thumb along the two rami for bony swellings and missing teeth.
- Compare the thickness of the rami with each other, but also with a normal young animal – bilateral thickening may be missed if you are unfamiliar with the normal, though it is common for only one side of the mandible to be involved which allows comparison between them.
- Note whether there are discharging maxillary or mandibular sinuses.
- Note abdominal distension for ruminal 'impaction' and/or pregnancy (likely to develop pregnancy toxaemia).

Now look inside if you really need to but remember sheep cannot open their jaws widely and it may

cause discomfort to force them apart. Make sure the animal is facing the light (have a good torch) and also have a good gag (e.g. block of bevelled hardwood 12 × 2 × 2 cm or a sheep gag). With the gag in place, note any gaps (particularly common in the lower jaw), irregularities, loose teeth, food impaction and spikes. Look particularly in the mid-third region (cheek teeth three and four): if there are gaps, the corresponding upper (or lower) tooth lengthens through lack of wear, making it even more difficult and painful for the sheep to chew properly.

- Be very careful in inserting a finger since the edges of the teeth are usually very sharp and it is easy to sustain a painful cut.
- We have found increasingly that we can determine the presence of molar tooth problems by external palpation and rarely resort to the use of a gag to examine inside the jaw.

Treatment

- Assess whether it is worth doing anything other than cull. Some action usually must be taken on grounds of welfare as well as economics, but dentistry provides only temporary relief and may only be indicated in late pregnancy in order to allow the ewe to produce valuable lambs which will probably have to be reared apart from the ewe.
- Very loose incisors are often best removed rather than left and can usually be removed without anaesthetic. Remove obvious loose molar teeth under sedation or light anaesthesia and inject long-acting (LA) antibiotic twice at four-day intervals. Ewes can thrive, given a chance, without any incisors ('gummers') providing their

Peers Davies and John Graham-Brown

cheek teeth are healthy. Molar rasping may have a short-term benefit but is very difficult to do effectively.

- Feed high-quality concentrates and roughage that are comfortable to eat and separate from greedy competitors. Proprietary nuts are usually too hard. A useful mix is 40% whole barley, 40% sugarbeet pulp, 17% soya and 3% minerals.

Control

Check feeding and breeding. A fault in Ca/P, vitamin D, copper and fluorine levels in the feed should be considered, as well as generally inadequate feeding which may lead to excessive soil eating (which compounds the problems of mineral deficiencies and gum irritation). Check for feeding blocks or molasses. Feeding blocks and roots may not promote incisor loss, but certainly require healthy teeth. The prevalence in a flock may suggest genetic factors, in which case the ram(s) or even the breed needs changing.

Parasitic Diseases

Whilst lambs are the primary risk group for the majority of parasitic diseases, there are some notable exceptions which also affect adult animals. In the context of thin ewes, chronic forms of fasciolosis and haemonchosis are of particular importance and should be considered as part of the broader list of differential diagnoses. Although acute fasciolosis and acute haemonchosis do not cause thinness in sheep, they are included in this section to give a better overall picture of the epidemiology, treatment and control of these diseases. Rumen fluke are included because of the similarity in life cycle to liver fluke and are an increasingly common finding.

Fasciolosis

Fasciolosis, specifically infection with *Fasciola hepatica* (liver fluke), is of immense importance to UK sheep farmers (and most other sheep-producers across the world). Damp and muddy areas of land form ideal habitats for the mud snail, which is key to transmission of the disease (Fig. 4.6). Infected animals can present with a range of clinical signs depending on parasitic burden and stage of infection. Sheep develop no effective natural immunity to *F. hepatica*, hence animals of all ages can become infected and, without effective treatment will remain so for months.

Control of fasciolosis is challenging. Resistance to triclabendazole, the only licensed flukicide with activity against all stages of fluke is widely reported across the UK (and the rest of the world). No licensed flukicides have persistent activity, meaning the timing of dosing must coincide with disease risk. An integrated control programme should therefore use diagnostics and other management tools to reduce reliance on flukicides and inform treatments in terms of both product choice and timing of administration.

Acute fasciolosis

Caused by profound tissue damage and blood loss associated with the migration of large numbers (typically thousands) of juvenile flukes through the liver parenchyma, acute fasciolosis may occur in sheep of all ages although, in general, this presentation is most common in lambs (Fig. 4.7A). Mortality can be very high in affected groups, with sudden death (no prior clinical signs) in very heavily infected animals; sometimes referred to as peracute fasciolosis. Otherwise, affected animals typically present with extreme weakness, abdominal pain, ascites, and a non-regenerative anaemia with packed cell volume (PCV) as low as 10% resulting from acute hepatic haemorrhage. At post-mortem, the liver appears enlarged with numerous haemorrhagic tracks caused by the migrating juveniles.

Chronic fasciolosis and subclinical infection

Caused by the accumulation of adult flukes (hundreds to thousands) in the bile ducts, chronic fasciolosis typically presents with progressive loss in body condition proceeding to emaciation. Blood-feeding adult flukes cause chronic regenerative anaemia (PCV ~15%), whilst impaired liver function can lead to hypoalbuminaemia. Clinically, these changes may present as pale mucous membranes and ascites. The nictitating membrane may appear pale and oedematous ('flukey-eye'), whilst the classical sub-mandibular oedema ('bottle-jaw') may also be observed. However, such signs are not always apparent and can occur with other clinical conditions (e.g. haemonchosis). At post-mortem examination (PME), the liver is often reduced in size, pale and cirrhotic. The bile ducts are often substantially enlarged with thickened walls and packed with mature adult flukes measuring 2–3 cm (Fig. 4.7B).

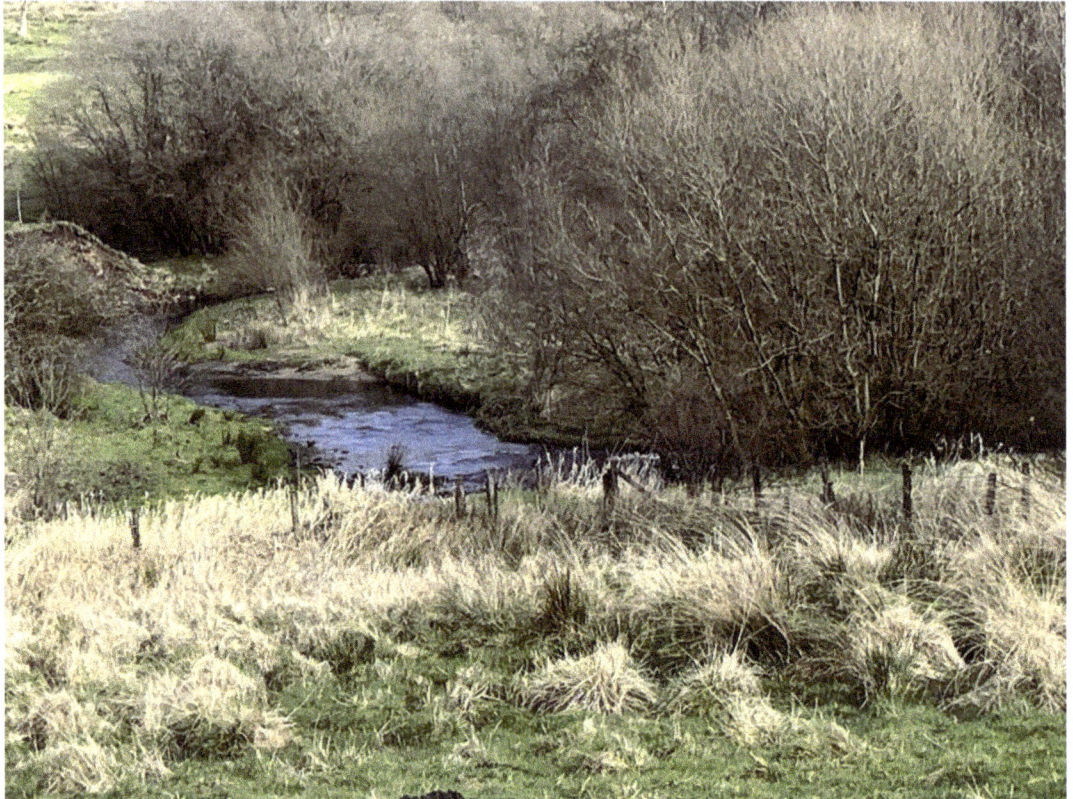

Fig. 4.6. This damp area with rushes adjacent to a stream is a typical habitat for fluke infection (photo Agnes Winter).

Whilst chronic fasciolosis is the clinical manifestation of adult fluke burdens, lighter infections may remain subclinical. It is not uncommon for sheep farmers selling direct to abattoirs to receive feedback of active fluke infection in groups of animals that may have otherwise appeared healthy. Subclinical infections are important from both a productivity and disease management perspective: subclinical disease can have profound long-term impacts on animal welfare and productivity and, in ewes, fleece growth, fertility and milk production may be affected. Without appropriate management subclinically infected animals are also an important source of fluke eggs for ongoing pasture contamination and transmission.

Epidemiology

Fasciola hepatica has a complex life cycle that is influenced by local environmental and wider climatic conditions. This means disease risk varies greatly from one farm to another and, where it is present, over both the course of the grazing season and from one year to the next.

At the farm level, disease presence and risk are principally dependent upon the presence, distribution and degree of interaction stock have with the habitat of *F. hepatica*'s intermediate host, the mud snail *Galba truncatula* (other species of Lymnaeid snails may serve as intermediate hosts in different countries, though all have similar habitats). These snails are small (up to 10 mm in length) and are typically found in muddy areas at the edges of streams, ditches and ponds as well as permanently wet, boggy ground (identifiable through the presence of water-loving plant species, e.g. rushes). The amount of suitable snail habitat present may also vary considerably by season and year. Temporary habitats can be established through flooding, broken ground caused by livestock movement and/or

Peers Davies and John Graham-Brown

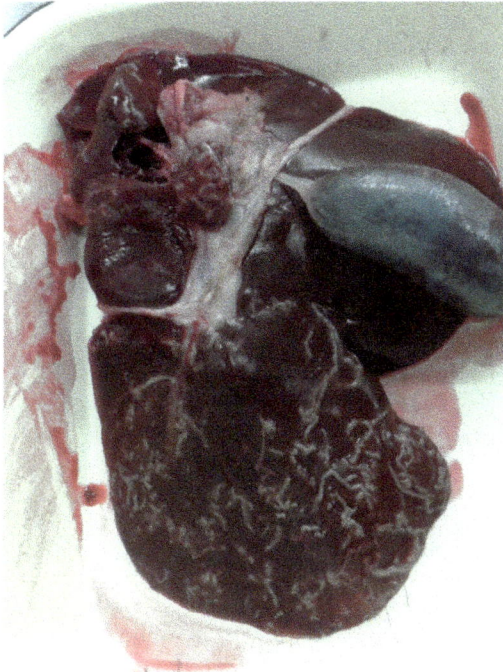

Fig. 4.7A. Acute liver fluke – juvenile flukes may be observed on the cut surfaces of affected parenchyma measuring anything from a few millimetres in length up to 0.5 centimetres depending upon their stage of maturation. Migratory tracks caused by juvenile flukes are visible within the parenchyma (photo University of Liverpool).

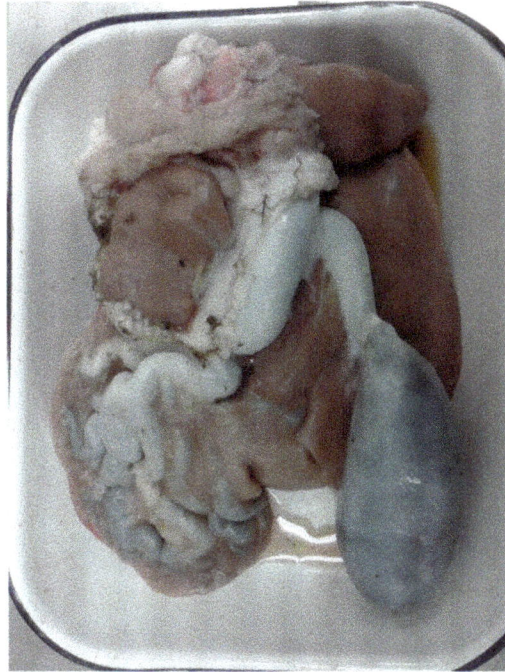

Fig. 4.7B. Chronic fasciolosis – the liver is cirrhotic with thickened bile duct walls with many visible flukes present. Chronic infections are characterized by adult fluke in the bile ducts, which appear distended. Note also the pallor of the tissue, indicating chronic anaemia resulting from extensive blood-feeding of adult parasites. (Photo University of Liverpool).

vehicle tracks, whilst agri-environment schemes encouraging wetlands may inadvertently introduce or increase more permanent snail habitats. *Fasciola hepatica* has a wide host range including wild mammals (e.g. deer, rabbits), which can further complicate disease control and biosecurity. It is also worth noting that *F. hepatica* is a zoonosis. Whilst uncommon in the UK, it is an important (re-) emerging food-borne trematodiasis in many developing nations. People become infected through the same route as livestock, namely the consumption of infective herbage, classically watercress in the UK – a word of caution therefore to aspirational foragers.

More broadly, the development and replication of both *F. hepatica* and its snail intermediate host are heavily influenced by climate. The key components which facilitate fluke (and snail) development are ambient temperatures exceeding 10°C and an abundance of moisture. The development and

emergence of infective-stage metacercariae on pasture from eggs shed in faeces usually takes 8–12 weeks, meaning long periods of warm, wet weather are required. Conventionally, the majority of this development is thought to occur over a single grazing season with snails becoming infected in the early part of the grazing season (May), with subsequent emergence of metacercariae beginning in late summer, continuing into the autumn (September–November) when pasture infectivity peaks. Whilst this period of external development is considerably longer than other parasitic helminths, it is important to bear in mind that during this development, *F. hepatica* undergoes clonal expansion within the snail; one fluke egg will produce one miracidium capable of infecting a single snail, but one infected snail may produce hundreds or even thousands of infective metacercariae. The consequence of this is that whilst development times are long, under optimal conditions the burden of pasture infectivity and therefore degree of disease risk arising from this can be profound when it finally arrives.

In addition to its reproductive potential, fluke transmission can be carried forwards from one season to the next in a number of different ways:

1. Metacercariae are hardy and can survive for several months on pasture, continuing to pose an immediate infectious risk to animals grazing over the winter and into the early part of the next season.
2. Fluke-infected snails may hibernate and re-emerge the following season and continue shedding metacercariae from early in the subsequent grazing season – sometimes referred to as winter snail infection or summer fluke risk.
3. Fluke eggs shed towards the end of the season typically do not develop once temperatures drop, instead overwintering to hatch and infect snails the following year.
4. Chronically infected animals may contaminate pastures through faecal egg shedding over winter and at spring turnout.

Given this epidemiology, it is unsurprising that fasciolosis is a particular problem in wetter regions of the UK (e.g. west coast, Scotland, Wales and Northern Ireland). Outbreaks of acute disease are normally seen in animals grazing 'flukey' pastures at or soon after the peak infectivity period in the autumn. In years where conditions have been favourable, acute fasciolosis can be widespread, with large numbers of animals affected. Chronic fasciolosis typically presents several weeks after initial exposure once a substantial proportion of the fluke burden has reached adulthood.

Due to the importance of climate in determining fluke development on pasture, the degree to which this risk varies from one region to another, and from year to year, can be quantified through a fluke-risk forecasting model. This uses monthly weather data (temperature and moisture abundance) from across the UK to give risk prediction reports for both the summer and autumn fluke-risk periods in a given geographic region (https://www.nadis.org.uk/parasite-forecast/ - accessed 29/2/24). Whilst this conventional view of fasciolosis in the UK is helpful, in the longer term it is also important to be aware that changing climate and weather patterns are altering the geographic and seasonal distribution of disease. Increasingly variable and extreme conditions (prolonged periods of dry

weather and heavy rainfall) experienced in the summer months are making prediction of the subsequent fluke risk in endemic regions more challenging, whilst milder winters may allow both fluke and mud snails to stay active and extend acute fluke risk much later into the season than would previously have been expected.

Diagnosis

Aside from PME, there are, broadly speaking, three diagnostic options available for *F. hepatica* infection:

1. Serological testing. Presently in the form of a serum antibody ELISA, fluke-specific antibodies can reliably be detected 4–6 weeks post-infection. Comparatively, this option offers a high sensitivity and is particularly valuable when considering risk of acute (pre-patent) fasciolosis. However, following seroconversion, antibodies can remain elevated for months, even after infection has been cleared. An antibody-positive result in an animal with long-term fluke exposure (over multiple grazing seasons) and previous treatment events therefore provide little clarity in terms of true infection status. Serology is of greatest value in animals with no prior fluke exposure or treatment history, i.e. first-season lambs. Such animals may be used as 'sentinels' for infection; repeated (monthly) testing of ten lambs over the expected risk period for acute fasciolosis will allow identification of when exactly exposure occurs and allow more accurate timing of effective flukicide treatments. At the time of writing, a lateral flow assay for the detection of fluke antibodies is also under development that will allow more immediate on-farm diagnosis.
2. Fluke egg sedimentation. Whilst highly specific, this diagnostic method has a relatively low sensitivity. Test methodology and equipment are sufficiently simple to set up and perform in-house, which, combined with the ability to test at the group/flock level through pooled faecal samples, makes this testing method a relatively quick and cost-effective option. By definition, fluke egg sedimentation only detects patent infection (10–12 weeks post-infection), making it of little or no use in the context of acute fasciolosis. Consequently, its deployment becomes more useful later into the fluke risk period (late winter/early spring) and/or in cases where chronic infection is suspected. A fluke egg sedimentation-based protocol has also

been developed and validated for use as a treatment efficacy test in sheep: collect and test pooled faecal samples prepared from two groups of ten sheep pre- and 21 days post-treatment. In addition to conventional fluke egg sedimentation techniques, new technologies are becoming available that aim to streamline sample preparation and automate the screening process through digital image capture and web-based diagnostic platforms. N.B. Fluke eggs cannot be detected through the standard flotation methods used for detection of roundworm infections.

3. Copro-antigen ELISA. Offered by some UK laboratories, this method detects fluke-specific antigen within faecal samples. In theory, the copro-antigen ELISA has an increased sensitivity compared to faecal egg sedimentation and is capable of detecting prepatent infections 6–9 weeks post-infection, although results vary between studies. As an antigen-based test, a positive result can generally be considered indicative of current fluke infection making interpretation straightforward compared with serology. At the time of writing, this test is only validated for use with individual samples.

In summary, serological testing is most informative in the diagnosis and treatment of acute fasciolosis in lambs, egg sedimentation is useful as a simple screening method for chronic fasciolosis and treatment efficacy testing, whilst the copro-antigen ELISA is a useful alternative where circumstances make these other two tests undesirable.

Sustainable fluke control

Flukicides are an inevitable component of fasciolosis control. However, for the reasons already discussed, their use should not be considered in isolation. In addition to diagnostics, there are several other measures relating to parasite epidemiology and on-farm management that can further reduce exposure and disease risk. Where treatment is indicated, there are a number of effective products licensed and available in the UK with varying characteristics and indications for use. One characteristic they all share, however, is a lack of any residual activity. Consequently, prophylactic administration ahead of exposure are not recommended as animals can become re-infected immediately after treatment. Aside from this, appropriate

product choice is largely determined by the stage of infection and whether there is any evidence of drug resistance and/or treatment failure on-farm.

The summer and autumn fluke-risk forecasts and timed press releases from experts (generally issued by SCOPS 2–3 times each year: https://www.scops.org.uk) can help determine how big an issue fluke is likely to be in a given year and area. Such information is particularly useful when considered alongside on-farm conditions and implementation of pasture management (where this is possible). Identification and avoiding grazing of 'flukey' pastures during peak risk periods will help to reduce exposure. Similarly, limiting the degree of overlap between sheep grazing and mud snail habitats year-round through fencing of wet areas, water bodies etc. will reduce likelihood of both snail and sheep infections occurring and therefore overall transmission. Whilst such grazing strategies are most effective when employed in a preventative manner, they are also beneficial in the face of active infection. Taking animals off infectious pastures at or following treatment will prevent their re-infection and reduce the likely need for further treatments. Since the metacercarial stage can remain infective on pastures for months, sheep should not be returned to high-risk pastures again in the same season and, ideally, avoided in the early part of the following season. If animals can be moved to 'non-flukey' (dry, well-drained) pasture post-treatment, this will minimize the risk of drug-resistance selection since any further eggs shed by resistant flukes onto such pastures will not complete their external development.

When faced with acute fasciolosis, triclabendazole is normally the drug of choice due to its high level of efficacy (>90%) against early juvenile flukes (from 2 days post-infection). However, treatment failures and triclabendazole resistance are widely reported across the UK (and globally). On farms where resistance to triclabendazole has been identified, an alternative option is to use two doses of closantel at an interval of at least 6 weeks. Closantel has some efficacy against early stages of fluke infection (23–91% 3–5 weeks post-infection). The rationale behind this latter approach is that the initial closantel treatment will act as a therapeutic dose in the face of clinical disease, killing a significant proportion of the juvenile flukes, with the second treatment intended to kill the remainder of the surviving burden, since closantel is 91–95% effective against juvenile flukes 6–9 weeks post-infection. It should be noted that whilst this treatment interval is partly to ensure a high level of efficacy is achieved with the second dose, it is also important from a pharmacokinetic perspective to prevent over-dosing. Acute cases showing overt and unambiguous signs of clinical disease should be treated without delay whilst seeking concurrent confirmatory diagnosis. Otherwise, implementation of routine diagnostic monitoring (e.g. serology) during key risk periods and actively planning a grazing strategy to further mitigate risk will help time treatments to have maximum impact and reduce the need for repeat dosing in the same season.

Whilst being a far less dramatic presentation, treatment of chronically infected animals is indicated from both an animal health and disease control perspective. As discussed, even animals harbouring subclinical infections suffer negative long-term effects on health, welfare and productivity and are also a potential source of pasture egg contamination. Whilst triclabendazole is highly effective against the adult stages of *F. hepatica*, it is generally recommended that an alternative product is used to treat chronic infections to ease selection pressure for resistance. Several alternative products are licensed for the treatment of chronic fasciolosis. Specifically, albendazole, clorsulon and oxyclozanide are 80–99% effective against the adult stages of the parasite from 12+ weeks post-infection and can be used where chronic (patent) infection is identified (by fluke egg sedimentation). It should be noted that albendazole requires administration at an increased dose (7.5mg/kg compared with 5mg/kg for treatment of roundworms). Since closantel has >90% efficacy from 5 weeks post-infection, it is also a useful option where animals are clinically affected by chronic fasciolosis and/or where animals have had ongoing exposure and are potentially harbouring fluke burdens of varying levels of maturity. Where clinical disease is not the principal concern, treatment of chronic fluke infections with an 'adulticide' can be carried out in mid-winter or early spring following a positive diagnosis by FEC or copro-antigen measurement. If sheep are housed over the winter, treatment can be delayed until 2–3 months post-housing, thus ensuring maximum treatment efficacy since the majority of fluke will be mature adults at this time.

A final point to consider in relation to treatment and control is that of quarantine and the risk posed by bought-in animals. Flocks without liver fluke should aim to prevent its introduction, and flocks with fluke should aim to prevent the introduction of drug resistance. Such measures should be considered as part of a wider quarantine policy and flock health plan. On farms with well-drained and dry pastures, risk of introduction is likely to be low, although periodic review of changes to land management and practices that may provide snail habitats are a worthwhile consideration to avoid complacency. It is currently recommended that, where there is doubt, assume bought-in sheep are harbouring triclabendazole-resistant parasites. All bought-in animals should therefore be treated on arrival with either triclabendazole or closantel and tested by pooled fluke egg counts at 21 days post-treatment. Where egg counts are negative it is assumed these animals can safely join the main flock without contaminating pastures. A follow-up treatment with closantel 6 weeks after the initial quarantine treatment is also recommended to eliminate any triclabendazole-resistant flukes or (where closantel was administered as the first dose) to eliminate flukes that may have been pre-patent juveniles at the time of initial treatment.

Where treatment failure is suspected in a flock, it is important not to jump to the immediate conclusion that this is caused by resistance. Poorly timed dosing, continued exposure and various other issues associated with incorrect administration (underdosing, poor/incorrect dosing technique, improper product storage and handling etc.) should first be considered and ruled out as possible explanations. Where other possibilities have been excluded a treatment efficacy check should be performed. As described, treatment efficacy checks are dependent upon the interpretation of fluke egg sedimentation counts from pooled samples, meaning these must be performed at an appropriate time of year on animals harbouring patent (chronic) infections. Ideally, pre-treatment egg counts should exceed 100 eggs per gram of faeces and dosing conducted in a controlled manner under veterinary supervision. Under such circumstances, pooled faecal egg counts at 21 days post-treatment showing <90% reduction compared to those observed pre-treatment are strongly suggestive of treatment failure resulting from drug resistance.

Rumen fluke

This fluke, *Calicophoron daubneyi*, has a similar external life cycle to the liver fluke and appears to share the same intermediate host, *Galba truncatula*, although other snail species may also be implicated.

It has been found in increasing numbers in sheep and cattle in the UK over the last 10 years and is thought to have been brought in from mainland Europe in imported cattle. Adults parasitize the rumen and reticulum and may be found in large numbers attached to the mucosal surface. Such adult infections are considered to be entirely harmless. There is some evidence to suggest that very heavy infections with juvenile-stage flukes may cause severe enteritis, with cases of fatal duodenitis reported in calves in Ireland, but the exact circumstances and processes which precipitate such clinical disease are presently unknown. Diagnosis of adult rumen fluke infections can be made through faecal egg sedimentation. Their clear, transparent fluke eggs closely resembling those of *F. hepatica*, lack the gold-coloured appearance of the latter due to an absence of staining with bile salts. Due to the overlap of external life stages, co-infections with rumen and liver fluke are common. Oxyclozanide is the only flukicide with efficacy against this parasite but, for reasons discussed, treatment based on the diagnosis of patent adult infection alone is probably unnecessary.

Haemonchosis

Caused by the 'Barber's pole worm' (*Haemonchus contortus*). Whilst, broadly speaking, the basic biology, life cycle and epidemiology of *H. contortus* is similar to those of other trichostrongylid parasites of sheep (see Chapter 9), there are a number of important distinctions to make.

Haemonchus contortus is a major pathogen of the tropics and sub tropics. Unsurprisingly, therefore, it thrives in warm, dry summers, but copes less well with cold winters. This is important from a UK (temperate) perspective as it means (unlike most other GI nematodes of clinical significance) this parasite is not found ubiquitously across the UK. Presently, it is more common in lowland systems and further south, but with changing weather patterns bringing warmer summers and milder winters it is likely it will become more widespread in years to come. Due to extremely high fecundity (a single female worm can produce as many as 15,000 eggs per day) combined with a short pre-patent period (14–21 days) and (under optimal conditions) rapid development from eggs through to infective L3 larvae on pastures (as little as 5 days), pasture build-up and disease risk can occur very rapidly. So, whilst winter survival on-pasture

of infective L3 *H. contortus* is poor, animals carrying subclinical and/or hypobiosed infections can quickly re-contaminate even clean pastures to dangerous levels by the early summer under suitably warm and moist conditions. As a consequence, whilst outbreaks of haemonchosis are often sporadic they can be severe, with high levels of mortality and morbidity in the absence of appropriate control measures. In particular, farms with no history of disease may be caught completely unaware should they inadvertently introduce *H. contortus* to their flock through purchase of infected carrier animals. The sporadic nature of disease risk also means protective immunity is usually not acquired, meaning both lambs and adult ewes can succumb to clinical disease, with ewes also acting as a major source of pasture contamination from one year to the next due to the effect of peri-parturient rise on faecal egg shedding.

Adult worms reside within the abomasum and are unique amongst the GI nematodes of sheep in terms of their blood-feeding behaviour; individual pre-adult and adult worms can consume up to 0.05 ml of blood meal per day. This is significant from the perspective of clinical disease. Acute haemonchosis occurs in animals that have accumulated large burdens (several thousand worms) in a short space of time, which can occur due to the parasite's enormous reproductive potential. Where burdens are very heavy (up to 30,000 worms), animals may present as sudden deaths due to rapid and severe blood loss and resulting cardiovascular collapse. At PME, large numbers of worms may be visible on the surface of the abomasum mucosa which will itself appear haemorrhagic. Adult female worms are large (2–3 cm) and easily distinguished from other nematode species of the abomasum due to the characteristic 'Barber's pole' appearance created by their pale-coloured uterus and blood-filled intestine winding around one another. Otherwise, animals bearing acute burdens of several thousand will appear listless, weak, lethargic and dehydrated with pale to white mucous membranes most noticeably over the conjunctiva and nictitating membrane and a marked non-regenerative anaemia. Chronic haemonchosis resulting from the cumulative effect of blood feeding by adult burdens over a longer period of time may similarly present with weakness, dehydration and pale mucous membranes alongside longer-term effects including loss of body condition, wool-break, poor fertility and submandibular oedema ('bottle-jaw'). Lactating ewes may have little to no milk resulting in hungry, malnourished and dehydrated lambs. Haemonchosis generally does not present with scours.

Diagnosis, treatment and control

Diagnosis of haemonchosis is relatively straightforward, although initial clinical presentation can potentially be mistaken for fasciolosis. Seasonal risk period and farm history can help distinguish these two conditions intuitively, but definitive diagnosis is generally advisable in the face of a clinical outbreak to ensure appropriate measures are taken. Where drug resistance is not a concern, all major anthelmintic classes used to treat roundworms are effective (see Chapter 9), although group 4-AD and 5-SI classes should ideally be reserved for use as late-season break drenches and/or quarantine treatments. Products containing closantel also carry a licence of efficacy against *H. contortus* and can be considered as a 'narrow spectrum' worming option where haemonchosis is the specific concern and there is a need to preserve the efficacy of other anthelmintic classes.

Due to their impressive fecundity, patent *H. contortus* infections are easily detected by standard faecal worm egg counts with such animals commonly registering counts in excess of 1000 eggs per gram. Whilst distinguishing the eggs of *H. contortus* from those of other strongyle species morphologically is challenging (this should not be relied on), the combination of clinical signs and presence of very high worm egg counts are often sufficient to make a diagnosis. Where there is still uncertainty, further specialist testing can be pursued. A fluorescent staining technique making use of peanut agglutinin (PNA) can be used to distinguish *Haemonchus* eggs from those of other strongyles, whilst recent advances in PCR and DNA sequencing technologies can allow precise reporting of species presence and abundance within samples. As is generally the case with gastrointestinal roundworms, in the face of outbreaks of clinical haemonchosis animals should ideally be moved on to a safe pasture shortly after treatment (usually 2–3 days), since the current pasture is likely to be heavily contaminated.

The concept of leaving a population *in refugia* is particularly important with respect to haemonchosis and anthelmintic resistance. The proportion of the total *H. contortus* population found within sheep (as opposed to the environment) is very high, particularly over winter, meaning blanket flock treatments will rapidly eliminate susceptible parasite strains and select for resistant ones. Where *H. contortus* is not already present on-farm, good biosecurity and quarantine measures for bought-in stock should be implemented to prevent its introduction (see Chapter 9). Where haemonchosis is already present on-farm, the use of targeted selective treatments (TSTs) is recommended to reduce selection for resistance. The aim of this is to use diagnostic and/or performance testing to identify and treat only those animals in need of treatment, thereby leaving a larger proportion of the total parasite population (within untreated animals) *in refugia*. As a general rule, at least 10% of the group should be left untreated. Where farms are already performing routine (monthly) faecal egg counts and/or performance monitoring with TSTs to control parasitic gastroenteritis (PGE) in their lambs (see Chapter 9) in most cases this will also control for haemonchosis effectively within this specific group.

However, it is important to remember this parasite also affects ewes (and rams). Where haemonchosis is a specific concern on-farm, either based on clinical presentation or a history of disease, additional monitoring and TSTs may also be indicated. These may take the form of additional faecal worm egg counts in these groups, or practical on-farm assessments such as BCS, or the FAMACHA card which has been specifically designed to gauge degree of anaemia caused by haemonchosis (https://www. researchgate.net/publication/11073441_The_ FAMACHAC_system_for_managing_haemonchosis_ in_sheep_and_goats_by_clinically_identifying_ individual_animals_for_treatment - accessed 6/3/24)

A final control option for farms with a history of ongoing problems with haemonchosis is a commercial vaccine which reduces both adult worm burden and faecal egg counts (Barbervax; Moredun Research Institute, https://barbervax.com). This vaccine raises antibodies to a 'hidden' gut antigen that ultimately kill adult worms when they take a blood meal. Since this immune response is directed towards a hidden antigen, protective immunity is not enhanced by natural exposure. Consequently, where implemented, it is recommended this vaccine is administered three times to previously unvaccinated animals in advance of initial exposure, and then every 6 weeks to at-risk groups over the grazing season. This vaccine is presently only available in the UK through a special import certificate under veterinary prescription.

Johne's disease (Paratuberculosis)

Johne's disease is found in older sheep in most sheep-producing countries of the world. In the UK and New Zealand prevalence studies have estimated between 65% and 80% of flocks are infected, and within infected flocks, prevalence may range from <1% to nearly 70% of individuals. However, it is not as frequently diagnosed by vets as might be expected or as well recognized by farmers; in both cases this is probably because of its insidious nature and subtle, non-specific presentation. In many ways it is the perfect example of an 'iceberg' disease, where the magnitude of the infected population is far larger than the small 'tip' of clinically obvious cases. The causative agent is *Mycobacterium avium* subspecies *paratuberculosis* (MAP; synonym *Mycobacterium johnei*) the same as in cattle, deer, rabbits and other species. In contrast to cattle, sheep frequently do not scour until much later in the course of the disease, if at all. The typical story is of a few dirty-tailed (Fig. 4.8) and broken-woolled ewes of about 3 years of age which are unaccountably thin (feed and teeth OK), often deteriorating soon after lambing, and they may have wool-break as a sign of metabolic stress as well. However, a far more common presentation of the disease occurs earlier in the production cycle where ewes in the earlier stages of the disease, still maintaining relatively good body condition whilst experiencing metabolic stress and thus a reduction in fertility, may be diagnosed as non-pregnant and are culled without further investigation of the cause. For this reason, screening for MAP should be part of a thorough investigation of poor fertility in a flock as well as for thin sheep.

Diagnosis

Diagnosis needs to be considered on either an individual or group flock basis. For individuals, scouring is not so obvious, often being intermittent with only soft faeces, so cannot be relied upon as a symptom. As with most debilitating diseases of sheep, the fleece pulls out easily (wool-break). In severe clinical cases the blood antibody ELISA tests are useful, inexpensive and accurate with two caveats: firstly, they cannot distinguish between diseased and vaccinated antibody titres so care should

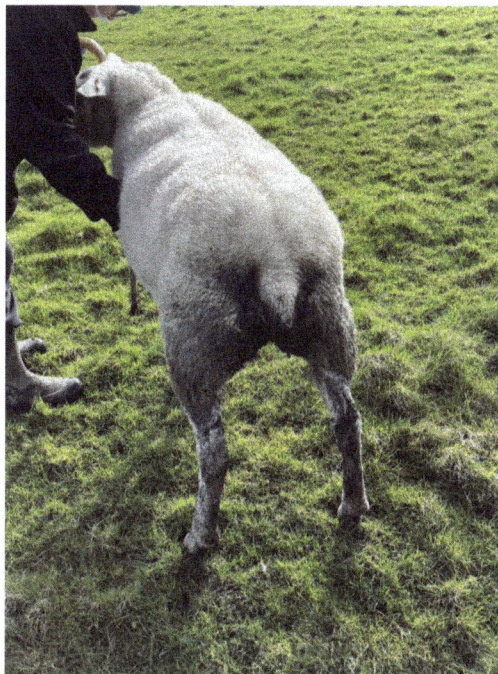

Fig. 4.8. This thin ewe with evidence of loose faeces was from a flock with known Johne's disease (photo Agnes Winter).

be taken to understand if the animal may have been vaccinated at any point in its life the ELISA is far too insensitive to be used for screening of animals that are not showing clear symptoms. For screening groups or flocks, including the screening of non-pregnant ewes, it is far preferable to test animals by PCR assay of faeces. This is also the only way to confirm the disease in vaccinated animals. Care should be taken in selecting the laboratory to run the PCR test as significant variability has been observed between diagnostic laboratories in their test sensitivity.

Control

- Cull clinical cases and fatten their lambs for slaughter rather than keeping them for breeding as infection occurs by ingestion of MAP by young lambs up to 6 months of age with clinical signs only developing 2–3 years later.
- Vaccination – live, attenuated vaccines are used in many countries including the UK. Vaccination

of lambs once with a single dose at about 3–4 months of age increases their resistance to the disease, slows shedding of bacteria and reduces incidence and severity of clinical disease. It does not prevent infection.

- Ensure good control of other debilitating conditions (e.g. lack of food, worms, fluke and cobalt deficiency) which appear to predispose to the development of the clinical disease and the shedding of large numbers of bacteria.
- Think carefully about the use of surplus colostrum in flocks which keep lambs for future breeding. Infection may be spread through this route although it is unclear how important this is in sheep in comparison to other sources of infection, but in problem flocks, use of commercial substitutes may be a wiser choice.

Chronic Respiratory Diseases

The two slow virus diseases affecting the lungs, maedi visna (MV) and ovine pulmonary adenocarcinoma (OPA, otherwise known as sheep pulmonary adenomatosis, SPA, or Jaagsiekte), can both lead to an increase in the number of thin young adult sheep, and be the cause of premature culling (see Chapter 13).

Caseous Lymphadenitis (CLA)

This chronic bacterial disease can also sometimes cause wasting in older animals but is more often seen as abscesses in external lymph nodes (see Chapter 12).

Tuberculosis (TB)

TB caused by *Mycobacterium bovis* occurs occasionally in sheep which have been exposed to high levels of infection, for example by close contact with an infected herd of cattle. It is usually spotted at slaughterhouse inspection rather than being suspected clinically. If suspected, APHA should be consulted as it is notifiable.

5 The Pregnant Ewe

EMMA FISHBOURNE*

Department of Livestock and One Health, Institute of Infection, Veterinary and Ecological Sciences, University of Liverpool, UK

Abstract

Correct management during the period of pregnancy (147 days) is vital to overall flock productivity and profitability. Fetal loss during early and mid-pregnancy reduces lambing percentages, whilst losses due to abortion agents in late pregnancy can have a devastating impact on a flock. Use of ultrasound scanning to predict fetal numbers is now a commonly used technique which can give previously unknown information about this stage of the production cycle. Housing pregnant ewes is also addressed in this chapter.

Ultrasound Scanning – Diagnosis of Pregnancy and Number of Lambs

Ultrasound scanning of pregnant ewes has become a widespread valuable technique in sheep husbandry throughout the world. In many situations it is sufficient to know if the ewe is pregnant or not, but the technique has the additional value in flocks with high lambing percentages, to distinguish the number of fetuses. Ewes can then be marked, separated and fed appropriately for their fetal burden. Commercial operators and veterinary surgeons have provided ultrasound services in Australia, New Zealand, the UK and in many other countries. Most operators offer a service which includes the determination of fetal numbers.

It is important that the operator scans a large number of ewes regularly to maintain expertise in detecting fetal numbers and accuracy will then be over 98%. An experienced operator can scan 80–120 ewes/h. Several veterinary practices with a large number of sheep clients operate scanning services which help in the introduction of sheep health programmes to farms.

Since the introduction of widespread scanning it has become possible to accurately determine fetal losses between scanning and lambing which were previously unknown. It has been estimated that losses of up to 30% may occur.

The value of the technique is that: (i) barren ewes can be sold when prices are high or fed less; (ii) ewes with single lambs can be fed less, saving feed and avoiding over-large lambs; and (iii) ewes with two or more lambs can be fed more concentrates which should reduce the possibility of loss of condition and pregnancy toxaemia (PT).

Ewes are scanned in the standing position without shearing and purpose-built handling systems allow large numbers of ewes to be scanned in a day. For accurate diagnosis of fetal numbers, the fetuses should not be less than 50 days and not more than 100 days gestation. Allowing for a 28-day period with tups in the flock, this means that the flock should be scanned between 80 and 100 days from the time that the tups were turned out with the flock.

The main alternative to ultrasound scanning is regular condition scoring and transfer of thin ewes to groups fed more concentrates. This avoids the need for pregnancy diagnosis but requires regular examination by good shepherds during late pregnancy.

Housing

The practice of housing pregnant ewes during the last 2 months of pregnancy or in wet, cold climates for longer periods has become adopted in the UK and many northern European countries, and in other countries such as the USA (Figs 5.1, 5.2 and 5.3).

*Email: emma.fishbourne@liverpool.ac.uk

© CAB International 2025. *A Handbook for the Sheep Clinician, 8th Edition*
(A.C. Winter and D. Grove-White eds)
DOI: 10.1079/9781800626355.0005

Advantages

- Housing prevents damage to the pasture by the sheep, which otherwise poach land during the wet winter and nibble young grass shoots in February and March. This is particularly important on wet, heavy land where removing the sheep in winter results in good grass growth in April when ewes are lactating heavily. This strategy allows an increase in stocking rate which is necessary if the costs are to be covered. Housing usually commences in December/January and sheep are turned out near the end of March, depending on the weather.

- Housing improves the working conditions of the shepherd and protects sheep (and newborn lambs) from extreme weather conditions and predators. Ewes are more carefully observed and shepherded during lambing which reduces lambing losses.

- Housing allows ewes to be sorted into different batches according to CS, number of lambs being carried (if ultrasound pregnancy detection is used), state of teeth, lambing dates, etc. The feeding of the ewes is more controllable and regular condition scoring allows appropriate adjustment to feeding to be made.

- Housing reduces the wastage of food, both forage and concentrates, if well-designed racks and troughs are used, whereas considerable wastage occurs in adverse weather if fed outside.

- Housing allows the winter shearing of ewes.

Disadvantages

- Capital costs: these depend on the type of building and whether existing buildings can be modified. The building does not need to be of complex design, the cheapest being the 'polythene

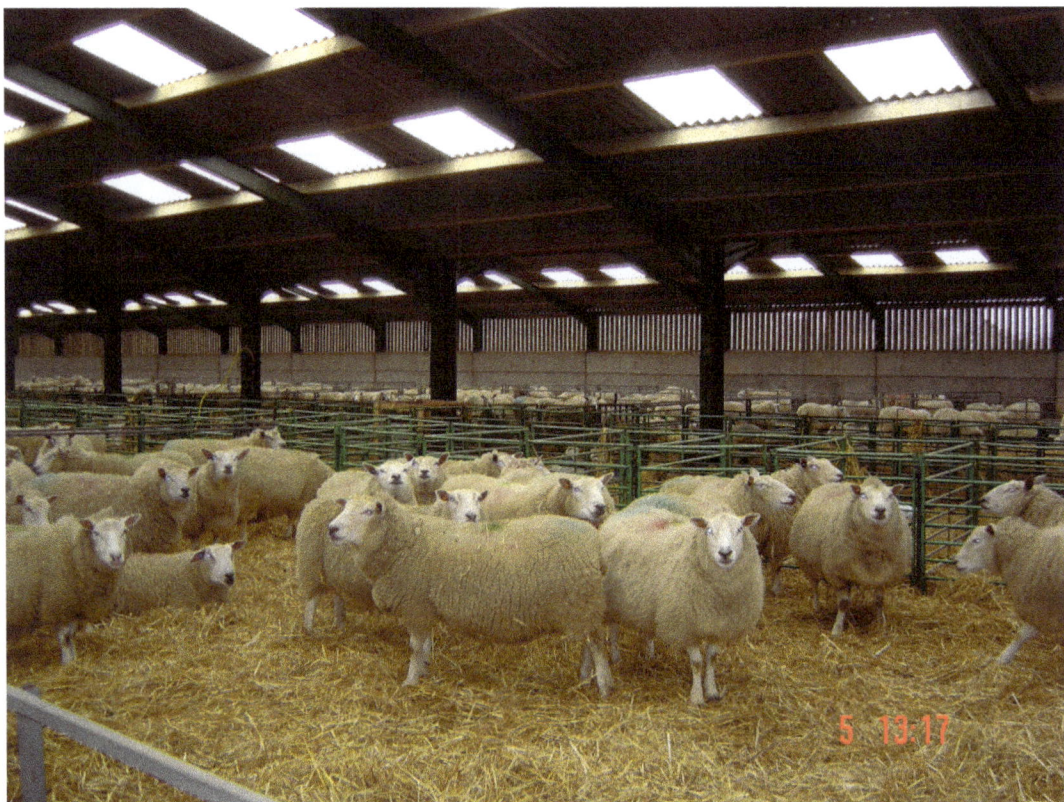

Fig. 5.1. This excellent shed holds a large flock of pregnant ewes divided into suitable groups (photo Agnes Winter).

Emma Fishbourne

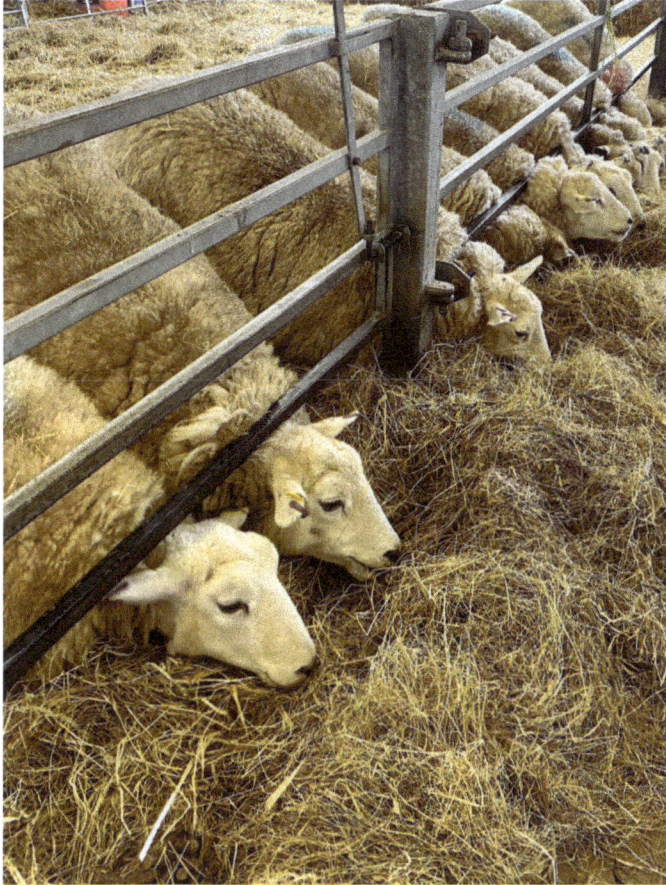

Fig. 5.2. Plenty of room for sheep to access feed at barrier (photo Helen Williams and Niall Connolly).

tunnel). The latter is composed of steel hoops covered with polythene and usually with walls of plastic mesh. The polythene covering must be replaced periodically, some types every 3 or 4 years, but some last 10 years. Most buildings may be used for some other venture (e.g. calves) during the summer and autumn.

- Disease risks: intensive housing may increase the risk of certain diseases such as neonatal scours, coccidiosis, FR and pneumonia but these can be controlled by good construction and management.
- Increased labour, food and bedding costs: food costs in March will be increased because the young grass is deliberately not made available to the ewes, but this will be beneficial in the long run. Straw is an additional cost and labour costs can be higher as they require more input.

Principles of design

Site

The house should: (i) be convenient for the shepherd; (ii) be sheltered from the prevailing wind and snow; and (iii) have ready access to water and electricity.

Design

It is usual to have a wide central passage, which allows access for feeding silage, or may hold hay and concentrate feed, and can be used for individual lambing pens later. Group pens to hold 30–60 ewes are sited on either side of the passage. The central passage should be concreted but hardcore is best for the pens to permit good drainage. The size

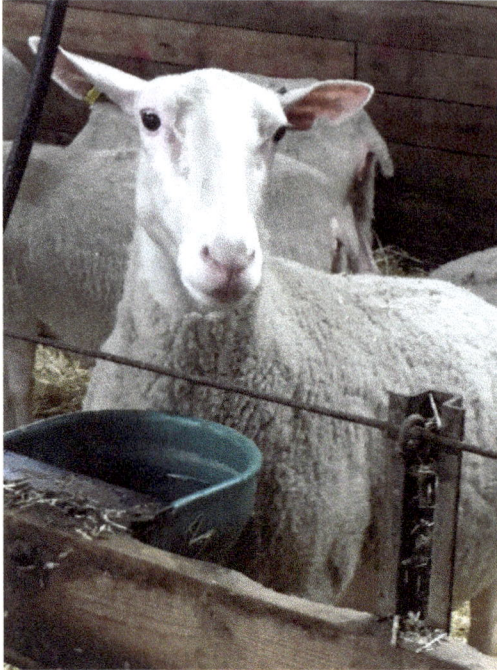

Fig. 5.3. A clean water supply is essential for housed sheep (photo Agnes Winter).

of the pens varies with breeds and shearing but should allow 1.0–1.4m² per ewe at least. It is most important that the ewe should have ample trough space (45 cm each). A useful design is to have removable, double-sided pen dividers, each side consisting of a lower food trough and an upper hay rack with a central walkway between the two sides. Ground-level 'walk-through' troughs are also often used for hay feeding. Alternatively, silage can be floor-fed in the passage with ewes reaching through a simple barrier, with concentrates also fed similarly, or scattered on the (clean) bedding. Straw bedding should be provided; about two bales of straw are needed for each ewe for a three-month period. Slats can be used, but ewes should not lamb down on them. The house must be well ventilated by Yorkshire (slatted) boarding, plastic mesh or open sides but be draught-proof at sheep level by having solid walls to a height of 1.0–1.2 m. Water may be provided in troughs, self-fill bowls or continuous flow along a rainwater gutter. The water should be at a height that the sheep can reach but not too low or it will become contaminated with

faeces, and thought should be given to the increase in bedding height which occurs during housing. It is important that the water sources are suitably placed in the pens to allow good drainage. Good lighting is essential as are power points for shearing and particularly for infra-red lamps over the individual lambing pens and for the shepherd's kettle! Individual lambing pens to house the ewe with lambs at foot up to 6 weeks of age should be between 1.8 and 2.2m² depending on the breed.

Shearing Housed Ewes

For many years in the UK, the winter shearing of ewes was done when the ewes were housed since this: (i) reduced heat stress and humidity which predisposes to pneumonia; (ii) enabled more ewes to be kept in the same space; (iii) increased food consumption and lamb birthweight; and (iv) enabled easy observation of lambing ewes without handling. It also provides some control of lice and keds since they breed more rapidly in thick wool. There are, however, disadvantages associated with the practice. If conditions are extreme, ewes became too cold and huddled together and it is necessary to allow at least 2 months' wool growth (15–20 mm) before turnout which may coincide with bad weather and delay turnout. There are increased feed costs and single lambs may be too large, causing dystocia and 'wool slip', associated with stress. In addition, the thick fleece which follows in the summer can cause ewes to be too hot and distressed. As a result of these disadvantages the practice seems to have died out and it is unusual to find sheared ewes in houses during the winter.

Abortion

The incidence of abortions in 'normal' flocks is usually quite low (1–2%) and is tolerated by the farmer without investigation. However, it must be remembered that many of these abortions are caused by pathogens or nutritional disturbances, which also cause: (i) apparently 'barren' ewes; (ii) fetal mummies; and (iii) very weak non-viable premature lambs. Abortions, therefore, even in small numbers should always be considered as only one part of the spectrum of reproductive losses and farmers should be questioned about these other aspects of reproductive loss before dismissing them as unimportant.

Emma Fishbourne

When, however, an infectious abortion agent is introduced into a fully susceptible flock, the incidence of abortions is often alarming and is recognized as a 'storm'. The cost of an abortion was estimated in 2018 to be between £123 and £177 per ewe depending on breed, number of aborted lambs etc.

Causes

All abortions should be regarded as infectious until proved otherwise. Although the prevalence of the different types of infectious abortion varies from year to year and from area to area, overall, the four most common causes of infectious abortion throughout the UK are:

- Enzootic Abortion of Ewes (EAE) caused by *Chlamydia (also known as Chlamydophila) abortus*
- *Toxoplasma*
- *Campylobacter* spp.
- *Salmonella* – various serotypes

Although these four infections are the most important in the UK, some do not occur in other countries and the relative importance of each will be indicated when dealing with each specific infection. In summary, these are the most common causes in countries in northern Europe. *Brucella melitensis*, which does not occur in the UK, where it is notifiable, is common in southern Europe and is an important zoonosis. Australia and New Zealand are, fortunately, free of EAE.

A number of other agents can cause abortions; these include:

- Schmallenberg virus;
- Bluetongue virus;
- Border disease virus (BDV);
- *Listeria monocytogenes*;
- tick-borne fever (TBF) – *Anaplasma phagocytophylum*;
- Q fever – *Coxiella burnetti*;
- *Trueperella pyogenes*;
- *Yersinia pseudotuberculosis*;
- Fungi.

Reports from diagnostic laboratories give useful figures to indicate the relative importance of the infections in different countries of the world. For the UK, a quarterly GB small-ruminant disease surveillance and emerging threats report is available, produced by APHA and SRUC (https://

www.gov.uk/government/publications/small-ruminant-gb-disease-surveillance-and-emerging-threats-reports - accessed 3/11/24). The latest report shows the frequency of diagnosis of the three most common causes of ovine abortion for the years 2019–2023 inclusive. EAE was the most common in 2019–22 followed by toxoplasmosis. However, in 2023, *Campylobacter* was most common although cases of toxoplasmosis and EAE were not far behind. Other agents, found in much smaller numbers, were *Salmonella* spp., *Yersinia* spp., *Listeria* spp., *B. licheniformis*, *T. pyogenes* and fungi. It must be recognized that these figures are derived from a relatively small proportion of total abortions as many are not submitted for laboratory diagnosis.

Often, around half the incidents reported do not result in a definite diagnosis, leading to the misconception that laboratory investigation of abortion outbreaks is unrewarding and not worth the costs involved. However, as a general rule, if there is a significant abortion problem and the laboratory receives sufficient useful material, the cause will be identified, allowing the appropriate specific control to be instituted and perhaps allowing treatment of the ewes which have not yet aborted. The most likely reasons for laboratories failing to arrive at a diagnosis are that the material submitted is unsuitable and incomplete and may be just the 'odd' abortion from the 'normal' flock. In addition, laboratories may only test for a limited number of infectious agents, though all will look for the four main agents.

In order to allow the laboratory the best possible chance of finding a causal agent, the following materials should be submitted as soon as possible after the abortion incident:

- fresh fetal membranes with cotyledons (if these are not available then supply swabs from the wet skin of the fetus or of vaginal discharge)
- fresh fetus(es)
- information, which will include:
  ○ size and nature of flock (e.g., Is it self-contained? Are the abortions in a particular group such as purchased, yearlings?);
  ○ feeding of the flock;
  ○ previous abortion history, including any laboratory reports;
  ○ dates of lambing;
  ○ facilities for isolation;

○ possible reasons for the abortion(s), for example handling and dosing, predisposing diseases such as fluke and PT and chasing by dogs (though the evidence for the latter is slight!).

- It may also be useful to submit a clotted blood sample (red tube) to test for serum antibodies for *Toxoplasma* or EAE (it is worth tagging aborting ewes so that they can be identified later). However, it is best to leave this for 1–2 weeks and only submit the sample if no diagnosis is reached from the fetal membranes or these were not available.

Remember that some ewes can produce twins, one of which is apparently normal, and the other abnormal and infected. A flock may be infected with more than one pathogen (e.g. *Toxoplasma* and EAE) so that it is worth continuing to submit aborted material to the laboratory even after the first positive diagnosis has been established (perhaps 10% of subsequent abortions).

General advice

- Isolate the aborting ewe and retain the fetus(es) and membranes for laboratory investigation; treat these as infectious (use polythene gloves and bags), not forgetting the zoonotic risks from *Chlamydia, Salmonella* spp., *Listeria,* Q fever and (less directly dangerous) *Toxoplasma* (since oocysts are the most dangerous stage).
- *Chlamydia* is particularly dangerous for pregnant women and their unborn children and they should not be involved with the lambing flock, since abortion may arise in a clean flock without notice. Keep aborting ewes in isolation until a positive diagnosis has been made and until obvious vaginal discharge has ceased (up to 3 weeks) and tag so they may be identified later, if necessary, for blood sampling or culling. If the ewe is ill, antibiotic therapy should be given but only after vaginal swabs have been obtained to submit to the laboratory.
- Do not use aborting ewes or ewes producing premature lambs as foster mothers until it is known to be safe to do so.
- It is usually better to retain aborting ewes and not sell them because, in general, they will now be immune to at least one pathogen and not abort again.

- For *Campylobacter*, it may be worth allowing the aborted ewes to mix with the ewes which have already lambed, and so induce general flock immunity (i.e. 'move on' rather than 'move back'). It is essential, however, to be absolutely certain that *Chlamydia* is not also present before recommending this practice. (Mixing ewes that have aborted with *Chlamydia* will increase the number of latently infected animals which may then abort the next year.)
- It is no longer sound advice for bought-in sheep to mix with the resident sheep, the general farm environment and on-the-farm food before tupping, for a variety of biosecurity reasons. They should, where possible, lamb separately in their first season on the farm, in case they are infected with *Chlamydia* and introduce EAE into the whole flock.
- An abortion 'storm' is usually not repeated in subsequent seasons and subsequent fertility is good, unless a different pathogen is introduced.
- At the time of abortions, those ewes yet to lamb should be kept apart from the infected group and spread out, and the possibility of therapy (see specific infections) should be considered. Where possible, they should not lamb in the same area as the infected group, or at least the lambing yard should be re-strawed.

Enzootic Abortion of Ewes (EAE)

EAE is caused by *Chlamydia (Chlamydophila) abortus*, a highly specialized bacterium which parasitizes host cells, in which it undergoes a complex life cycle involving the formation of reticulate and elementary bodies. Although chlamydiae are bacteria and are susceptible to certain antibiotics, they require 'virological' (tissue-culture) techniques for their isolation and propagation so cultural confirmation of diagnosis is not routinely available.

Veterinary surgeons have responsibilities to the health of their clients as well as the livestock under their care. Infection of pregnant women causes death of the fetus and abortion and a very serious life-threatening disease in the mother. Although only a small number of cases have been reported, you should reiterate the zoonotic potential and advise that pregnant women should not be involved with lambing flocks or handle live *C. abortus* vaccine. Flu-like illness has also been documented following *C. abortus* infection.

Clinical signs

Abortion occurs in the last 2 or 3 weeks of pregnancy with no evidence of illness in the ewes. The pathology of infection is essentially a necrotic placentitis so lambs usually appear fresh and show little or no gross pathology, although the abdomen is sometimes distended with blood-stained fluid. In addition to aborted fetuses, premature and weak live lambs, and even apparently healthy lambs but with infected membranes, are seen. Fetal membranes are sometimes retained, which may lead to metritis, but usually no clinical signs are seen in the ewes. At a flock level, outbreaks of EAE can be devastating with up to 30% of ewes in a naïve flock aborting the following year after incursion. Between 5% and 10% may abort annually in subsequent years if no preventative measures are put in place.

Epidemiology

- The most important source of infection is from aborting ewes since the organism is mainly excreted at the time of abortion and in subsequent vaginal discharges, which resolve in a maximum of 3 weeks. Infection is, therefore, mainly spread at lambing time and the rate of infection and the development of flock immunity is usually slow. Ewes become infected by ingestion or inhalation. Few 'storms' occur but the incidence of abortions tends to persist for years unless otherwise controlled. The disease is almost unknown in hill flocks where the management at lambing is less intensive than lowland, whereas it represents a serious and increasing hazard for sheep lambing under intensive, housed conditions.
- Infection is introduced to a 'clean' farm by the purchase of ewes which are latently infected. The chlamydiae are mobilized during pregnancy, giving rise to abortions etc. in the following year after the ewe became infected. No serological response can be detected during the 'latent' infection and there is no method of deciding whether purchased ewes are infected. Since only a few purchased ewes may be infected and abort, material may not be submitted for diagnosis and the disease is not recognized until a much greater number of ewes abort at the next lambing season.
- The characteristic picture, therefore, is that the first season of infection shows itself as a few purchased ewes aborting or producing premature

lambs; the next one or two seasons, abortions and stillbirths occur in all age groups and the following seasons abortions etc. are mainly confined to yearlings and bought-in sheep, since the older ewes will have acquired immunity, which is dependent on infection of membranes.
- Lambs can be infected at birth from their mother or other ewes and produce infected lambs and membranes at their first lambing (which may not be until they are shearlings) and then become solidly immune.
- Ewes infected for the first time in late pregnancy do not usually abort then but may abort during their next pregnancy. It takes about 40–50 days from infection to abortion which means that infection and abortion can occur within the same lambing season if batch lambing is practised. Ewes with lambing dates of more than 6 weeks apart should not be mixed close to lambing.
- Once a ewe has aborted due to *C. abortus* she is immune to further chlamydial abortions. Evidence is weak that they may continue to shed the bacteria in vaginal discharges at subsequent lambings.
- Intestinal chlamydiae are common in sheep but the majority of these are now described as a separate species, *Chlamydia (Chlamydophila) pecorum*. The intestine may also act as a reservoir of the abortion chlamydia, *C. abortus*, but there is little evidence that uninfected ewes become infected by these intestinal chlamydiae.
- Rams can become infected and may show epididymitis, but it is generally accepted that there is little likelihood that infection will be introduced into a flock, or transmitted within a flock, by rams. However, it seems unwise to purchase rams from flocks which are known to be infected.
- Chlamydiae are not transmitted in the milk of infected ewes but vaginal discharges may contaminate the udder and teats.
- Recently, *Chlamydia* of the vaccine strain have been isolated from a few cases of abortion but it is accepted that this is no reason to cease vaccination as a control method.

Diagnosis

There is usually an obvious placentitis with thickening and necrosis, but the gross pathology is indicative rather than pathognomonic. The lesions of abortion caused by *Y. pseudotuberculosis* are very similar and the membranes should be stained for chlamydiae and subjected to bacteriology for this agent. Modified Ziehl-Neelsen staining of smears from chlamydia-infected cotyledons will usually show large numbers of intracellular inclusion bodies. However, infection may not be very obvious in the placenta when organisms are few and tissue culture has revealed organisms where smears have been negative. If no membranes are available, smears can be made from the wet skin/fleece of a recently aborted fetus or from the vagina of the ewe for 24 h or so after abortion. The Moredun Research Institute has developed a highly sensitive blood test (MVD-Enfer *Chlamydia abortus* specific ELISA test) which is available through veterinary diagnostic laboratories (see https://moredun.org.uk/wp-content/uploads/2021/10/chlamydia-flyer_moredun_2017.pdf - accessed 3/11/24).

Treatment

Aborting ewes rarely require any treatment other than isolation until their discharges cease. It is wrong to mix these sheep with lambed ewes until discharges cease since the lambed ewes may become latently infected and abort the following year. A decision has to be taken immediately after a positive diagnosis has been made as to whether it is worth treating the ewes yet to lamb. This decision will be influenced by the size and value of the flock as well as a guess as to what the subsequent abortion incidence is likely to be. Oxytetracycline (20mg/kg given intramuscularly) is effective against chlamydiae and injection of an LA preparation will maintain pregnancy until nearer the expected lambing date. Injection could be repeated 2 weeks later for ewes which appear not to be close to lambing. Oxytetracycline does not sterilize the infection so membranes are still infective. You should also warn the farmer that, despite treatment, some ewes may still abort or produce weak lambs. Although overuse of antibiotics is discouraged, it may be appropriate to use this treatment in the face of an outbreak and in the following lambing season.

Control

If EAE has been diagnosed

The following measures should be employed:

- Reduce transmission to other ewes.
  - Remove and destroy all membranes, whether believed infected or not (on-farm burial is now illegal, therefore they should be burnt or disposed of with dead lambs).
  - Attempt to clean up the area in the lambing shed and cover with clean straw.
  - Do not use colostrum from aborted ewes as their teats may be contaminated from the uterine discharge.
  - The use of aborted ewes to foster lambs should be discouraged but, if practised, the lambs must be sent for slaughter and females not retained for breeding since it is highly probable that they will have become latently infected or only foster castrated males onto these ewes.
  - Ewes which abort should be kept since they will be immune, but keep them isolated (along with any surviving lambs) for 3 weeks.
- Protection of ewes by vaccination. In the UK there are currently two live *Chlamydia* vaccines available which provide immunity for up to 4 years. There was an inactivated vaccine which is no longer available at the time of writing, although there is a dead combined Chlamydia and *Salmonella* Abortusovis vaccine available; however, uptake is low as *Salmonella* Abortusovis occurs rarely in the UK. Vaccination not only protects against abortion but also reduces the number of chlamydiae shed at lambing. You should refer to the individual data sheets for information on timing and administration.

If EAE is not present on the farm

The following strenuous efforts should be made to prevent its introduction:

- Maintain a self-contained flock. No female breeding stock or lambs for fostering should be purchased except from known clean flocks and although it is generally believed that rams are of little risk, it is preferable to use the same precaution in their purchase. The penalty for introducing EAE is so severe that no sheep is a bargain!
- Purchase replacements from flocks which are monitored free from EAE as part of the Premium Health Scheme of the SRUC (https://www.sruc.ac.uk/media/0v4isdnj/eae_rules.pdf) or on other well-attested evidence.
- Lamb purchased ewes separately from, or later than, the 'home' flock for the first year and investigate all abortions and apparently barren ewes carefully.

Toxoplasmosis

Caused by *Toxoplasma gondii*, a coccidian protozoan, in which tissue cysts are found in virtually all mammals including man, and in birds, and in which a sexual cycle is completed only in cats and other Felidae, to produce resistant oocysts. When susceptible sheep ingest sporulated oocysts (*Toxoplasma* resemble *Isospora* oocysts, with two sporocysts each containing four sporozoites), the sporozoites penetrate the epithelial cells of the small intestine and are distributed to many organs, including muscles, brain and, in pregnant ewes, the placenta. Multiplication occurs and cysts develop in these sites, which remain viable for the life of the sheep but are not mobilized. This means that adverse effects are only seen in pregnant ewes soon after the ingestion of oocysts. A solid life-long immunity develops about 4 weeks after infection.

Infection of susceptible pregnant women by oocysts or from tissue cysts in undercooked meat may result in abortion or fetal abnormalities including hydrocephalus. Infection from handling cat-litter trays or soil where cats defaecate is the most likely source rather than from aborting sheep.

Clinical signs

These depend on the stage of gestation at which infection takes place.

- If oocysts are ingested in the first 60 days of gestation, fetal death and resorption occurs. If the rams have been removed, the ewes will then appear to have been barren or, if the rams are still present, the ewes will be served again.
- Infection between day 60 and day 120 results in the typical signs – abortion in late pregnancy, often with mummification of one or more fetuses, or with one or more stillborn lambs, or the production of weak lambs.
- Infection after day 120 results in an infected normal lamb which becomes immune.

The ewes are not obviously ill, though they do have an increased temperature and lose appetite a few days after infection. Abortion usually occurs about 30–50 days after ingestion of the cat oocysts.

Epidemiology

- Sheep become infected by oocysts passed in cat faeces. Infection and abortion can result from infection with as few as 200 oocysts. The most likely sources of infection to sheep are by contamination of stored grain or hay or from pasture, by the spreading of manure containing cat faeces or by cats defaecating on the pasture. The oocysts are very resistant and remain viable for many months.
- Immunity following infection is strong and ewes never abort more than once. If infection occurs outside pregnancy, the ewe will become immune, without showing any clinical signs.
- Although it is known that rams can excrete the organism in their semen for a short time after infection, this does not seem to be of importance and infection at this time, of course, would not result in abortion.
- Ewes do not become infected by eating infected membranes, that is direct ewe-to-ewe transmission at lambing does not occur.
- As mentioned above, vertical transmission occurs if susceptible ewes ingest oocysts after 120 days of gestation. However, although infected ewes have viable *Toxoplasma* cysts in their tissues for life, their mobilization and vertical transmission probably occurs very rarely.
- Young cats first become infected when they commence to hunt, particularly from mice, and shed many millions of oocysts over a few days about a week later. Infected cats develop an immunity which partially suppresses oocyst excretion; thus, young cats pose the greatest risk compared to mature adults.

Diagnosis

- Fresh fetal cotyledons often show small (2 mm) white necrotic or calcified foci – 'white spot placenta' or 'frosted strawberries' – often attached to brown, dry mummifying fetuses. The white foci are often easier to see if a microscope slide is placed on the cotyledon, or the cotyledon pressed against the side of a clear polythene bag.
- Direct immunofluorescent antibody techniques on sections or smears of cotyledons show brightly fluorescing tachyzoites or cysts.
- Serology (IgM) may be performed on pleural or peritoneal fluids of stillborn lambs, or blood in the case of live lambs prior to ingestion of colostrum. Antibody positivity demonstrates there was active infection of the ewe during pregnancy.
- Histology or smears of placenta and histology or squash preparation of fetal brain may show *Toxoplasma* cysts or a specific cell reaction.

- The detection of specific antibody by various techniques (e.g. indirect haemagglutination, latex agglutination, ELISA) is useful in epidemiological studies but antibody persists for years and serology is of little value in individual aborting sheep. Paired sera taken at abortion and 2 weeks later with a marked increase in titre may be helpful.

Treatment and control

- During an outbreak of toxoplasmosis, aborting ewes are not dangerous to other ewes, nor useful in transferring infection and therefore immunity, so there is no obvious justification in continuing to isolate them once the diagnosis has been established. However, the farmer can easily become confused with this exception to the rule, and one must also always be aware of mixed infections, especially with *C. abortus*. Abortions and fetal membranes should therefore be handled with disposable gloves due to the zoonotic risk.
- During the outbreak there is usually little to be done other than to grin and bear it, although it is prudent to look for the possible ways that sheep could have ingested cat faeces containing oocysts and postpone feeding any potentially contaminated material until after lambing. Keep cats away from cereals, hay and bedding likely to be available to pregnant sheep (pelleted concentrates are likely to be safe since they are subject to high temperatures).
- After lambing, retain the aborters and maintain within a closed flock, or introduce bought-in replacements to the farm environment for as long as possible before tupping so that they are exposed to material likely to contain cat oocysts.
- Cats perform a useful role in rodent control on farms. In the event of diagnosis of toxoplasmosis abortion, it is sensible to neuter all adult animals to prevent further production of young cats, which represent the greatest risk. It may not be advisable to cull all cats since this may result in rat-associated problems in the future.
- A commercial vaccine developed at the Moredun Institute has been used widely in the UK and elsewhere. It consists of live attenuated tachyzoites and is injected into non-pregnant ewes at least 3 weeks prior to tupping and can be given at the same time as an EAE vaccine but at a different site. The vaccine is given via the intramuscular (IM) route, multiplies in the sheep for a few days but does not give rise to tissue cysts in the muscles. It is infectious to humans, as are the live EAE vaccines, thus strict precautions against self-injection or contamination should be taken. It is assumed that immunity is boosted by natural exposure so it is usual to only vaccinate the animal once.
- Chemoprophylaxis with decoquinate given in pregnancy at a concentration designed to produce 2.0 mg/kg bodyweight is effective in reducing abortion and is palatable. The problem is that it is unusual to feed concentrates during the susceptible period (60–120 days gestation) increasing costs and there are practical problems of feeding ewes at this time. Under most circumstances, vaccination is the better option, but this must be planned before tupping.
- Prior to the availability of a vaccine, deliberate exposure of young sheep prior to their breeding was advocated as a means of 'naturally vaccinating' young sheep, with mixed results.

Campylobacteriosis (Vibriosis)

The organism causing this form of sheep abortion was originally classified as *Vibrio fetus*, leading to the disease being called vibriosis but it is now agreed that it belongs to the genus *Campylobacter*. Sheep abortion is caused by *Campylobacter fetus* ssp. *fetus* and *Campylobacter jejuni* but occasionally other isolates may be found. It is particularly important in New Zealand and North America and in 2023 was the most common cause of abortion in GB with *C. fetus* accounting for 91% of *Campylobacter* abortions. *Campylobacter* spp. are common intestinal commensals of sheep and likely found in all flocks. The underlying reason why this commensal may cause abortion in some flocks but not in others is unclear although recent work has demonstrated specific abortion-associated clones of *C. jejuni* in the USA, whilst it has been postulated that the lowered immune response of the ewe may play a role.

Clinical signs and epidemiology

- Infection typically results in late-term abortions.
- Infection is ingested and is primarily intestinal. It is therefore excreted in the faeces from symptomless carriers, which often introduce infection into a susceptible flock.
- Ewes are rarely ill at the time of abortion.

- Birds (e.g. crows and magpies) and voles may introduce the infection to a flock as well as introduced carrier sheep; the infection is then spread from sheep to sheep via faeces, abortions and personnel.
- Early fetal loss is rare as ewes appear to be resistant in the first 3 months of pregnancy; campylobacter infection is therefore not associated with 'barren ewes'. Bacteraemia follows infection in later pregnancy followed by placental infection which results in abortion 7–25 days after infection.
- Immunity following infection is strong to a particular serotype, of which there are three in the UK and many more in other countries like New Zealand, and subsequent fertility is good. Outbreaks may re-occur every few years because of lack of immunity in replacement stock, but usually abortions are few in number after the initial year of introduction.

Diagnosis

There are no visible lesions in the placenta though visible focal necrosis of fetal liver is sometimes present, but the organism can be identified in smears or cultured from cotyledons, fetal stomach or liver. *Campylobacter* is not difficult to culture, but exact typing is complicated. Serology is not helpful.

Treatment and control

- Usually the individual aborting ewe does not require any therapy. Once the diagnosis is confirmed, such ewes should mix with the ewes which have already lambed, but not with the pregnant sheep.
- The remaining pregnant sheep must be kept away from the infection as far as possible and spread out, although the number and spread of abortions may not make this possible. Consideration can be given to antibiotic treatment of in-contact groups of pregnant ewes, with, for example, LA oxytetracycline.
- The farmer should consider keeping a closed flock, although infection can be introduced by birds. Aborting ewes should not be sold. If replacements are bought then they should be mixed with the resident flock for as long as possible before mid-pregnancy, but separated in late pregnancy.

- Effective vaccines are not available in the UK but are used in other countries such as Australia and New Zealand where the disease is more common.

Salmonellosis

One sheep-specific salmonella, *Salmonella* ser. Abortusovis, causes abortion as do a number of other less specific serotypes including *Salmonella* ser. Typhimurium, *Salmonella* ser. Dublin and *Salmonella* ser. Montevideo. *Salmonella* ser. Abortusovis is now rarely reported in the UK but is found elsewhere. Abortion is the only clinical sign with some serotypes like *S.* ser. Abortusovis and *S.* ser. Montevideo but some serotypes are much more pathogenic for ewes, resulting in severe illness and death. This is particularly true for infection with *S.* ser. Typhimurium and *S.* ser. Dublin.

Clinical signs and epidemiology

- Abortions occur mainly in the latter half of pregnancy, although apparently barren ewes may reflect earlier fetal loss.
- Ewes may also be ill at or before the time of abortion: some scour, some die, some have an offensive smelling vaginal discharge for a week or more.
- Except for *S.* ser. Montevideo, lambs are often ill at or soon after birth, and develop a fatal septicaemia or pneumonia.
- Symptomless carriers are found in both ewes and lambs though the serotypes which cause the more severe disease in ewes often result in a solid immunity without carrier status in those ewes which do recover.
- A measure of immunity to a particular serotype is apparently induced because it is uncommon for ewes to abort the next season.

Diagnosis

- There are no obvious lesions in the placenta.
- *Salmonella* is usually easily cultured from membranes and fetus, providing faecal overgrowth is avoided (a possibility if only vaginal swabs are provided).
- Blood testing and rectal swabs provide little worthwhile information.

Treatment and control

Salmonella is frequently found to be sensitive to a range of antibiotics *in vitro* and, theoretically, treatment of individual sick animals is indicated. In practice, such treatment frequently fails to cure the sick or sterilize the carrier. Consideration must be given in any *Salmonella* outbreak to the risks of infecting humans and to producing drug-resistant organisms.

The principal aim in the control should be to:

- reduce the weight of infection by the isolation of aborting, scouring and sick sheep;
- prevent further infection of pregnant sheep, as far as possible, by keeping the aborting group (usually the nearest to term) separate from other groups yet to lamb;
- upset the flock as little as possible and make sure food (hay or concentrate) is always available, particularly immediately following flock movement
- try to ensure that most of the flock becomes immune after lambing by spread from carrier ewes to non-pregnant ewes (i.e. mix recovered aborters with ewes that have lambed).

Avoid reintroduction of the disease from sources such as: (i) 'foreign' slurry; (ii) bought-in sheep and other grazing stock; and (iii) infected feed (including bird faeces). Attempts should be made to prevent birds, especially magpies, entering sheep houses and feeding from the sheep troughs.

If *Salmonella* Abortusovis is diagnosed, there is a dead vaccine combined with *C. a bortus*.

Q Fever (Coxiella burnetii)

This has been a problem in Germany and The Netherlands where there have been many outbreaks of disease in sheep and goats and associated human disease. A vaccine is available to aid control.

Schmallenberg Virus (SBV)

SBV is a teratogenic virus transmitted by *Culicoides* biting midges and causes abortions, stillbirths and fetal malformations in naïve ruminants. The disease was first reported in northern Europe in autumn 2011 and transmission appears to be cyclical in nature. Mating start dates and lambing season seem to impact the occurrence of the disease with farms mating in the summer seeing more disease compared to farms mating later in the autumn, probably due to activity of the vector. The vulnerable period of gestation for fetal deformities appears to be ~ 28–56 days of gestation. Control measures include vaccination, if available (not in UK at time of writing, March 2024) and coinciding mating with colder periods.

Bluetongue Virus (BTV)

Bluetongue virus, of which there are 24 serotypes, has a widespread distribution globally; however, it is not yet endemic in the UK and outbreaks have been associated with windborne spread from mainland Europe. At the time of writing there is evidence of BTV-3 in the UK. As with SBV, BTV is transmitted by *Culicoides* biting midges. Unlike SBV it can cause serious morbidity in adult cattle and sheep. However, as with SBV, if the period of virus transmission coincides with mating or early pregnancy, it may cause abortions, stillbirths and fetal malformations.

6 The Periparturient Ewe

NIALL CONNOLLY* AND HELEN WILLIAMS

Department of Livestock and One Health, Institute of Infection, Veterinary and Ecological Sciences, University of Liverpool, UK

Abstract

This chapter covers care and problems of the ewe at lambing time, when most veterinary attention is sought. It covers the three main metabolic diseases – pregnancy toxaemia, hypocalcaemia and hypomagnesaemia–as well as different types of prolapse and dealing with obstetric problems.

This is the time of the production cycle when sheep clients are most likely to request veterinary support. Most commercial farmers and smallholders, depending on experience, will be able to give 'first aid' for many individual ewe problems and should have equipment, consumables and first-line medicines available to do this on-farm (Fig. 6.1).

Remember RCVS guidance for prescribing POM-V antimicrobials and anti-parasiticides in production animals:

'When prescribing antibiotics, antifungals, antiparasitics or antivirals for production animals, farmed aquatic animals and game, veterinary surgeons should ensure they have an in-depth knowledge of the premises, including its production systems, the environment, disease challenges and the general health status of the herd, flock or group. Veterinary surgeons should have attended and inspected the premises and physically examined at least one representative animal prior to prescribing, or recently enough to ensure they have adequate current information and knowledge to prescribe responsibly and effectively, taking into account any available production data and diagnostic laboratory results' (RCVS Guidelines 1/9/2023).

Therefore, this is a suitable time of year to conduct a flock plan to review parasite control and antibiotic usage to ensure best practice when prescribing.

Important Periparturient Ewe Problems

The major problems seen in periparturient ewes are:

- abortions (see Chapter 5)
- metabolic diseases
- prolapses
- obstetrical problems

Metabolic Diseases–a Clinical Approach

Metabolic diseases in ewes can be difficult to differentiate clinically because they share many clinical signs and sometimes coexist. The clinical signs can be similar to other diseases, e.g. listeriosis, CCN. A further complication is that animals will often have already been treated by the farmer with veterinary advice only being sought in the case of treatment failure or when multiple cases have occurred. The clinical signs and any blood results from treated sheep in such cases may not be representative of the initial presenting problem.

In many cases, especially those with pregnancy toxaemia, response to treatment can be disappointing. This makes it difficult to ascertain whether the diagnosis and treatment was incorrect or whether the sick ewe was severely affected and unable to recover despite appropriate treatment. Therefore, when faced with a ewe which you suspect as having metabolic disease it is useful to take a systematic clinical diagnostic approach.

*Email: conno11y@liverpool.ac.uk

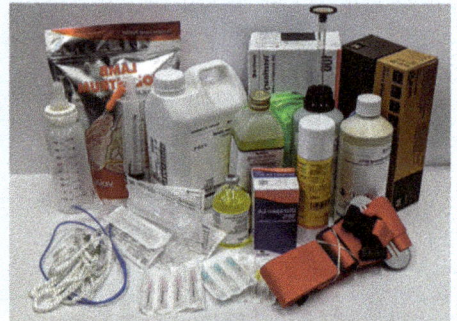

Farmer's First Aid Kit

Treatments/medication

For metabolic disease in ewes:
- Calcium borogluconate injection
- Glucose 50% injection
- Oral twin lamb disease treatment, either propylene glycol or commercial preparation

For newborn lambs:
- Commercial dried colostrum
- Frozen colostrum (in 200ml lots, ideally from ewes from the same flock; can be cows but carefully consider biosecurity)
- Strong iodine for navel dipping or alternative.

For disease or injury in ewes or lambs:
- NSAID injectable, e.g. meloxicam
- First-line antibiotic with farm-specific advice on its use
- Antibiotic aerosol

Consumables
- Lubricant
- Arm-length and short disposable gloves
- Paper towels
- Cotton wool and surgical spirit or medicated teat wipes
- Needles 16G x1″, 18G x 1″ 19G x 1″, 21G 5/8″
- Syringes 50, 10, 5 and 2ml

Equipment
- Thermometer
- Prolapse harnesses
- Lambing ropes and snare
- Lamb stomach tube and syringe or funnel

Fig. 6.1. Items that most experienced farmers should have in preparation for lambing season (photo Helen Williams and Niall Connolly).

Clinical diagnosis

It is useful to take a pre-treatment blood sample (red or green top for Ca, Mg, P and beta hydroxybutyrate (BOHB). This is then available if the animal(s) does not respond to treatment and to facilitate a definitive diagnosis. Treatment needs to be prompt for all three conditions, otherwise the prognosis is hopeless; hence initial therapy by the farmer is usual, with the vet being called if their treatments fail or many animals are affected. It is important to emphasize the necessity to treat early – delay leads to permanent damage (especially with pregnancy toxaemia) or death, with loss and dissatisfaction all round.

If the diagnosis is uncertain

A 'rough-and-ready' approach is:

1. Take pre-treatment blood sample (red or green and grey tubes) for Ca/Mg/BOHB estimations.

2. Give 20ml of 40% calcium also containing magnesium hypophosphite diluted with 30 ml glucose 50% in a 50 ml syringe slowly i/v plus 20 ml of glucose 50% i/v (i.e a total of 50 ml of 50% glucose).

3. Give 50 ml $MgSO_4$ 25% subcutaneously in several separate locations.

4. Give electrolyte and/or propylene glycol orally.

5. If there is no response, send the blood samples for analysis and review your diagnosis, checking particularly for signs of listeriosis.

Pregnancy toxemia (twin-lamb disease, ketosis)

Pregnancy toxemia is a metabolic disease affecting ewes in late gestation which occurs in the last month of pregnancy. It usually affects ewes at either end of the condition score spectrum, i.e. thin ewes (condition

Niall Connolly and Helen Williams

score 2 or less) or fat ewes (condition score 4 or more). It often occurs when insufficient quantity or quality of food (particularly in rations lacking concentrates) is provided or when feed access is limited in housed sheep. This undernourishment may have gone on for some weeks but could be sudden (e.g. following harsh weather or movement). Ewes with pregnancy toxaemia are usually old and may have broken mouths with molar problems or other comorbidities, however it can also occur in shy young ewes with inadequate access to limited feed. The affected ewes will typically have a large abdomen with two or more lambs present. In pregnant sheep, insulin secretion decreases and cortisol increases; these differences are more apparent in twin-bearing ewes. Over-conditioned ewes will have reduced insulin sensitivity. As a result, these ewes are unable to maintain an adequate energy balance, becoming hypoglycemic and ketotic.

Clinical signs

The first sign of the disease is often refusal of feed. Affected ewes become quiet and separated from the rest of the flock. These ewes can present with blindness, are often easy to catch with some standing motionless and some with ataxia. Fine tremors of the face may be observed, some sheep develop neurological signs such as head pressing, opisthotonos and convulsions on excitement and handling. If not treated, the condition progressively **worsens over days** and the animal dies.

Diagnostics

Most practitioners carry portable ketone meters; a sheep-side blood sample will often show beta hydroxybutyrate reading >3 mmol/l confirming the diagnosis. Ketones levels may also be measured semi-quantitatively in urine with Rothera's reagent or urine dipsticks.

Treatment

Treat as soon as refusal of feed is noticed – don't 'wait until tomorrow to see what happens', it may be too late!

For ewes that refuse feed, in the first 24 hours treatment can be administered by the farmer. A number of proprietary oral pregnancy toxemia treatments are available; the main constituents of these are typically glycerol and propylene glycol, otherwise 50 ml propylene glycol (given orally)

should increase dietary energy. This should be repeated in a few hours. These sheep should be individually penned and offered good-quality hay and a little high-energy palatable concentrate (e.g. flaked maize). Some ewes will begin to feed on their own at this stage but others will require hand feeding and oral rehydration before an improvement can be seen. If housed, turning out for a few hours on to good grass, if available, may help to stimulate appetite.

Veterinary intervention often involves administration of 50ml of glucose 50% plus 20 ml calcium borogluconate 40% intravenously (use the cephalic, saphenous or jugular vein and inject very slowly to avoid adverse effects on the heart) in addition to the oral treatments outlined above. Calcium borogluconate is given as the reduced feed intake predisposes to hypocalcemia. Treatment with intravenous glucose 50% can be repeated after a few hours if required. If there is no response, review your diagnosis (see hypocalcemia below) and consider the prognosis of the ewe. Sheep with concurrent diseases such as lameness or infection should be treated appropriately to remove any other causes of reduced appetite. This treatment should include nonsteroidal anti-inflammatory drugs (NSAIDs), since as well as pain relief, there may be an underlying benefit in all cases of pregnancy toxemia associated with reducing underlying inflammatory pathways.

The next day, if the ewe is improving, continue with oral propylene glycol until the ewe is feeding well, then monitor carefully. Avoid prolonged therapy (more than 2 or 3 days) as it can lead to diarrhoea. If the ewe is not improving, consider euthanasia to avoid welfare compromise. If less than 1 week before term, aborting the lambs may help (16–25 mg of intramuscular dexamethasone), or perform an elective caesarean section. Unfortunately, the outlook is considered poor for these ewes; it often takes 36–48 h for an induced lambing to take place; the lambs are often dead or have very low viability and the ewe has deteriorated further in this time. A dose of 375μg of cloprostenol may increase steroid sensitivity and facilitate induction. A caesarean may save the ewe if she is not in an irreversible stage of disease, but it is unlikely to yield viable lambs. Neither would be beneficial if the ewe is comatose.

Control

The sheep should be condition scored approximately 8 weeks before lambing is due to start and split into feeding groups, based on fetal number (when sheep are scanned) and condition score. Body condition score (BCS) will help guide feeding, e.g. thin ewes scanned for a single lamb would perform better within the twin group and thin, twin-bearing ewes are better placed in the triplet group. It is also important to consider which group will best suit the needs of shy feeders or older ewes with broken mouths. The provision of high-energy self-help blocks in the triplet and twin groups is sensible. Top dressing forage with molasses may improve forage intake in these groups. Where nutritional problems arise shortly after housing, consider giving access to green grass, if available, with additional feed outside and re-house when eating well. When ewes already outside present with pregnancy toxaemia, consider moving the whole group to more sheltered fields if available.

Pre-lambing flock assessment

See Chapters 1 and 4 for information on feeding the pregnant ewe. However, summarized below are some basic checks and assessments that can be made.

- On farm nutritional assessment should involve observing the sheep at the feed barrier. During concentrate feeding, all ewes should be able to feed at the same time with trough space of at least 45 cm per ewe. *Ad lib* forage access should be at least 15 cm per head allowing at least a third of the group to feed at any one time.
- Good-quality forage should always be available and concentrates should be fed to all sheep below BCS 3, preferably giving two feeds daily avoiding feeding more than 500 g per feed.
- Farmers should avoid increasing concentrate amounts too quickly as this may lead to acidosis. Feeding concentrates within a total mixed ration will improve feed intake and reduce the risk of acidosis.
- A pre-lambing laboratory assessment of forage quality is sensible to guide feeding based on available metabolizable energy. The best available forage should be given to ewes expecting twins or triplets, aiming to reserve the absolute best of this forage for late pregnancy.
- Farmers should monitor BCS when the clostridial vaccination is given. Loss in condition is often masked by fleece growth, hence the need to handle the sheep. Thin sheep at this point should be assessed for endoparasite burden and treated accordingly (see Chapter 4).

- Blood sampling a representative sample of ewes (n = 5 per group) from each group (single, twin, triplet) 2–3 weeks prior to lambing and conducting metabolic profiles is sensible and allows ewe assessment for energy (BHOB), protein (albumin, urea), minerals (magnesium) and trace elements (copper) to be analyzed. This information can help guide nutritional adjustments for the final stages of gestation and allow improvements to be made for the following year.

Hypocalcemia (trembling, lambing sickness)

In contrast to cattle, hypocalcemia is most common in late pregnancy rather than early lactation; however, it can occur, albeit less commonly, during lactation. Often there is a history of recent movement (e.g. the ewes have been gathered for vaccination or housing) and a delay or sudden change in feeding, therefore multiple ewes may be affected simultaneously.

Affected ewes can be in any body condition score. They show typical signs of 'milk fever' – ataxia, leading to recumbency, depression and atony (bloat, no faeces, etc.) and loss of consciousness. In the later stages, saliva or regurgitated rumen contents may trickle down the nose. It is easy to assume this is a nasal discharge and to misdiagnose it as pneumonia. If not treated, the condition progressively worsens over hours and the animal dies. The blood sample shows total serum calcium concentration is <2 mmol/l.

Hypocalcaemic ewes may go on to develop pregnancy toxemia following initial successful treatment, especially if they have not eaten for several hours.

Treatment

At present, 20% calcium borogluconate solution is unavailable in the UK. Most calcium borogluconate preparations licensed for cattle are 40% providing 29.7 mg of calcium per ml although a slightly less concentrated preparation licensed for sheep is available in the EU which provides 21.5 mg calcium per ml. Any calcium product given intravenously needs to be given very carefully to avoid a fatal cardiac dysrhythmia. Farmers can begin treatment by giving 60–80 ml of 40% calcium borogluconate under the skin in several places to aid absorption. However, as absorption from the subcutis may take several hours, intravenous administration is often needed to

Niall Connolly and Helen Williams

prevent death. The authors' preferred option is to give 20 ml of 40% calcium diluted with 30 ml glucose 50% in a 50 ml syringe slowly i/v. You expect the ewe to respond like a cow with milk fever, eructating, defaecating and even 'walking off the needle'. If there is no response to treatment, review your diagnosis consider the possibility of listeriosis.

Control

- Watch the flock after movement and have a calcium injection at hand.
- If the flock is being moved any distance (walking or by trailer) provide hay and concentrates before leaving and on arrival.
- In theory, keeping the calcium content of the diet a little below requirement until the last month of pregnancy then increasing the content in the ration should help in control, but this method is much more difficult to achieve than with cattle, because of the spread of lambing.

Hypomagnesaemia (grass staggers)

Hypomagnesaemia nearly always occurs after lambing, when the ewe is rearing twins and is at peak lactation (i.e. there is a big metabolic drain on the ewe). It is most often seen when the animal is grazing lush grass (low in magnesium, low in fibre), but occasionally when on bare pastures (insufficient food). Clinical signs develop very rapidly, the ewe becomes excitable with tremors leading to convulsions. If not treated, the condition progressively worsens over minutes and the animal dies, so often the animal is simply 'found dead'. Blood sampling affected ewes reveals a serum Mg concentration <0.6 mmol/l, sometimes coexisting with hypocalcemia. Aqueous humour from the eye can be sampled for Mg and Ca concentrations in ewes found dead.

Treatment

Give 50 ml $MgSO_4$ 25% subcutaneously immediately in several separate locations to aid absorption. However, often intravenous therapy is required. At present there is no 20% calcium solution containing magnesium available to give intravenously and unfortunately there is little evidence on the safety or efficacy of combining products. The authors' preferred option is to give 20 ml of 40% calcium also containing magnesium hypophosphite diluted with 30 ml glucose 50% in a 50 ml syringe slowly i/v. You hope that the ewe will quickly become less excitable and behave normally within an hour, but some equally quickly die.

Remember, don't give $MgSO_4$ 25% intravenously!

Control

Since magnesium levels in the blood reflect dietary intake and absorption (there is little storage in the body), it is likely that other sheep in the flock have low blood concentration of magnesium and are at risk of clinical disease. Analysis of blood from other apparently healthy sheep in the flock will help determine the level of risk. Consider supplementing the remaining flock with magnesium to prevent further cases/deaths. The cost of supplementation should be weighed against probable losses, based on previous flock history or estimated risk.

Options for supplementation include:

- boluses;
- adding to concentrate feed (and giving extra food to any animals underfed);
- adding to water; and
- lick buckets (less reliable as not all sheep will take in the same amount).

Recommend that the farmer watches the flock closely, especially after movement on to lush or bare fields and have a magnesium sulfate injection handy. If already on lush pasture, consider moving the animals to poorer grass, until a magnesium supplement is added. Avoid using high levels of fertilizer containing potassium earlier in the season.

Prolapses

Vaginal prolapse (eversion of the vagina/cervix)

Vaginal prolapses (which often involve the cervix) usually occur in the last 3 weeks of pregnancy, particularly during the last week, although they may occur as early as 6 weeks pre-lambing. The UK incidence is considered low at 1% and even lower in hill sheep. However, there is large variability between flocks, some having an incidence of 5–10% which will have a significant impact on welfare and profitability. Minor prolapses may not cause much disturbance, popping in and out as the ewe gets up and lies down, but if left, severe complications often arise which endanger both the ewe and the lambs; the condition must therefore always be taken seriously and treated quickly.

The evidence base regarding risk factors for vaginal prolapse is sparse and it is likely to be a multifactorial problem. Prolapses tend to occur in ewes carrying multiple lambs and it has been shown that obesity is a risk, although thin ewes can also be affected. There is evidence to suggest that lack of exercise and lameness are predisposing factors as well as steep terrain. Low serum calcium concentration (subclinical hypocalemia) and high plasma cortisol concentration have also both been associated with the risk of the disease. Other suggested risk factors include genetic predisposition (i.e. certain breeding lines), variations in rumen fill, acidosis, short tail docking and coughing.

Ewes that prolapse the vagina invariably do it again next year. Cases in commercial flocks should be marked for culling; however, in the case of individual valuable pedigree ewes or pet animals it is possible to keep them, providing that a suitable external support is put on at the first sign of the prolapse reappearing the following year.

Treatment

If treated in the initial stages, replacement of the prolapse is typically easy. If there is a delay, damage and subsequent swelling provokes further straining. The urethra may become occluded, preventing urination, resulting in a vicious cycle of yet more straining. The prolapsed tissue is prone to damage and contamination. If the prolapse is spotted early and swelling is only mild, non-invasive methods can be used to keep it in place. Often this will be done by the farmer. Farmers should be advised that when the prolapse is swollen and/or the ewe is persistently straining, the ewe should be assessed by a veterinary surgeon so suitable local analgesia and treatment can be provided. Before any prolapse is replaced it should be cleaned and examined for viability, and for the presence of fetal membranes, indicating lambing has started.

Epidural anesthesia should be used in all cases that are straining, i.e. all but the mildest cases. This will facilitate replacement, prolong retention as well as allow suturing if necessary. Epidurals can provide prolonged relief from severe straining by adding xylazine to the local anaesthetic.

It is often easiest to replace the prolapse in a standing ewe. In a recumbent ewe, carefully raising the hind end will help with replacement. A word of caution urine will usually be passed as soon as the prolapse is replaced and the urethra is repositioned!

Suitable methods of retention:

- Commercial harness (truss) – several varieties are available which work well when fitted correctly (Fig. 6.2). This is the method of choice.
- Intravaginal devices ('spoon') – these support the cervix but can cause irritation themselves and may be pushed out.
- Suturing (under epidural anaesthesia) – using broad nylon tape, there are several patterns including purse string, mattress sutures and Buhner suture (Fig. 6.3). It is worth noting these can cause tearing if excessive straining recommences. Farmers will need to be advised on how best to remove the suture at lambing.

Non-steroidal anti-inflammatory drugs (NSAIDs) should be provided for all cases of vaginal prolapse. Those with oedema, damage or signs of infection should

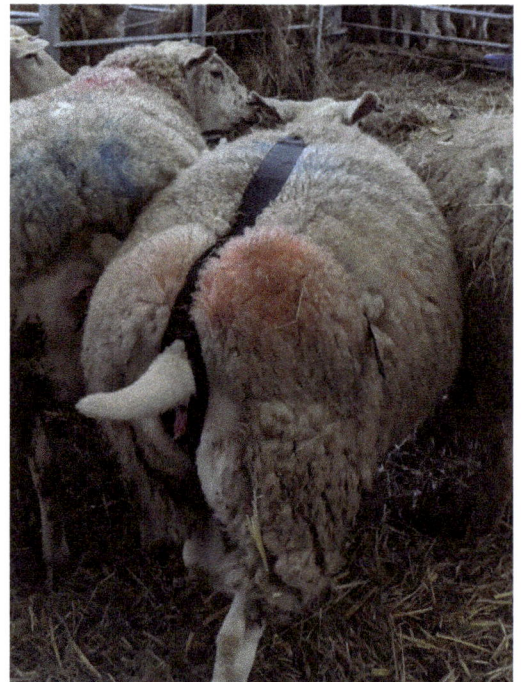

Fig. 6.2. Harnesses are a good and humane way of retaining a vaginal prolapse (photo Helen Williams and Niall Connolly).

Niall Connolly and Helen Williams

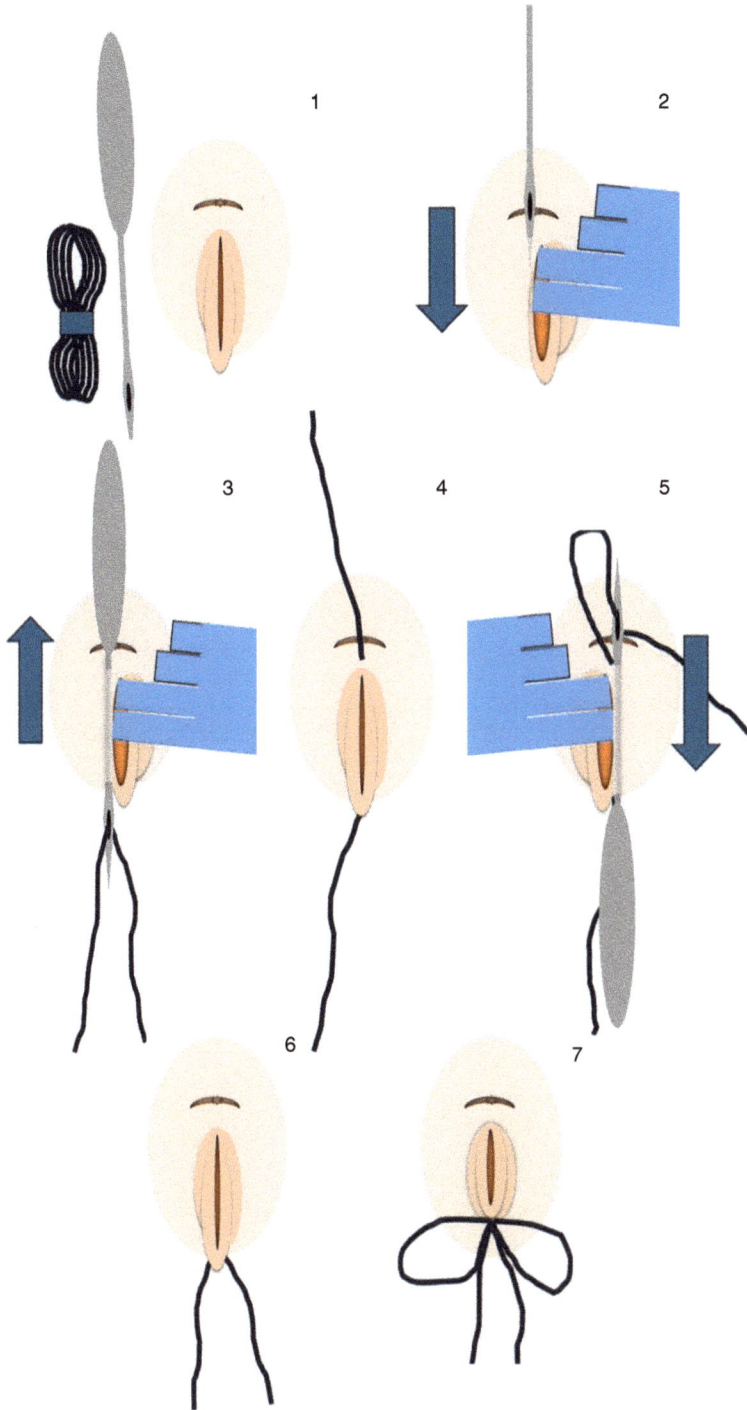

Fig. 6.3.1–7. Placing a Buhner suture. The arrows indicate the direction of the Buhner needle.

receive suitable antibiotic cover. Complications following vaginal prolapse are common, such as persistent straining, ringwomb and dead lambs, these ewes will require additional observation.

Treated ewes must be observed carefully for the onset of lambing – if a harness or suturing has been used, these will need to be taken off once lambing is underway.

Control (difficult when the cause is not clear)

It is worth assessing the ration, in particular the quality and quantity of the roughage in relation to the ewes' body condition score and fetal load. Metabolic profiles can help assess diet suitability. Look at the feeding arrangements – too little feed space leads to pushing which may increase intra-abdominal pressure. Since inactivity has been suggested as a predisposing factor, ensure housed ewes have sufficient space. It is also important that there is good lameness prevention and cases are treated promptly. Ewes that prolapse need marking, recording and selecting for culling before the next breeding season. Records should be reflected upon, and susceptible breed lines should be monitored more closely or not used.

Vaginal rupture/intestinal prolapse

This catastrophe follows a rupture of the vaginal wall near the dorsum of the cervix, with loops of intestine prolapsing through the vaginal wall and vulva. Death from shock is rapid. If the ewe is found alive, and within the final 2 weeks of pregnancy (which is almost always the case) an attempt can be made to salvage the lambs; however, the chance of survival is poor. The preferred method for salvage would be to euthanase with a captive bolt and immediately remove the lambs via caesarean. Alternatively, an emergency caesarean can be carried out followed by immediate euthanasia. The cause for this is unknown but concurrent uterine torsion has been noted in some cases.

Post-lambing prolapse of the cervix

This can occur several days or even weeks after lambing and usually follows damage at lambing, particularly when cervical tearing has occurred. The healing cervix remains swollen and inflamed and this can trigger straining. These can be difficult to replace, because the pelvic ligaments have tightened up, and difficult to keep in place – suturing the vulva will be necessary, with the suture left permanently in place until culling, which is indicated.

Uterine prolapse

Uterine prolapse less common than vaginal prolapse and usually occurs is immediately after lambing. In the initial stages after prolapse of the uterus, where the uterus has not been damaged, the ewe may not present as sick. However, these cases should be seen as a veterinary emergency. The uterus should be cleaned, and contaminated fetal membranes carefully removed from the caruncle or trimmed if still adhered. With the aid of epidural anaesthesia and with the ewe standing or hind end raised, the uterus can be gently replaced. Care needs to be taken not to damage it and ensure the horns are fully everted into their correct position. A truss/harness or suture should be used to prevent a recurrence. Provision of calcium and oxytocin is sensible in these ewes after replacement. Some prolapses can occur a few days after lambing, if unnoticed these ewes can suffer shock, and death is common. Unlike vaginal prolapses, ewes that have suffered a uterine prolapse are not at risk of relapse the following year.

Caudal epidural anaesthesia

As described above, epidural anaesthesia is a valuable technique which should be utilized when dealing with vaginal and uterine prolapses, difficult lambings or any other condition causing excessive abdominal straining.

Control of straining can be achieved for 2–36 h by the correct choice of drugs:

- Local anaesthetic – 1–4ml of procaine (40 mg/ml) will give analgesia for 2–4 h; the hindlimbs will become affected if more than 2 ml is used in smaller sheep.
- Local anaesthetic plus 2% xylazine – the addition of xylazine will prolong the action for up to 36 h and is particularly useful to control straining associated with prolapses. Keeping the volume the same, draw up 1.75 ml (70 mg) of procaine and add 0.25 ml (5 mg) xylazine.

- 2% xylazine – given alone this takes up to 1 h to produce an effect, but then can last up to 36 h. A dose of 0.25 ml (5 mg) is made up to 2.5 ml with sterile water.

Epidural technique

The best site is the sacrococcygeal space (locate the first intercoccygeal space which is easily identified by manipulating the tail, and then feel forward for a depression indicating the sacrococcygeal joint which has little mobility). The site should be clipped and surgically prepared. For sheep, a 20G × 1–1.5″ needle is inserted in the midline with the bevel facing cranially (a 21G × 5/8″ needle is required for lambs). The needle usually needs to be angled with the hub caudal to the vertical at an angle of 10–45° to the skin (this can be variable). Position a 'hanging drop' of epidural agent within the needle hub. Advance the needle slowly until a loss of resistance is noted. This indicates entry of the needle into the epidural space. Due to the negative pressure within the epidural space the drop gets drawn in confirming correct positioning (the ewe may wag its tail at this point). Before administration of your agent, draw 0.5–1 ml of air into the syringe, then *slowly* inject the liquid contents of the syringe. The air bubble should not compress on administration. If resistance is felt or compression is noted, consider repositioning the needle and repeating the hanging drop technique. Success is indicated by loss of tone in the tail and loss of sensation in the perineal area. The first intercoccygeal space may be used if difficulty is experienced in finding the sacrococcygeal space, but results are not as reliable.

Abdominal Muscle Rupture

The rupture may involve any part of the abdominal wall although it most commonly affects the left side, presumably because of the weight of the rumen. It occurs in late pregnancy in lowland ewes carrying twins or triplets and although the ewe is not usually distressed or disturbed at first, complications may arise from entrapment of abdominal contents and it may interfere with lambing. Surgical correction is usually impossible. Affected ewes need assistance lambing (rolling onto their back may make reaching the lambs easier) but a caesarean may be needed. Old ewes are most prone, particularly if they are too thin, and perhaps if they are squeezed or knocked during handling and housing.

Obstetrical Problems

The seasonal pattern of lambing presents problems, with: (i) sudden numbers and lack of practice; (ii) a large susceptible population; and (iii) very intensive conditions.''

In most cases the shepherd will have already attempted to lamb the ewe and the lamb(s) can often be dead when the vet's assistance is sought. However, valuable pedigree ewes may be presented for a caesarean sooner rather than later, particularly if carrying a large single or for a large lamb in posterior presentation, and smallholders may also seek assistance earlier.

When approaching a lambing, keeping the following considerations in mind will help with success.

Maternal considerations

- Ewes do not withstand prolonged vaginal and uterine interference; a sick ewe often becomes a dead ewe!
- Uterine, cervical and vaginal tears are common following rough handling and inadequate lubrication.
- Clostridial infections are common after vaginal interference if vaccination is inadequate and/or antibiotic is not injected.
- Unlike cattle, retention of the fetal membranes is rarely a problem.

Fetal considerations

- Often there is more than one lamb – a sorting out job – be patient. Remember how to differentiate front and back legs by feeling the direction of flexion of joints.
- Head and leg deflections are common. Ensure the head is aligned before traction is applied to the legs.
- The head is the major cause of obstruction and there is rarely sufficient room in the pelvis for the lamb's head and legs plus your hand, so using a snare over the head will permit traction.
- Tight lambings can lead to fractured ribs, ruptured liver or intra-cranial haemorrhage and death of the lamb.

- If lambing is prolonged and the lamb survives, it is often weak and very susceptible to hypothermia so good aftercare is needed.

Equipment for lambings

Ensure that you have the equipment listed below.

- Gel hand disinfectant or soap and water
- Lubricant
- Disposable arm-length polythene gloves (although these can tear or get in the way in difficult lambings)
- Snares (nylon cords with loops or plastic-coated wire – a clean piece of baler twine will do in an emergency)
- Injectable first-line antibiotics
- Injectable non-steroidal anti-inflammatory drug
- A scalpel blade and a guarded knife

History

Some pertinent questions are:

- Is the ewe at full term?
- Has the ewe a history of prolapse?
- How long has the ewe been lambing? The normal range is approximately:
  - o change in temperament – 2–4 h
  - o cervical dilatation – 0.5–2 h
  - o delivery – 0.5–2 h
- Have any lambs been born or delivered?

Examination

Take special note of the following when examining the animal.

External inspection

- Does the ewe look ill or exhausted?
- Are there signs of shepherd interference? Note bleeding and bruising.
- Presence or absence of lamb or membranes at vulva, strings attached to legs or head.
- Smell – putrefaction implies poor prognosis and indicates embryotomy rather than caesarean.
- Udder – check that colostrum is present (if not, may indicate prematurity) and whether there is mastitis.

Internal examination

EWE

- Note the size and shape of the pelvis.
- Observe any damage to the vagina and the degree of dryness.
- Consider the extent of softening and dilatation of the cervix. If the cervix is not fully dilated, particularly if unruptured membranes are palpable, re-examine in about half an hour, rather than risk manual dilation. It may just be too early. Be careful if attempting to dilate manually – tearing and haemorrhage may result.

LAMBS

- Are they dead or alive? (It is not always easy to be certain; assume alive if not sure.)
- How many? A jumble of legs and heads implies at least two, probably more.
- Presentation – anterior? posterior? transverse? breech?
- Ankylosed joints may indicate other deformities.

Delivery

- Aim to complete delivery within 15 minutes or make a quick decision about doing a caesarean.
- Consider giving a caudal epidural – this makes things more comfortable for the ewe and easier for you.
- Lubrication is very important – use plenty. Adding warm water to the lubricant and filling the uterus may help in a difficult dry case.
- Positioning of the ewe can sometimes help; raising the ewe's hind end (but carefully and not for too long) can help to avoid straining and allow repulsion of a lamb; however, this should not be used in place of epidural anaesthesia.
- Where the uterus is contracted down, consider giving clenbuterol. This is not licensed for sheep but can make a difficult case easier and can be used under the 'cascade'.

Ringwomb

Ringwomb is a failure of the cervix to fully dilate leaving a ring of constriction varying from a narrow band less than a centimetre thick to the full depth of the cervix, preventing parturition. Depending on the size of the opening the membranes may or may not present at the vulva and rupture and it can trigger a malpresentation with head or one limb back. The underlying cause is not known but may relate to hormone imbalance or stress blocking oxytocin release and progression at a critical time in the parturition process. A lack of calcium may cause uterine inertia, but as it is a focal area that is not dilated rather than no progression whatsoever, this suggests it may be something localized.

Depending on size of the opening, gentle dilatation with fingers and copious lubrication may be possible. Caudal epidural and clenbuterol (Planipart; authorized on cattle and used under the cascade) may improve fetal viability and reduce straining to allow time for dilation. This needs to be patient to avoid tearing and damage to the cervix.

Sensiblex (Denaverine hydrochloride 40.0 mg/ml; authorized for cattle and used under the cascade) is indicated to promote dilation of the soft tissues of the birth canal in cases where the birth canal is insufficiently opened in cattle. Data in a clinical trial in cattle suggest a reduced duration and force was needed in assisted calving but these were not clearly ringwomb-like in cause. Anecdotal reports of its use in ringwomb in sheep show a variable impression of efficacy. It probably will not cause harm so, until better data are available, remains a possible treatment.

Anterior presentation

HEAD ONLY   It is common for only a swollen head to be presented outside the vulva, with both front legs retained.

- If the head is not swollen, put a snare on, then carefully replace, find the legs, and deliver normally.
- If the lamb is dead (no suck or blink reflex), then decapitate. If uncertain, treat as if alive.
- If the lamb is alive, lubricate well and insert a small hand beside the head and neck and try to find a limb and extend it. It is often then possible in ewes (but not ewe lambs) to withdraw the lamb with only one limb extended – twisting the lamb while pulling will help to prevent the shoulder becoming locked.
- When the lamb is large or ewe is tight, get one leg up, put a rope on, replace, and repeat with the other leg before using both ropes to pull both legs.

HEAD AND NECK DEFLECTIONS   These are common and often made worse by pulling on the legs,

expecting the head to follow. The head is the main bulk, so put a loop on the head first, then straighten the head, and then find the correct legs before pulling.

Posterior presentation

Large lambs in posterior presentation are very vulnerable to hypoxia and to physical damage such as broken ribs. Provided both hindlimbs and tail are present, withdraw with gentle traction. Be aware of the possibility of stifles locking under the pelvic brim – lift and extend the legs before pulling.

Breech presentations

It takes a good shepherd to spot a breech presentation early; often the only sign is wetness down the back of the udder (indicating rupture of membranes). Gently repel the lamb and search for the hind legs, then bring them up one at a time into the pelvis by flexing/extending the limb joints.

Embryotomy

For ewes with dead smelly lambs, this is a better option than a caesarean as the survival rate is only 50% compared with ewes with live or freshly dead lambs.

For known dead lambs: with a swollen head, decapitate; for other anterior presentations, find a front leg and pull so you can cut around the skin above the knee *outside* the vulva with a sharp knife, then use your fingers to undermine the skin and break down the muscles holding the shoulder blade to the chest. Both forelegs can be removed leaving the head to pull. The more decomposed the lamb, the easier it is. Remove any detached membranes and general debris.

Caesarean operation

Indications for a caesarean are listed below.

- Non-dilatation of the cervix (ringwomb) after one or two examinations at approximately half-hour intervals
- Fetal oversize
- Large (valuable) lambs in posterior or breech presentation
- Noncorrectable malpresentation
- Deformities

- Uterine torsion (rare – try 'unrolling' first and check carefully for uterine tears).
- Elective due to pregnancy toxemia or intestinal prolapse – rarely get viable lambs.

The operation is relatively quick and easy, compared with other species, and needs to be considered early in the proceedings. The most common site is the left flank, with linear local infiltration anaesthesia or inverted L block or paravertebral injection. Remember that sheep are more susceptible to overdose of local anaesthetic than cows, so take care with the total amount of local anaesthetic injected especially in smaller sheep (should be less than 20 mg/kg procaine).

Paravertebral anaesthesia

This is easy and satisfying to perform in lean ewes but can be difficult in fat animals. The technique is as in cows: (i) prepare the skin over the posterior thoracic and lumbar transverse processes; (ii) identify the first lumbar vertebra; (iii) inject 1–2 ml 2% local anaesthetic subcutaneously and into the muscle about halfway between the midline and the end of the process; and (iv) 'walk' the needle off the front edge of the transverse process to catch T13 and inject 3–5 ml just below the level of the process. Repeat off the posterior edge of L1, then the posterior edges of L2.

Caesarean technique

1. Make an incision in the centre of the left flank, being careful not to cut too deep, accidentally cutting into the rumen – the abdominal wall can be surprisingly thin.
2. Palpate the uterus, identify the extremity of the lamb and carefully exteriorize, holding it through the uterine wall.
3. Incise over the extremity along the greater curvature.
4. Grasp the lamb and remove.
5. Check the uterus for more lambs – it can sometimes be difficult to reach a lamb in the other uterine horn – feel down towards the cervix before 'turning the corner' and entering the far horn. Remove any remaining lambs carefully.
6. Remove the fetal membranes if they are detached, trim and leave *in situ* if still attached.
7. Repair the uterus with an inverting suture making sure no membranes protrude.

8. Replace the uterus in the normal position.
9. Suture the flank incision in two or three layers.

The survival rate of a ewe undergoing a caesarean with live or freshly dead lambs should be high.

After delivery

Revive the lamb, clear the mouth and nose and stimulate breathing by rubbing the chest. If the lamb does not initiate breathing, artificial respiration may be attempted. A stomach tube can be used to inflate the lungs by positioning it in the pharynx and blocking off the oesophagus and nose, and then blowing down the tube. Once the lamb is breathing, return it to the dam quickly for licking. If the lamb is slow to revive, has reduced consciousness and lacks a suckle reflex, consider giving 10 ml of 8.4% sodium bicarbonate solution intravenously to reverse a metabolic acidosis. Alternatively, consider employing the Madigan Squeeze technique as developed to treat dummy foals and calves (https://doi.org/10.1080/00480169.2019.1670115).

Finally, carry out the following:

- Re-examine for:
  - the presence of other lamb(s) both internally and by ballotting;
  - damage – tearing, haemorrhage.
- If there is bruising or tears or if there has been prolonged manipulation or contamination, then consider the administration of a long-acting antibiotic injection.
- The authors give an NSAID routinely to almost all sheep presented to them for a lambing, as by default these cases will have been a more difficult lambing and have been lambing for a prolonged time. Studies in cattle have shown a benefit to welfare and mobility when all calved cows received an NSAID. As yet there is no licensed NSAID for use in sheep; however, it can be used following the cascade.
- Check the udder – milk off some colostrum and give it to the lamb(s) using a stomach tube; if there is none, give a substitute.
- Check and treat the lamb's navel with strong iodine or antibiotic aerosol.
- Check for defects such as entropion – correct immediately by everting the affected eyelid(s).
- Put the ewe and lamb(s) in an individual pen so bonding can occur and the group can be closely observed (Fig. 6.4).

Niall Connolly and Helen Williams

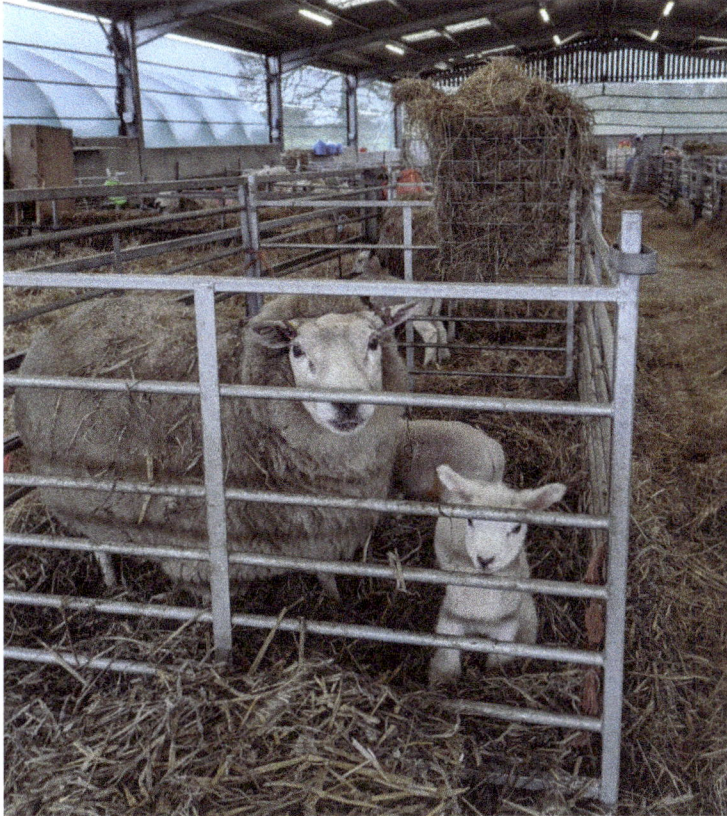

Fig. 6.4. Individual pens should be used to separate ewes with newborn lambs or ewes or lambs which require extra care (photo Helen Williams and Niall Connolly).

7 Neonatal Lambs

JENNIFER DUNCAN* AND JOSEPH ANGELL

Department of Livestock and One Health, Institute of Infection,
Veterinary and Ecological Sciences, University of Liverpool, UK

Abstract

Maximizing lamb survival is one of the most important factors affecting flock profitability. This chapter covers the main factors affecting survival of newborn lambs and describes the major causes of mortality. Key areas are the health and nutritional status of ewes, adequate and skilled supervision of lambing ewes, hygienic lambing conditions, and rapid and adequate intake of good-quality colostrum by lambs.

The neonatal period is the highest-risk period for lamb losses, with important animal welfare, economic, and sustainability issues for sheep farms. The main causes of lamb disease and death during this period are hypothermia, starvation, infection, trauma, congenital defects and predation. The majority of these are preventable by excellent flock health management practices throughout the sheep production year.

Recent farm-based estimates suggest about 8% of lambs will die in the neonatal period. This means that in a flock of 1000 lowland ewes anticipating 1800 lambs, over 135 lambs may be lost in the first seven days of life. Based on finished lamb prices of £100, this equals an estimated loss of £13,500 per year. Estimates like this for a farm can act as a good motivator for change and provide a budget for interventions.

In this chapter, much of what is discussed is relevant for both intensively, and extensively farmed sheep. Clearly, there are major differences between sheep lambed outside and those lambed indoors. It is important to bear in mind that investigating issues and incorporating interventions should always be managed in the specific context of each farm and the systems in place. Some issues will occur more readily in the extensive context over the intensive (and *vice versa*), and the application of some interventions will be more or less relevant, or possible, depending on the context.

Therefore, for vets to help farmers improve neonatal survival, interventions need to be both problem- and farm-specific. This requires a good understanding of the causes of neonatal losses together with a farm investigation and plenty of discussion with the farm team.

Lamb Survival

Farmers (and sometimes vets) are inclined to place too much significance on the pathogens that cause infections in this age group and therefore on therapy with antibiotics and other drugs. The main problems more often stem from: (i) poor ewe health; (ii) poor ewe nutrition; (iii) high infection challenge because of dirty, unhygienic conditions; (iv) inadequate observation; (v) lack of early intervention; and (vi) inadequate treatment of individual cases.

Ewe health and nutrition

Ewe health and nutrition are paramount to lamb survival. If a ewe is in poor health (e.g. due to liver fluke or lameness) or has an inadequate diet, it may produce small lambs with low birthweight, inadequate colostrum (quality and volume), inadequate volume of milk, and show poor mothering ability. These are all key risk factors for lamb morbidity and mortality. Therefore, ensuring good ewe health

---

*Email: jsduncan@liverpool.ac.uk

© CAB International 2025. *A Handbook for the Sheep Clinician, 8th Edition*
(A.C. Winter and D. Grove-White eds)
DOI: 10.1079/9781800626355.0007

and nutrition throughout the production cycle needs to be the priority for all flocks to ensure high lamb survival rates.

Key points for ewe nutrition (see also Chapters 1 and 4) are:

- Regular body condition scoring all-year-round so ewes lamb at an appropriate BCS: lowland ewes at 3.0–3.5, upland ewes at 2.5–3.0, hill ewes at 2.0–2.5.
- Periparturient nutrition should be based on *ad lib* excellent-quality forage/grass with additional supplementary concentrates as required (max 0.5 kg per feed). A forage analysis should help with an accurate estimate of requirements.
- Group according to scanning numbers and maximum 50 sheep per pen.
- Stocking rates pre-lambing (1.2–1.4m² per ewe).
- Ensure adequate feed/trough space (concentrates: 45–60 cm per ewe, *ad lib* forage: 15–20 cm per ewe).
- Monitor and suplement relevant trace elements in the ewes such as iodine, copper, selenium and zinc.
- Manage ewe lambs separately.
- Cull ewes that are thin and have faulty teeth and/or udders.

For more information see AHDB Feeding the Ewe https://ahdb.org.uk/knowledge-library/feeding-the-ewe (accessed 4/11/24).

Colostrum

Optimizing colostrum quantity, quality, and the timing of administration (quickly) is crucial to maximizing lamb survival (Fig. 7.1., Fig.7.2. and Fig. 7.3). Lambs needs 200–250 ml colostrum/kg BW in the first 24 h, with 50ml/kg BW given in the first 2 hours; this is to satisfy energy demands and will provide plenty of protective IgG and IgA if the ewe has been correctly vaccinated. Target birthweights for lambs born to lowland ewes are as follows: single 4.5–6.0 kg, twin 3.5–4.5 kg, triplet >3.5 kg.

Ewe colostrum

This is by far the best colostrum for a lamb. It can be stored in a freezer for at least a year. Surplus from milky ewes can be hand milked or milked out using a commercial hand pump. Oxytocin (1 ml intramuscularly) can be given to help letdown. It can be beneficial to use even small aliquots, e.g. 50 ml from ewes with large volumes of high-quality colostrum to supplement lambs from ewes with less superior-quality/lower-volume colostrum.

Cow colostrum

Cow colostrum (the first milking) can be used as a substitute feed (though less energy-dense than ewe colostrum). The cow can be vaccinated with sheep

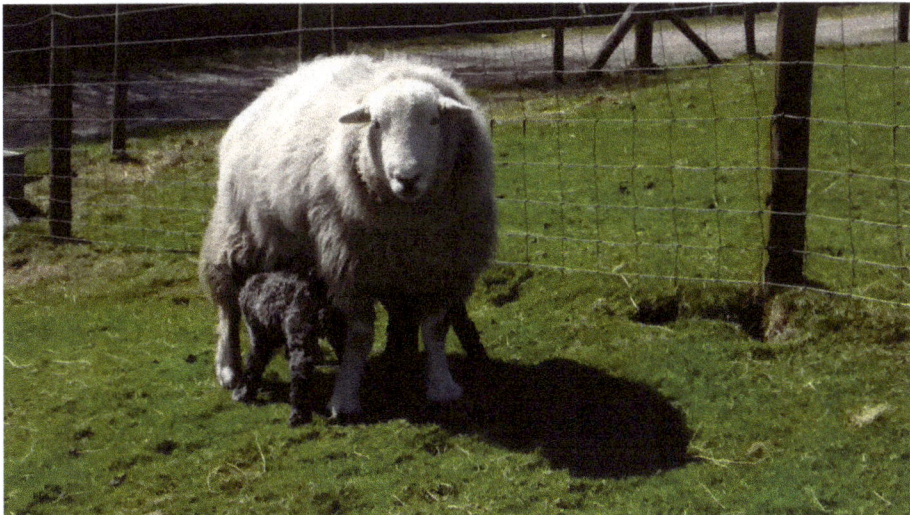

Fig. 7.1. Newborn lambs need a good feed of colostrum as soon as possible after birth to provide energy and antibodies (photo Agnes Winter).

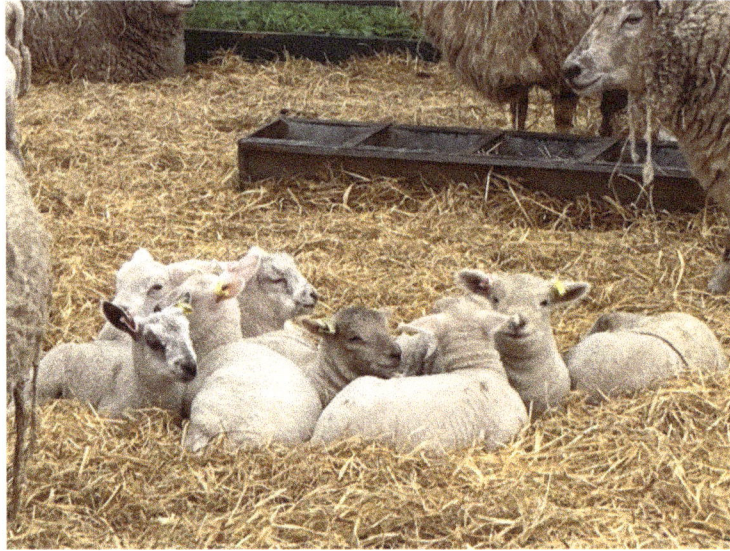

Fig. 7.2. Thriving and content young lambs (photo Agnes Winter).

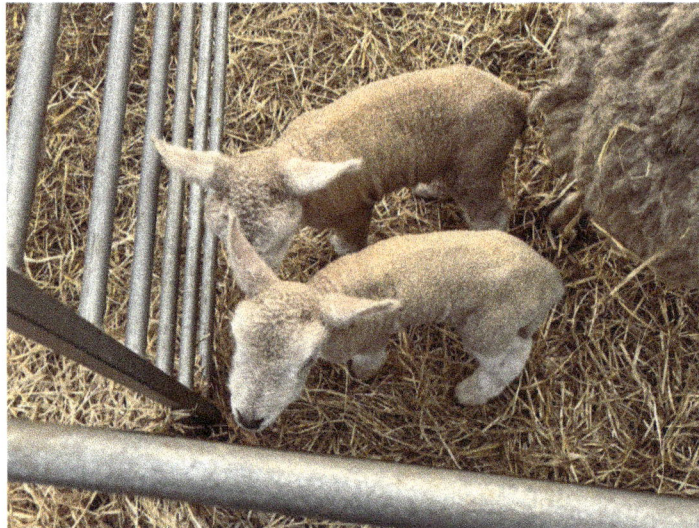

Fig. 7.3. A pair of two-day-old twins where one (nearest the camera) is not thriving as well as its mate (photo Agnes Winter).

8-in-1 clostridial vaccine (3 months before calving and again at 1 month and 2 weeks before calving). Mix colostrum from several cows before feeding to lambs to reduce the possibility of haemolytic anaemia caused by feeding cow colostrum. Some cows produce a factor in their colostrum which, because of an immunological reaction in some lambs, leads to the rapid destruction of the recipient lamb's red blood cells together with the precursors in the bone marrow. This causes lambs of about 10–14 days old to become suddenly weak and to stop sucking; they show extreme pallor (PCV <0.10), and they urgently require a whole-blood transfusion. This can be supplied by taking blood from a ewe in a

Jennifer Duncan and Joseph Angell

large syringe containing a drop of heparin and giving it intraperitoneally (10 ml/kg) as for a glucose injection. Corticosteroid and antibiotic injections are also indicated both to these lambs and to other lambs which may have received that batch of colostrum. A response is expected within a day, although some die and reveal very watery blood and creamy white bone marrow on PME.

Goat colostrum

Colostrum from goats is like ewe colostrum in composition and antibody content if the goats have received clostridial vaccines. There is a risk of caprine arthritis encephalitis (CAE), border disease virus (BDV), and Johne's disease transmission.

Commercial colostrum substitutes

These are variable in both energy and antibody content when compared with ewe colostrum. None is a true substitute and may have lower than ideal immunoglobulin concentration. They can be a useful energy source and are most effectively used to 'extend' a limited amount of ewe colostrum so that lambs get some of each.

Feeding by stomach tube

Check the tube length against the position of the lamb's stomach and mark at the appropriate point. Lubricate the tube by dipping in colostrum/lubricant, then introduce it into the lamb's mouth and push gently. In most cases the tube will enter the oesophagus and can then be advanced into the stomach. Check that the tube is not in the trachea by allowing the lamb to suck/swallow the tube, and carefully watch the neck as the tube is passed and see or feel it as it passes down inside the oesophagus. You can then be confident in giving colostrum or milk (1 × 50 ml syringe for a small lamb, 2 × 50 ml for a medium lamb and 3 × 50 ml for a large lamb). This is a quick and easy method of ensuring that weak lambs or multiple births get a good start and do not quickly succumb to hypothermia.

Key points for colostrum management:

- Create a specific colostrum policy for each farm to which all team members agree.
- Ensure optimal ewe nutrition.

- Measure colostrum quality of the first 20 ewes to lamb using a Brix refractometer (target >26%) to help monitor effectiveness of nutritional plan, and to have early warning of colostrum density issues. Increase concentrates/energy/protein in pre-lambing ewes if needed.
- Monitor colostrum intake (check lamb bellies, watch lamb sucking, check ewe udder).
- Decide which lambs will routinely need supplementing (e.g. triplets, ewe lambs, sick ewes, dystocia cases).
- Ensure adequate colostrum stores (store from ewes with high-density colostrum (>26% on Brix refractometer).
- Clean feeding equipment/stomach tubes between lambs. Use Milton baby bottle sterilizing fluid to disinfect.
- Measure lamb plasma proteins in 10–20 lambs at 2–7 days of age using refractometer (<45g/dl low, >60g/dl adequate).

Key points for hygiene practices:

- If housing pre-lambing, plan to clean the shed out in the week prior to lambing so ewes are lambing onto a clean surface without a build-up of manure.
- In large flocks, plan a break in the lambing sequence (batch lambing) to allow cleaning out of the buildings and lambing pens and recovery time for shepherds.
- Dag ewes pre-lambing.
- Wear gloves when lambing ewes.
- Clean all lambing and feeding equipment between uses.
- 1 lambing pen (1.5m × 1.5m) per 8–10 ewes, change bedding and clean and disinfect pen between ewes.
- It may be advantageous to use shavings as bedding rather than straw if diseases such as joint ill are a problem.

Key points for lamb care:

- Employ 1 lamber per 250 ewes.
- Ensure adequate colostrum (quantity, quality, and quickly).
- Dip navels with strong veterinary iodine within 15 minutes of birth and again 2–4 hours later.
- Do not try to lamb outdoors at inappropriate times of the year and be prepared for harsh weather even during normal outdoor lambing times.
- Provide adequate shelter if lambing outdoors (even a zigzag of straw bales in the field is helpful).

- Ensure early detection, isolation and treatment of sick lambs.
- Vaccinate ewes against clostridial disease and pasteurellosis pre-lambing.
- Avoid creating wounds in lambs, e.g. tagging, castrating and tail docking, as much as possible. If carried out, delay until the lamb is at least 24 hours old and disinfect wounds in strong veterinary iodine and keep equipment clean.

Common Neonatal Lamb Conditions

A decision should always be taken about the outcome of sick lamb cases. If the outlook is poor, the lamb should be humanely euthanized rather than being allowed a lingering death.

Hypothermia

This occurs when heat loss is greater than heat production. Use of plastic jackets can help to protect lambs against developing hypothermia (Fig. 7.4).

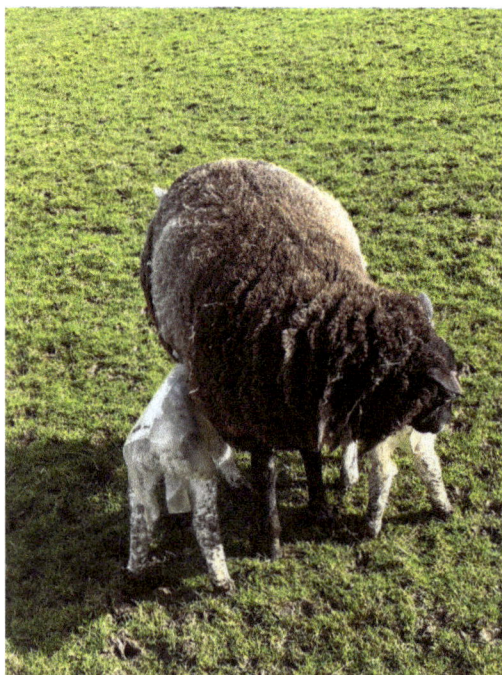

Fig. 7.4. Plastic lamb jackets help protect very young lambs in adverse weather and also help to protect from attack by crows (photo Agnes Winter).

Hypothermia is indicated by a body temperature lower than the normal:

- 39–40°C (102–104°F) is normal.
- 37–39°C (99–102°F) is mildly hypothermic.
- Below 37°C (<99°F) is severely hypothermic.

Newborn lambs (<5 hr old) which are still wet can suffer from exposure (high rate of heat loss); they usually have brown fat reserves and will respond to drying, warming, then feeding, by stomach tube if necessary (50 ml/kg BW colostrum).

Slightly older lambs (>2 h old) suffering from hypothermia, may have no brown fat reserves left; if warmed without being being given energy, they will develop hypoglycaemic fits and die. Energy can be supplied as follows:

- If the lamb can hold its head up, feed it by stomach tube (50 ml/kg colostrum), then warm, then re-feed.
- If the lamb cannot hold its head up, it is dangerous to feed (will regurgitate, inhale and die). Therefore, give an intraperitoneal injection of glucose before warming the lamb.

Technique for intraperitoneal glucose injection

- Use 10 ml/kg of warm 20% glucose/dextrose solution (if using 40% solution, use an equal volume of freshly boiled water to dilute and to bring it to body temperature).
- Holding the lamb by the front legs and, using a 19G × 1″ needle directed backwards at 45°, inject it into the abdominal cavity just below and to one side of the navel (see Fig. 7.5).

Then put the lamb to warm, preferably in a warming box with a fan heater under wire mesh. An infrared lamp can be used, but great care must be taken to avoid overheating the lamb. When the lamb's temperature returns to almost normal and it is conscious and able to swallow, feed 50 ml/kg colostrum via a bottle or stomach tube and return it to the ewe as soon as it can suck the ewe vigorously. If the lamb is one of twins, remove the other from the ewe and return them together when ready. If it cannot be returned to its mother, it will need to be reared artificially or mothered onto another ewe.

N.B. Do **not** give an intraperitoneal injection to a lamb with scour or watery mouth.

Jennifer Duncan and Joseph Angell

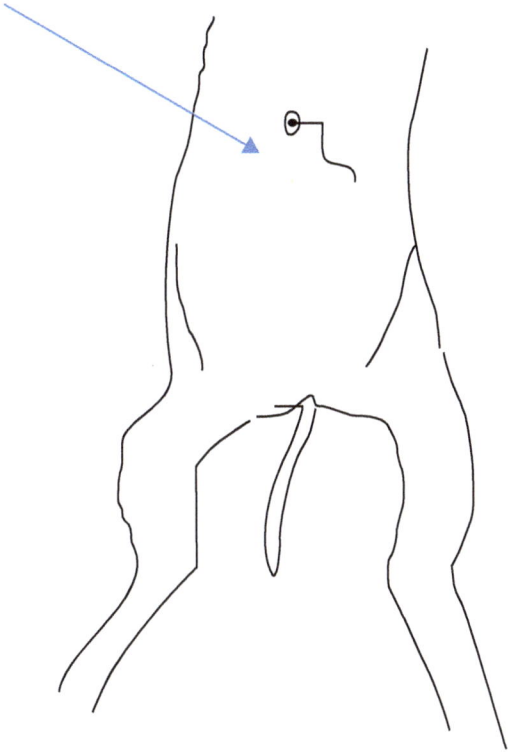

Fig. 7.5. Intraperitoneal injection site.

Watery mouth (slavers, rattle belly)

These are common terms used to describe a condition which affects young lambs (up to 7 days old, but most cases are seen within the first 72 hours). The condition is characterized by the following:

- Lambs rapidly become dull and weak, recumbent and unwilling to suck.
- They have cold, wet lips and muzzles from drooling saliva (but note that terminally ill lambs dying of other causes often drool saliva).
- Often (but not exclusively) no faeces (meconium) are visible, and the tail is dry.
- The temperature is at first normal, but hypothermia follows from a lack of feeding.
- The abdomen is relaxed at first and looks full, but later there is abomasal tympany (which may be visible as right-sided swelling) and tenseness which may cause 'rattling' when tapped or shaken, and the distension may cause distressed breathing or recumbency.

- Without treatment, they usually die within the day, but some live long enough to develop scouring and even joint ill, just to complicate the picture!
- The incidence can be frighteningly high (>20%) and is most common in twins or triplets from ewes with CS <3 and lambed indoors.

Cause

Watery mouth is an endotoxaemia which develops following ingestion of large numbers of 'non-pathogenic' *E. coli* from a heavily contaminated environment before they have sucked colostrum. The bacteria are not destroyed in the abomasum (pH is 7 after birth) and they pass into and colonize the small intestine in the absence of colostral antibodies and other putative anti-infective molecules derived from colostrum. There is subsequent passage of bacteria across the intestinal wall, via the normal pinocytotic mechanisms designed to absorb the colostral antibodies, resulting in a bacteraemia and further bacterial proliferation. The end result is the production of endotoxin (lipopolysaccharide LPS) as the bacteria die *en masse* in the blood system resulting in fulminating endotoxic and death. It is unclear whether endotoxaemia produced within the intestinal lumen is absorbed, contributing further to the endotoxaemia. One early effect of the endotoxaemia is gut stasis with an accumulation of saliva and gas, giving the bloated rattling effect.

Treatment (must be early)

- Systemic antibiotic injection (broad spectrum e.g. amoxicillin) repeated daily for 5 days.
- Oral antibiotic with activity against *E. coli* (aminoglycoside).
- 50 ml/kg BW of glucose/electrolyte solution administered by stomach tube, repeated four times daily. Do not feed milk until recovering.
- NSAID such as meloxicam (anti-endotoxin). Meloxicam can be given at a dose of 1mg/kg under the cascade; careful weighing and dosing is required to ensure dosing is accurate.
- If retained meconium, warm soapy-water enema (10–20 ml administered via a cut-down stomach tube).
- Leave the ewe and lamb(s) together if possible and keep warm.

Control

This disease is a race to the guts between colostrum and gram-negative bacteria. Infection may occur within 15 minutes of birth. Make sure lambs get plenty of colostrum early (within minutes, not hours):

- Optimize ewe nutrition so that BCS at lambing is at least 3.
- Supplement colostrum quickly to at-risk lambs (weak lambs, triplets, etc.). Use ewe colostrum wherever possible due to its increased density compared to commercial alternatives.
- Ensure good bonding (avoid moving a ewe and its lambs too soon after birth).
- Ensure the lamb(s) suck well (avoid early castration and have good shepherding).
- Reduce the weight of infection: review hygiene – housing bedding, pens, equipment, and udders, muck out, use lime etc.

Neonatal diarrhoea

While *individual* scouring lambs can be dealt with without resort to laboratory diagnosis, it is important in an outbreak to establish, if possible, if there is one dominating causal organism. To do this requires submitting up to ten faeces samples from healthy and diseased lambs (not swabs), as well as any terminally ill untreated lambs and/or fresh carcasses. This should provide sufficient information to prescribe appropriate treatment and control measures. Irrespective of cause, oral fluid therapy is key to treatment, whilst control involves hygiene and ensuring adequate colostrum intake. If outbreaks occur at grass, it is worth considering the age range of lambs within the group and the overall group size. Ideally, lambs should not be kept in groups with an age range greater than 7–10 days, since the older lambs will act as a source of pathogens for the younger lambs within a group.

General treatment of lambs with diarrhoea

- Leave with ewe if possible but isolate them to prevent further spread.
- Wash hands after handling sick lambs to reduce transmission of infective organisms to other lambs.
- Provide additional warmth, e.g. heat lamp.
- Give 50 ml/kg BW (~200 ml) oral electrolyte solution four times daily.

- Administer broad spectrum antibiotics if a bacterial cause is suspected.
- Encourage to suckle or provide colostrum or ewe milk by stomach tube four times daily.

Specific causes of neonatal diarrhoea

- Lamb dysentery – can occur in an outbreak with high mortality; there may be a range of symptoms from found dead to dull and depressed with tenesmus and a haemorrhagic diarrhoea (dysentery). Treatment of infected lambs may be attempted with a penicillin-based antibiotic, NSAIDs, and electrolytes. It is invariably associated with an absence or a breakdown in ewe clostridial vaccination. Control is aimed at a review of vaccination, colostrum and hygiene practices. Vaccinate any ewes remaining to lamb and, for the next season, implement an effective ewe clostridial disease vaccination policy.
- Salmonellosis – can occur as an outbreak; a range of symptoms may be observed from being found dead to being dull and depressed with haemorrhagic diarrhoea and/or signs of septicaemia. Often ewes and lambs are affected together. Transmission is rapid between animals with a low infective dose required and large volumes of highly infective diarrhoea produced. Antibiotic sensitivity testing should be undertaken to establish the appropriate treatment. Antibiotic-resistant strains are common. Control is aimed at reviewing hygiene and colostrum practices. Other species on the farm may be involved, therefore check cattle (source/subsequent infection), and keep separate if possible. Risk of zoonosis. Vaccination of in-contact cattle for some serovars is possible.
- Enterotoxogenic *E. coli* – use antibiotic sensitivity testing to establish the appropriate treatment, review hygiene, colostrum provision.
- Rotavirus – review hygiene, colostrum.
- *Cryptosporidium parvum* – typically affects lambs from a week of age, particularly orphan lambs reared in groups on milk feeders. Prevention is through optimizing hygiene and colostrum. Halofuginone has been used preventatively under the cascade, but care is needed with dosing due to the low toxic threshold. Treatment can be given using paromomycin at 100 mg/kg given daily for 3–5 days. This treatment is used under the cascade. In addition, electrolytes and other supportive measures can be beneficial.

Neonatal Infectious Arthritis (Joint Ill)

Neonatal infectious arthritis or 'Joint-Ill' is a commonly observed infection of the neonatal lamb. It can be caused by a number of bacterial species including *Streptococcus dysgalactiae, Staphylococcus aureus, Erysipelothrix rhusiopathiae. Pasteurella multocida*. Different bacteria have different risk factors associated with them; therefore, it is helpful to obtain a bacterial culture from cases to ensure appropriate antibiotic therapy and control measures are advised.

Streptococcus dysgalactiae:

clinical signs

Lambs with *Streptococcus dysgalactiae* joint-ill typically present at less than 4 weeks old, with one or more swollen joints and associated lameness. If the intervertebral joints are affected, they may also present with paresis, paralysis, a hunched appearance or recumbency. The source of the infection of *Streptococcus dysgalactiae* in the flock is primarily the ewe. The bacteria have been identified in the reproductive tract, udder, nasal and oral cavities, and faeces. The bacteria can persist in indoor and outdoor lambing environments and the infectious challenge is thought to build up over the lambing period. The known routes of entry to the lamb are the navel and other wounds (ear tagging) and the oral route via the tonsil.

Treatment

Early and prolonged treatment is required to prevent chronic infection and damage to joints. Lambs should receive a *minimum* seven-day course of systemic antibiotics (not oxytetracycline) such as penicillin or amoxicillin, wounds should be cleaned and disinfected. NSAIDs such as meloxicam may help. Penning the lamb and ewe can facilitate the lamb feeding, avoiding it needing to keep up with its mother. Euthanasia should be considered in severe or unresponsive cases.

Prevention

Prevention should focus on improvement of farm hygiene, wound management and colostrum policy. If an outbreak is occurring in a particular lambing environment, consider moving to a fresh field or clean shed. Lambing pens should be cleaned and disinfected between sheep and all hygiene measures reviewed. Consider the use of shavings rather than straw bedding. Lamb navels should be dipped in strong veterinary iodine, within 15 minutes of birth and again 2–4 hours later (as often the ewe licks off some of the iodine). Avoid creating management wounds in lambs (ear tagging, castration, tail docking) during the risk period (less than 4 weeks old); if such wounds are necessary, implement iodine treatment of wounds and ensure hygiene of equipment.

Staphylococcus aureus and *Erysipelothrix rhusiopathiae*

Staphylococcus aureus is a commensal of the skin of most animal species and joint infections are typically (but not always) associated with tick bites (tick pyaemia or cripples), therefore control should focus on minimizing exposure to ticks in the young lamb. *Erysipelothrix rhusiopathiae* can be found ubiquitously in the farm environment and can persist in soil. Prevention should focus on improvements in farm hygiene. Some practitioners report anecdotal success using a vaccine licensed for pigs, given to ewes pre-lambing, under the cascade. Adverse reactions have been reported so always consult with vaccine manufacturer before off-licence use.

Omphalophlebitis (Navel Ill)

Omphalophlebitis may be confined to external infection of the navel tissue or extend into the abdomen resulting in complications such as infection of the urachus, septicaemia, peritonitis or hepatic necrobacillosis.

The conditions occur due to opportunistic bacterial infections of the untreated navel and/or poor indoor or outdoor environmental hygiene.

Clinical signs

The clinical presentation will vary depending on the extent of infection. The navel will be swollen, wet, and may show purulent discharge. If there is accompanying peritonitis or hepatic necrobacillosis, the lambs will be dull, depressed, inappetent, and standing with an arched back.

Treatment

Treatment of an uncomplicated navel infection should be by cleaning the navel with iodine disinfectant and a prolonged course of broad-spectrum antibiotics (at least 7 days).

The prognosis for peritonitis, necrobacillosis and septicaemia is very guarded, and euthanasia should be considered.

Prevention

Prevention is by ensuring optimum colostrum management, instituting a strict navel-dipping policy, and improved environmental hygiene.

Pneumonia

Pneumonia due to pathogens such as *Mannheimia haemolytica* is common in lambs less than 4 weeks old, especially when housed.

Clinical signs

Dull, depressed, inappetent, increased respiratory rate and effort, fever, sometimes with nasal discharge. Diagnosis is usually based on clinical signs but confirmed, along with bacterial etiology and antibiotic sensitivity, by PME.

Treatment

Broad-spectrum antibiotics such as oxytetracycline, and supportive care such as NSAIDs, supplementary feeding and warmth.

Prevention

Review underlying risk factors such as air hygiene, bedding hygiene (elevated levels of ammonia at lamb level can be measured using a handheld ammonia meter), failure of passive transfer and ewe vaccination.

Neurological Problems

In addition to the central nervous system (CNS) diseases of young lambs which may follow any post-partum bacteraemia or septicaemia, there are three specific conditions which originate pre-partum: (i) swayback; (ii) border disease; and (iii) daft lamb disease. These need differentiation and whilst at first the clinical signs may appear non-specific or confusing, careful history-taking and clinical examination should give you the confidence to arrive at a provisional diagnosis; this usually needs biochemical and histological support before flock control measures are introduced.

Bacterial meningitis

Bacterial meningitis occurs as a result of bacteraemia from infection with opportunist organisms such as *Escherichia coli, Mannhaemia haemolytica, Staphylococcus pyogenes* and *Truperella pyogenes* multiplying in the CNS. Failure of passive transfer is also likely to play a role in disease pathogenesis.

Clinical signs

These will vary depending on stage of disease; however, affected lambs will be dull with congested mucous membranes, show neck extension and pain, recumbency, hyperaesthesia, opisthotonus, seizures and death. Diagnosis may be confirmed with a cerebrospinal fluid sample or brain histopathology.

Treatment

Treatment with intravenous potentiated sulphonamides, supportive care and corticosteroids may be attempted but euthanasia would be warranted in all but the earliest cases with efforts made to address underlying risk factors of hygiene and failure of passive transfer.

Septicaemia

Septicaemia is defined as bacteria present in the bloodstream which are multiplying and causing systemic disease. Several opportunist bacteria can cause septicemia in the neonatal lamb and include *Escherichia coli, Mannhaemia haemolytica, Bibersteinia trelahosi Staphylococcus pyogenes* and *Trueperella pyogenes*. Failure of passive transfer and inadequate hygiene are likely to play a role in disease pathogenesis. Clinical signs such as anorexia, tachycardia, increased respiratory rate, fever and depression will be observed. In addition, specific organ involvement such as pneumonia or gastro-intestinal symptoms may be present. Diagnosis and specific bacterial causes are confirmed at PME.

Treatment

Treatment with intravenous potentiated sulphonamides and supportive care may be attempted (including intravenous fluid therapy in valuable animals), but euthanasia would be warranted in all but the earliest cases with efforts made to address underlying risk factors of hygiene and failure of passive transfer.

Swayback (enzootic ataxia)

This is one of the most important of the many CNS diseases of lambs and is caused by faulty development and degeneration of nervous tissue, particularly myelin sheaths, in the brain and spinal cord of lambs whose mothers had low copper concentrations in the blood in the latter part of pregnancy. The cause can be associated with an absolute deficiency in the diet of the ewe, or induced by an excess of molybdenum, sulphur and iron.

It is important to remember that copper still heads the list of poisons in sheep, so copper supplementation should *never* be given without a clinical reason, backed up with confirmatory tests. Note that it is illegal to add copper to sheep feeds or minerals.

Diagnosis

Diagnosis is based on a combination of history, clinical signs and laboratory tests.

HISTORY

- Swayback has been diagnosed clinically on the farm before.
- Copper has not been given to the ewes during pregnancy.
- It has been a mild winter. This influences the quality and quantity of the grass and the amount of soil eaten. Minerals such as molybdenum and sulphur can combine with copper to form thiomolybdate, rendering the copper unavailable to the ewe. Additionally, minerals such as iron ingested with soil, or via water with a high iron content, can block the absorption of copper. Consideration also needs to be given to the quantity of concentrates consumed by the ewes (although no copper is added there is inevitably a 'background' concentration of copper, and the cereals present can serve to increase the rate of absorption of copper from the available diet).
- Housing reduces the risk because ewes are prevented from ingesting soil and are fed concentrates.

Forecasts of likelihood of swayback, based on weather, are published in the farming and veterinary press.
- The grazing is lush. Improved, fertilized (high-sulphur) and reclaimed pastures with single-sward grasses, high molybdenum (often land prone to flooding) are particularly likely to give rise to swayback.

Clinical signs may be present at birth, within a few days of birth, or delayed until lambs are several weeks old.

- Congenital – lambs at or within a few days of birth show varying degrees of ataxia, paresis, and inability to stand. Some may be born dead or die within a few hours. Some will be able to suck if permitted and most appear alert and aware. The signs are, at best, only suspicious and can easily be confused with the other CNS disturbances of young lambs, in particular primary hypoglycaemia. It has been shown that lambs in flocks suffering from subclinical copper deficiency (i.e. no obvious cases of swayback) have increased lamb mortality rates. The main differential diagnosis for lambs of a few days to a few weeks old is spinal abscess and joint ill.
- Delayed – seen in lambs a few weeks old, which were normal at birth, develop varying degrees of hind-leg weakness, ataxia (swayback) and paresis. The signs are more obvious when the lamb is chased about and turns quickly. It looks like a spinal rather than a brain condition and the lambs can suck and graze normally; some will fatten because they learn how to cope with the disability.
- Acute delayed – rapidly developing signs in lambs a few weeks old which die within a few hours. This type is uncommon.

Incidence

This will depend upon the control measures adopted and the weather, but it is common for a swayback-prone farm to have a few years with very few cases, followed by a calamitous 'storm' (50%). Fortunately, the advent of housing and safer copper supplementation has reduced these incidents.

Pathology

Material required for diagnosis should include:

- Formalinized brains and brainstems.
- At least ten clotted (red tubes) and heparinized blood samples (green tubes) from pregnant ewes

that have not recently had supplementary copper. Plasma copper concentrations below 9 µmol/l suggest an acute copper deficiency problem.

- Liver samples, if available – copper concentrations below 1124µmol/kg DM are suspicious, with concentrations below 225µmol/kg DM deficient.
- Herbage analysis – the following are suspicious: Cu – below 5 ppm DM, Mo – above 1 ppm DM, S – above 0.20% DM.

Treatment

Because swayback can be a progressive condition, it is worth treating those young lambs which are not too severely affected with a single injection of copper (no more than 5 mg) to stop the condition getting worse, although no improvement should be expected. Severely affected lambs should be euthanized.

Control

1. During an outbreak – all the remaining pregnant ewes (unless the breed is susceptible to copper toxicity, e.g. Texel, in which case liver tissue analysis is essential to establish safe copper supplementation) should be treated with a suitable copper preparation, together with those healthy lambs already born out of ewes not previously dosed, to prevent delayed swayback.
2. Next year – consider housing the ewes during the last half of pregnancy, thus removing them from the source of the problem. If housing is not practicable, dose all ewes in early pregnancy with copper (capsules containing copper oxide needles are the safest) but also then remove other known sources of copper such as licks or minerals that contain copper and proprietary cattle and pig concentrates.

If there is a problem of ill-thrift, poor-quality fleece and multiple fractures in lambs due to copper deficiency, then the lambs also require dosing, but not before other causes have been eliminated and copper deficiency established.

COPPER PREPARATIONS

- Beware of copper toxicity! Some breeds, especially continental ones, are very susceptible.
- Check very carefully for the recommended dose of the product to be used.

Injectable (copper heptonate) and oral preparations (copper oxide) are available. The safest and most reliable preparations are in the form of capsules containing copper oxide needles, or in the form of a soluble glass bolus delivered orally by an administration gun. Ewes are dosed once, either prior to tupping or in mid-pregnancy, and lambs as required when they are over 5 weeks old. Combined multimineral boluses are available containing varying combinations of copper, selenium, cobalt, iodine and zinc either in a compressed composite form or as a soluble glass bolus.

Short-acting drenches are sometimes used, but they require repeat dosing and risk toxicity. Copper sulfate on its own (1.0 g in 30 ml water) is still used prophylactically by farmers, but it is a risky material to have about on sheep farms.

Toxicity through overdose can occur within hours of injection or weeks after dosing/administration of a bolus. To avoid this:

- Make sure copper is necessary.
- Conduct a detailed mineral audit after weaning and prior to tupping, considering sources of copper and any antagonists (forage, concentrates, water, all supplements) and the animal's response to the inputs using blood and liver tissue analysis. Monitor the animal's response to any interventions through follow-up blood and liver tissue analysis.
- Reduce the dose in small sheep, e.g. mountain or small traditional breeds, ewe lambs etc.
- Remove any other obvious source of copper, particularly if the animals are housed and fed concentrates.
- Treat ewes with care and follow makers' recommendations.

Individuals and breeds vary in susceptibility to copper deficiency and toxicity. For example: (i) Scottish Blackface and Swaledales are more prone to deficiency; (ii) Texels and other continental breeds are prone to toxicity; and (iii) the North Ronaldsay, whose natural diet is seaweed, which is very low in copper, is extremely susceptible to toxicity, often succumbing on diets which would be deficient to other breeds. A change in breed might be considered, or an alteration in the lambing date, or special precautions for selected breeds, or cull those ewes that produce swayback lambs (there is familial variation as well as breed variation). Remember that high sulphur, molybdenum and iron concentrations in the diet are known to

Jennifer Duncan and Joseph Angell

decrease copper 'availability,' hence the term 'conditioned' copper deficiency, and hence also the use of ammonium tetrathiomolybdate and sodium sulfate in attempts to control chronic copper toxicity.

Border disease (hairy shakers)

This is a congenital disease, first reported from the English–Welsh border counties but since recognized throughout the world. It is caused by infection with a pestivirus (BDV) related to bovine viral diarrhoea virus (BVDv). Antigenic differences can be recognized between BDV and BVDv, and sheep strains will infect cattle and *vice versa*, though it is unclear how much spread occurs between the two species under natural conditions. Sheep which are immune to one strain are susceptible to the others. Both the pathogenesis and epidemiology of BDV in sheep and BVDv in cattle are very similar such that diagnosis and control in both species follow the same principles.

Clinical picture

BDV infection produces clinical signs, though they do not all occur in every flock. One or more of the following pictures may be seen:

- Several lambs showing a typical long hairy coat, or coats with colour changes (e.g. brown patches), some of which are also ataxic with fine rhythmic tonic/clonic contractions of skeletal muscles ('hairy shakers'). These signs are usually evident at birth, although in the naturally long-woolled breeds, the abnormal birth coat is not obvious. The incidence of border disease in lambs is variable but 'storms' are reported. Gimmers produce the highest percentage of border disease lambs, indicating progressive immunity.
- Many affected lambs survive for a time, but their growth rate is poor, and they appear stunted with domed heads and lag behind the rest of the flock. In addition, persistently infected lambs occur, many of which do not show early clinical signs, but some show chronic unthriftiness and scouring. Some survive to breeding age, and though their fertility is reduced, they can produce infected lambs in successive pregnancies. Persistently infected rams can transmit virus in semen.
- There is a high prevalence of barren ewes, abortions or weak lambs. This means that the disease

may present as an abortion and infertility problem rather than as a disease of young lambs.

Pathogenesis

- Infection of healthy non-pregnant sheep produces no obvious clinical signs and gives rise to the production of neutralizing antibodies and an immune sheep. It is 'antibody-positive, virus-negative'. Immunity is believed to be life-long.

Infection of pregnant ewes leads to a similar course of events in the ewe, but the virus crosses the placenta and leads to the various clinical pictures, depending on virus strain and breed of sheep, but most importantly, on the stage of gestation:

- Infection prior to 60 days, at a time when the fetus has no ability to mount an immunological response, will result in fetal death in a high proportion of cases, leading to resorption and barren ewes or mummification and abortion. Virus strains vary in virulence and these early infections may allow some infected fetuses to survive with virus particles in every organ. Infection of the CNS leads to myelin deficiency and 'shaker' lambs whilst infection of the hair follicles leads to 'hairy' lambs and sometimes pigment changes. Weak or apparently healthy infected lambs may be produced. Such lambs will be immunologically tolerant to BDV and 'antibody negative, virus positive' at birth, and although they will acquire antibodies in the colostrum, this will wane and they will be 'virus positive' for life. These lambs are persistently infected carriers, and as such represent a severe risk if purchased into naïve flocks
- If infection occurs after about 85 days, the fetus mounts an immunological response and destroys the virus. Most will be normal at birth and will be 'antibody positive, virus negative', like the dam.
- If infection occurs between 60 and 85 days, when the fetus is becoming immunologically competent, either of the above responses may occur with either clinical outcome.

Epidemiology

Most flocks become infected by the purchase of persistently infected lambs as breeding replacements. It has been suggested that, rarely, infection may be introduced by pestiviruses from other species such as cattle, goats or deer, or even by a contaminated live vaccine.

Diagnosis

The following list indicates the tissues needed for laboratory confirmation of clinical diagnosis:

1. From 'hairy-shaker', weak, scouring lambs, or suspected persistently infected sheep – clotted and heparinized blood (red and green tube) from live lambs for virus isolation and serology. In dead animals, viruses can be detected by immunofluorescence and virus isolation from fresh tissues put in transport medium (e.g. kidney, spleen, thyroid; plus brain and spinal cord in formalin for histology).
2. From aborting or barren ewes – clotted and heparinized blood for virology and serology, and placenta for virus isolation.

Treatment and control

There is no treatment and there are dangers in attempting to support weak or hairy shaker lambs which will be excreting large amounts of the virus.

- Ideally, a closed flock should be maintained, or replacements obtained from a flock which is serologically negative (this may form part of a sheep health scheme in the future). Maintaining replacements as a separate flock from tupping to lambing will enable monitoring of lambing to be done.
- In a flock which has recently had border disease for the first time, the sheep suspected of introducing the infection may be identified as 'antibody negative, virus positive' from blood samples. They and their lambs should be culled before the next tupping season.
- In an endemically infected flock, all breeding ewes should be deliberately exposed to infection 2–3 months before mating by housing in close contact with persistently infected sheep for 3–4 weeks.
- Vaccines are available for BVD in cattle, so may eventually be produced for sheep.

Other congenital neurological problems

Several neurological diseases affecting newborn or young lambs with a particular breed association have been recognized.

- Hydrocephalus (Dandy Walker malformation) has been seen in Suffolks – this causes dystocia so needs to be considered if dealing with this breed. Sometimes the lamb's skull is so soft that it can be crushed, aiding delivery; sometimes a caesarean may be necessary. It is fatal.
- Daft lamb disease has been seen in several breeds – lambs are born with cerebellar abnormalities such as head nodding, ataxia and tremors and, as the name suggests, may appear mentally stupid, having difficulty finding the ewe's teat.
- Cerebellar abiotrophy has been seen in Charollais lambs – cerebellar signs appear during the first weeks of life with ongoing deterioration.
- Schmallenberg disease – although affected lambs are most usually born with abnormalities of the limbs and joints (arthrogryposis) some lambs appear normal but present with neurological signs.

Affected lambs should be euthanized and diagnosis may require PME and histological examination of the brain. Breeding records should be carefully examined since some of these diseases are often familial.

Lamb D-lactic acidosis syndrome/Drunken lamb syndrome/Lamb nephrosis syndrome

This has two presentations either seen in lambs aged 1–2 weeks of age or later at around 1 month or older.

In the younger age group, lambs are seen in the initial stages with a reduced flight response, ataxic, dull and depressed and, as the disease progresses rapidly, become recumbent. The neurological symptoms are because of a build-up of the D optical isomer of lactic acid, produced by abnormal fermentation of carbohydrate in the large intestine. This is thought to usually be because of another underlying cause of decreased gut transit time, e.g. rotavirus, E. coli infection, etc. The D-lactate is absorbed from the gut into the blood resulting in the neurological symptoms seen; it also causes damage to renal tubules resulting in nephrosis. Diagnosis is based on clinical signs, although assays for D-lactate may become more readily available. Detection of low blood bicarbonate concentrations together with clinical signs can give a strong suspicion of disease.

Treatment can be given using a single 50 ml dose of a 1 molar solution of sodium bicarbonate given

Jennifer Duncan and Joseph Angell

orally by stomach tube. This solution can be made by dissolving 35 g of sodium bicarbonate in 400 mls of tap water, from which 50 ml can be drawn to administer to affected cases. Unused solutions should be kept sealed and discarded after one week. Clinically affected lambs tend to make a rapid recovery (usually showing improvement within 1–2 hours). Investigation and treatment of the underlying causes should then be considered to prevent further cases.

In the older age group, lambs are typically detected later in the disease and may present with depression/dullness, without ataxia, but with polyuria and polydipsia indicative of renal failure. They may be seen standing by water sources and rapidly lose condition. The prognosis is hopeless so they should be euthanized. At PME the kidneys appear swollen and nephrosis is identified using histopathology. Again, an investigation into the possible underlying causes, e.g. coccidiosis, severe nematode parasitism, cryptosporidiosis etc., should be made.

Investigation of Neonatal Losses

When working with farmers and their team to reduce neonatal losses, targeted advice must be given, based on veterinary investigation. In addition, an estimate of the cost of the losses to the farm (number of lambs lost × finished price) can be a useful motivator and provide an estimate of the budget for any interventions. For example, how many lambs do you need to save to justify the intervention? It is often only one or two!

1. History
2. Data collection
3. Examination of relevant ewes and lambs
4. Examination of the environment
5. Laboratory tests

History

- Farmer's account of the problem, clinical signs/treatment.
- Numbers involved (size of problem).
- Problems in previous years.
- Is the problem confined to one group of ewes (e.g. replacement ewe lambs)?
- Breeding and lambing dates.
- Weather conditions throughout pregnancy.
- Feeding of ewes, vaccination, parasite control (e.g. copper, fluke).

Data recording

The data recorded and the methods of recording in flocks are variable. To estimate lamb losses from flocks the minimum useful data to collect are:

- Scanning data (number of fetuses scanned/ number of ewes put to tup)
- Rearing percentage (number of lambs reared/ number of ewes put to tup)

This will give an estimate of total lamb losses. Current estimates for *total* lamb losses (birth to sale) range from 5–30%, whilst AHDB recommends farmers to aim for less than 15% total lamb losses.

To provide further targeted advice, additional data collected could also include:

- lambing percentage (birth) = number of lambs born alive/number of ewes put to tup;
- lambing percentage (7 days) = number of lambs at 7 days/number of ewes put to tup;
- lambing percentage (weaned) = number of lambs weaned/number of ewes put to tup.

Benchmarking neonatal losses (<7 days)

- 5% or less indicates above-average management.
- 8% indicates average management.
- > 10% indicates definite room for improvement.

Further useful benchmarks for lamb losses:

- Pre-partum stillbirths (including abortions) – 2%. These could be due to uterine infections such as *Toxoplasma, Salmonella, Campylobacter*, enzootic abortion, border disease. Other causes include Tickborne fever, pregnancy toxaemia and swayback.
- Parturient stillbirths (dystocia) <5%. If the losses are due to lambing problems, then the quality and quantity of the workforce needs consideration, alongside the age, breeding and feeding of ewes (e.g. large singles, and ewe lambs that are CS 4 and crossed with a Texel ram!).
- Post-partum mortality – 8%. This includes some that were said to be born dead but died soon after birth and losses from neonatal diseases.
- Further benchmarking data may be found from AHDB website (https://ahdb.org.uk/knowledge-library/ewe-fertility-for-better-returns-accessed 4/11/24)

Farm observations

- Hygiene (ventilation, pens, ewes, at lambing, isolation)
- Stocking density, groups, pen sizes
- Outdoor shelter
- Ewe and lamb feeding
- Colostrum policy
- Dystocia management
- Shepherding quantity and quality
- Lamb care practices (navels, mutilations, tagging)

Clinical examinations

- Ewes – clinical examinations, BCS
- Sick/weak lambs

Laboratory examinations

Submit plenty of fresh material (including fetal membranes). It may include:

- Paired blood samples from marked ewes for EAE, *Toxoplasma,* and BDV, plus blood biochemistry (copper, plasma selenium, glutathione peroxidase (GSHPx), zinc; gamma glutamyl transferase (GGT) and BOHB from ewes yet to lamb). BOHB can also be measured on farms using a handheld ketone meter which can be useful in formulating rapid advice around feeding to correct subclinical/clinical ketosis (pregnancy toxaemia).
- Colostrum density can be measured using a handheld Brix refractometer on farms.
- Lamb blood serum total protein concentrations, an indicator of colostral antibody transfer, can be measured using a refractometer at the practice.
- Faecal material for diarrhoea and parasite investigations.

Post-mortem examination of neonatal lambs

Post-mortem examination is an extremely useful but under-utilized tool to investigate causes of neonatal losses. A full guide to conducting a lamb post-mortem is available from AHDB (https://projectblue.blob.

core.windows.net/media/Default/Beef%20&%20 Lamb/PM-Worksheet2564_190123_WEB%20 2019.pdf (accessed 3/11/24).

Some useful indicators:

- Decomposition – indicates pre-partum death.
- Clouding of cornea indicates pre-partum death.
- Weight – singles should be 4.5 kg, twins 3.5 kg (but allow for breed variations). Excessive weight indicates possible dystocia, underweight suggests a pre-partum problem (e.g. feeding of ewe, uterine infection, large litter size).
- Umbilical vessels – thrombus indicates that death is post-partum. In lambs dying immediately before or during parturition, the end of the artery is sharply pointed (because of contraction of the arterial wall), but if death occurred some time pre-partum, the ruptured end is square. If the end is shrivelled, death is at least some hours post-partum.
- Lung aeration indicates post-partum death (check to see if a piece of the lung floats or sinks in water).
- Presence of food in the stomach indicates post-partum death but does not rule out hypothermia if a stomach tube was used to feed shortly before death. Unclotted milk suggests recent feeding probably by stomach tube.
- Subcutaneous oedema of distal parts of the legs, tail or head indicates dystocia or hypothermia.
- Hepatic rupture, thoracic, abdominal or meningeal haemorrhage (open up cranium and spinal canal to check) indicate dystocia.
- Well-nourished lambs are born with brown fat reserves which support them during the first few days of life. In starvation, as the fat is metabolized, it is replaced by soft, red gelatinous tissue – look particularly around the kidneys and heart.
- Wear on feet indicates the lamb has lived for a few hours.

Checking for the presence or absence of the above features should enable you to decide if deaths are occurring mainly in one category. That is, if the deaths are mainly pre-partum, look for causes of death *in utero*; if at birth, then the shepherd's vigilance and availability may be inadequate; if after birth, then the lambs have probably not sucked adequately and have become cold.

8 The Lactating Ewe

JENNIFER DUNCAN*

Department of Livestock and One Health Institute of Infection, Veterinary and Ecological Sciences, University of Liverpool, UK

Abstract

The post-lambing period covered in this chapter is characterized by the ewes having to cope with the demands of lactation. Particular challenges include variable grass and nutrient supply and the increasing metabolic demands of fast-growing meat lambs. Ewe mastitis, teat lesions and, rarely, hypomagnesaemia are the main disease risks of this period.

Ewes rearing twins or triplets are likely to be in energy deficit in early lactation so they will lose weight. This is not a problem, providing they were in good condition at lambing and do not become less than body condition score 2, as they will regain body condition after weaning. However, depending on grass quality and quantity, ewes may need supplementary feeding. See https://ahdb.org.uk/knowledge-library/feeding-the-ewe (accessed 27/2/24) for much useful information.

This is especially important for young ewes, aged ewes, ewes rearing multiple lambs, and rearing fast-growing meat lambs such as Texel or Beltex cross lambs. In these situations, the ewes will be under increasing metabolic stress (Fig. 8.1) with hungry lambs suckling her, predisposing her to teat lesions which may lead to mastitis. These ewes should be managed separately with good grazing and lamb creep feed supplied so that the nutritional demand on the ewe is reduced.

The main problems of the lactating ewe are:

- mastitis
- teat lesions
- hypomagnesaemia.

Mastitis

Recent estimates indicate that mastitis prevalence is around 4–5% in lowland flocks, lower in hill flocks. It is also important in dairy sheep, in which knowledge about cattle mastitis can be usefully applied. Studies in the UK have identified ewe undernutrition, concurrent disease, triplet bearing, ewe age (older and youngest ewes), abnormal teat position, udder abscesses, teat lesions (orf, teat damage), breed differences and farm hygiene as important risk factors for disease, and vets should assess each farm for relevant risk factors when drawing up preventative advice.

Mastitis in the non-dairy ewe is commonly seen at three stages in the production cycle and is usually irreversible:

1. Acute, often gangrenous, at peak lactation – may be fatal; if not, euthanasia should be considered on welfare grounds as the animal should be culled when recovered. Note: ewes with active mastitis lesions cannot be presented at markets for welfare reasons.
2. Chronic, seen after weaning or at the pre-tupping examination; requires culling.
3. Blind teat at lambing – this is same category as (2) but was not detected at that time. Also eventually requires culling but would rear a single lamb if the other half is normal.

Organisms commonly involved are:

- *Staphylococcus aureus*, which is found on the skin.
- *Mannheimia (Pasteurella) haemolytica* which is found in the nasopharynx of healthy lambs.

*Email: jsduncan@liverpool.ac.uk

Singly or together, these bacteria cause 80% of cases (both acute and chronic forms) and invade the udder via the teat canal especially when the skin of the teat is damaged. Other bacteria sometimes found include streptococci, *E. coli*, coagulase-negative staphylococci, with occasionally *T. pyogenes* and *C. perfringens*.

Other causes of mastitis include:

- MV – this causes an indurative mastitis.
- *Leptospira hardjo* (sometimes also called *Leptospira interrogans* serovar *hardjo*) has been associated with sudden milk drop.
- *Mycoplasma agalactiae* is important in Europe, causing contagious agalactia, but this does not occur in the UK currently.

Acute mastitis

This occurs most commonly early in lactation, when the ewe is at peak milk production. The clinical picture is dramatic and typical: the ewe is obviously ill with a swollen udder (usually only one half), she walks stiffly and the lambs appear hungry. The teat and a portion of the udder skin often become cyanotic and cold, and oedema extends along the region of the mammary vein (Fig. 8.2). Death may occur within hours so the ewe may be simply found dead. If the ewe survives, the necrotic udder and, commonly, the skin and tissue surrounding the milk vein, slowly slough off with an extensive loss of abdominal skin, leaving tubes of mammary ducts and blood vessels exposed. Healing then takes many weeks and the ewe loses much condition. The ewe will also be at risk from fly strike.

Consider first whether treatment is justified on both welfare and economic grounds. If so, vigorous systemic treatment is indicated immediately, but the local pathological change is often already irreversible. Give a high dose of broad-spectrum antibiotic, repeated twice daily until the ewe shows improvement (a day or so) or dies. Fluids (1–2 l) given orally or intravenously and a NSAID are also indicated. Strip the secretion out of the gland each time the ewe is treated. Drainage may be aided by removal of the teat if it is gangrenous. Intramammary tubes are an option. Ensure the ewe is comfortable and has tempting food and water nearby. Her lambs will need to be fed with milk replacer unless old enough to manage on creep feed.

Control

- Ensure adequate ewe nutrition pre- and post lambing, prioritize young, aged and thin ewes.
- Don't turn out ewes with triplets.
- Control concurrent disease, e.g. fluke and worms
- Monitor and treat teat lesions.
- Prevent orf.

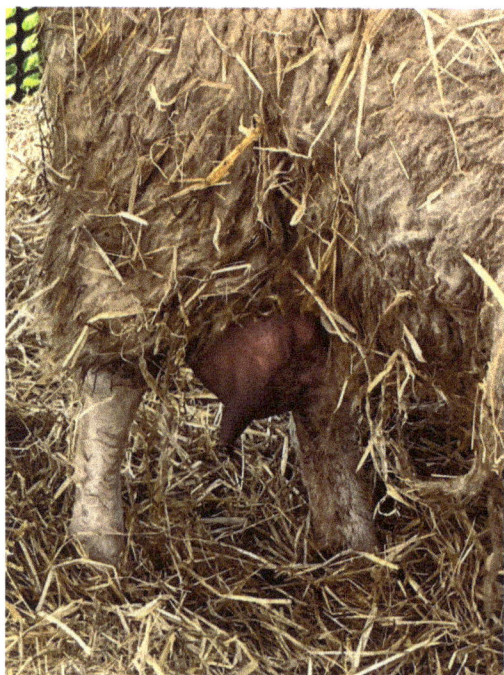

Fig. 8.1. Ewes at peak lactation are vulnerable to mastitis (photo Agnes Winter).

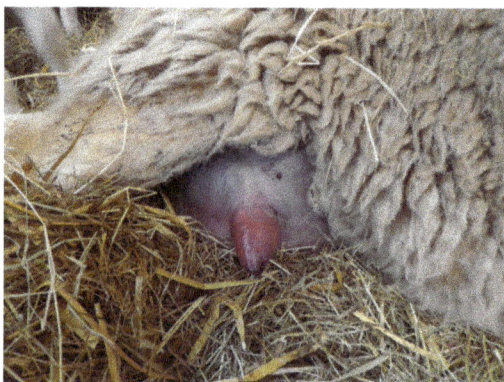

Fig. 8.2. Ewe with gangrenous mastitis of her udder (photo Jennifer Duncan).

Jennifer Duncan

- Ensure good lamb nutrition, especially with fast-growing breeds (creep feeding/grass).
- Wean lambs according to weights/growth rates/ewe BCS/ at 10-12 weeks of age maximum.
- Cull ewes over 7 years old, those with udder lumps, broken-mouthed, abnormal teat position.
- Ensure good bedding hygiene in sheds.
- Review breeding policies, especially if using fast-growing lamb breeds.
- Review lambing season turnout policy as cold weather may reduce grass growth and create extra demands on the ewe to feed cold, hungry lambs.

Chronic mastitis

This is usually discovered before tupping at a time when the ewes are selected for breeding or culling (e.g. because ewes are too thin, have problem teeth, are barren, or have a known disease). One half of the udder, less commonly both, is lumpy and distorted with palpable fibrosis or chronic abscesses. The flock prevalence varies between 1% and 15%. If cases are not obvious at this time, they become apparent at lambing and probably account for many of the ewes which lamb down with mastitis or only one functional gland, and for the problem of neonatal disease that this leads to.

Control

- Review risk factors for mastitis in general on the farm.
- Review weaning policy. Farms should wean based on grass availability, ewe BCS, lamb age and growth rates. Poor ewe body condition, poor grass cover and low growth rate in lambs (<200g/day) over 12 weeks of age should prompt weaning. Higher ewe body condition, good grass cover and better growth rates should allow lambs to remain with ewes for a couple of weeks longer.
- Place ewes on poor pasture at weaning and keep them well away from the sound and sight of their lambs, to reduce milk production. Do not restrict water intake.
- Mark mastitis cases for culling. Note: ewes with active mastitis cannot be presented for sale at markets.

Teat Lesions

These commonly predispose to mastitis (Fig. 8.3). Additionally, affected ewes may be reluctant to let their lambs suck, so they may be a cause of ill thriven or dead lambs.

The main causes are:

- *S. aureus*
- Orf

Staphylococcal infection

This produces very painful ulcerated and swollen lesions at the base of the teat, probably triggered by damage from the sharp incisors of lambs when sucking. It is crucial to treat these as soon as possible, otherwise the consequences of mastitis and starving lambs follow. Aggressive treatment with injectable antibiotic and NSAID, plus local application of antiseptic and local anaesthetic gel helps. While at first sight removal of the lambs might seem a good idea, it is better to allow them to remain with the ewe with additional supplementary feeding if required in the hope that rapid resolution of lesions will allow the ewe to suckle lambs comfortably again.

Orf infection

Orf is a highly infectious, zoonotic skin infection caused by a pox virus. Lesions may be seen on ewes' udders and around lambs' mouths. The lesions will eventually self-cure but as they are very painful, supportive care with local and parenteral antibiotics to help to control secondary infection is advised, as well as pain relief and isolation of affected cases to prevent spread. Lambs may also require supplementary feeding.

It can be difficult to prevent infection since orf virus survives well, especially in the indoor environment.

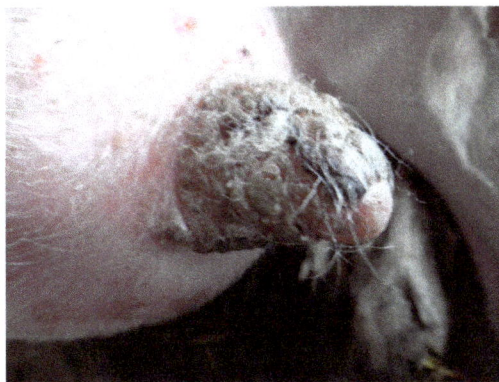

Fig. 8.3. Teat lesions are a high risk for mastitis (photo Jennifer Duncan).

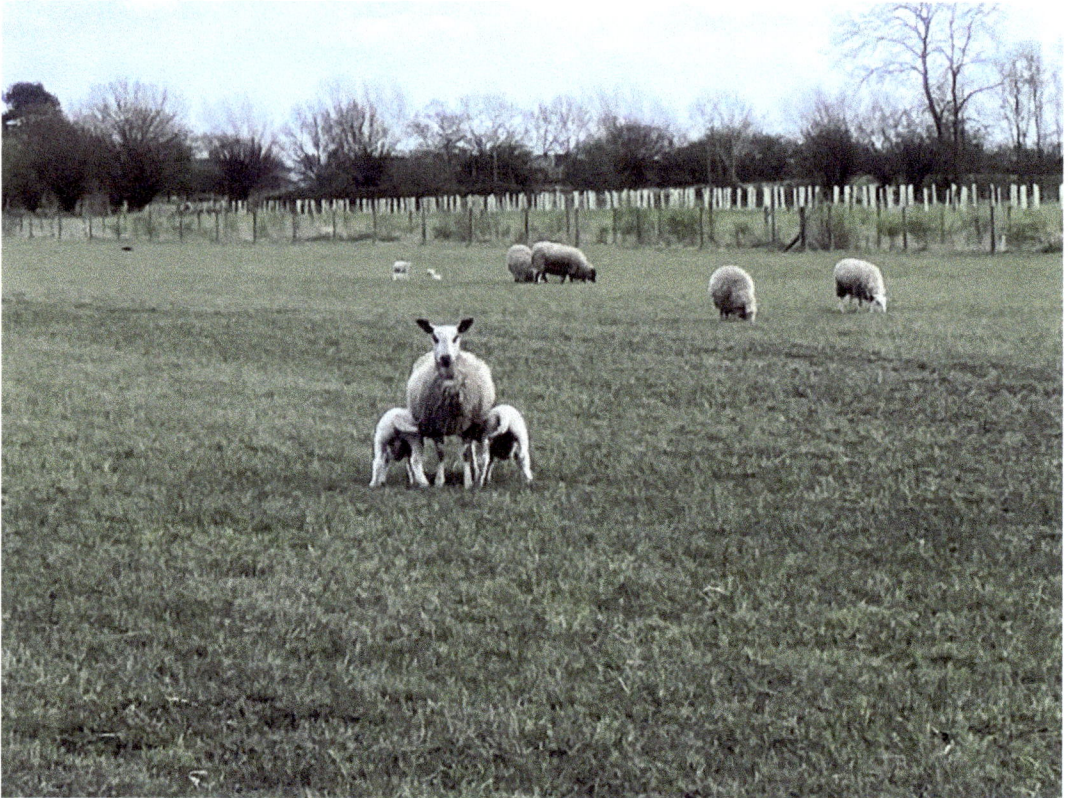

Fig. 8.4. Milky ewes suckling twins or triplets are vulnerable to hypomagnesaemia (photo Agnes Winter).

You can lessen the possibility of exposure by taking steps like these:

- Since animals with cuts or abrasions are most susceptible to infection, reduce the likelihood of this by removing thistle or harsh brush from pastures.
- Disinfect buildings, feed troughs and feed equipment with iodine-based Defra-approved disinfectant.
- Vaccination.

Hypomagnesaemia

As described elsewhere, this is most usually seen in ewes at peak lactation suckling twins (Fig. 8.4).

The stress of lactation, combined with grazing low-fibre, rapidly growing grass, often fertilized with nitrogen, trigger the disease. Most often, ewes are found dead, but may sometimes be seen collapsed and in convulsions. See Chapter 6 for treatment and control.

Jennifer Duncan

9 Growing Lambs

JOHN GRAHAM-BROWN*

Department of Livestock and One Health, Institute of Infection, Veterinary and Ecological Sciences, University of Liverpool, UK

Abstract

Poor growth rate in growing lambs is a common problem which has a major impact on welfare and flock profitability. Coccidiosis and parasitic gastroenteritis are by far the most common causes although mineral deficiencies, especially of cobalt, can also be implicated in some areas.

A common complaint made by farmers is that a significant number of the lambs are not growing as rapidly as expected (Fig. 9.1 and Fig. 9.2). The growth rate of lambs on lowland farms being raised for slaughter should be 250–300 g/day though single lambs and lambs being raised for sale as rams will manage higher growth rates than these. In the UK it has not been routine for farmers producing lambs for slaughter to weigh these regularly but with the increasing use of electronic tagging and data collection this is becoming more common.

If the growth rates are not known, these can be estimated by looking at lamb sales data and working out the times taken to achieve slaughter weight. For example, if we assume that the lambs are born in March and slaughtered at around 40 kg live weight in July, the weight gain will be 300 g/day whereas if they are sent for slaughter in September, the weight gain will only be 200 g/day. Many lambs grow well until some specific incident occurs, the timing of which will help in diagnosis.

Although many causes are possible, the most common reasons for a significant proportion of the lamb crop being thin are coccidiosis and parasitic gastroenteritis (PGE), and in some areas, mineral deficiencies, particularly of cobalt, which also predisposes to parasitic problems. It is highly likely that the poor weight gain will also be associated with scouring.

Coccidiosis

Coccidiosis is a considerable hazard for intensively reared lambs worldwide, with highly stocked lowland systems at particular risk in the UK. Coccidial protists are highly host species-specific. Several *Eimeria* species have been described in sheep, of which *Eimeria crandalis* and *E. ovinoidalis* are considered the most clinically significant.

Clinical signs and pathogenesis

The first signs a farmer may notice in a group of young lambs, typically around 4–8 weeks of age, include lost 'bloom' and an 'open' fleece (poor growth and condition) followed by mild scour and soiling of fleece around the animal's back end. Over time, these signs may become progressively more visible and widespread leading to considerable numbers of animals with diarrhoea, reduced weight gains and/or weight loss due to intestinal ulceration and villous atrophy caused by consecutive cycles of infection, exponential replication and subsequent egress of *Eimeria* parasites from the intestinal mucosa. Untreated cases with heavy infections may continue to deteriorate with extensive scouring, dehydration and even death. After treatment, lambs often continue to grow slowly as a consequence of protracted healing of the intestinal tract and ongoing issues with impaired nutrient and water absorption.

*Email: J.Graham-Brown@liverpool.ac.uk

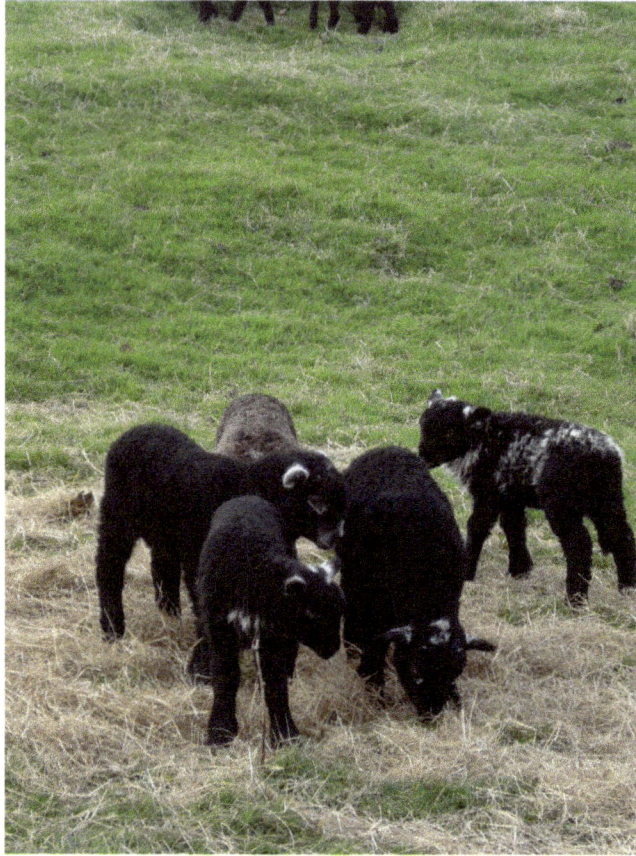

Fig. 9.1. These lambs are thriving but could be vulnerable to coccidiosis, nematodirosis or parasitic gastroenteritis (photo Agnes Winter).

Epidemiology

The life cycle of *Eimeria* follows a direct route of transmission. Following their ingestion as sporulated (infective) oocysts these parasites infect the epithelial and crypt cells of the intestinal mucosa (*E. crandalis* and *E. ovinoidalis* both have a predilection for the large intestine) where they undergo a number of rounds of asexual then sexual replication. Eventually this replication produces the next generation of oocysts which are shed in the faeces. A single infective oocyst may give rise to several thousand in the next generation. The pre-patent periods for *E. crandalis* and *E. ovinoidalis* are 15–20 days and 12–15 days, respectively. Once shed, these oocysts undergo a brief 2–3-day period of sporulation (development) to become infective,

after which they can remain viable in the environment for up to a year, including survival over winter. Oocysts can successfully sporulate and survive in both housed environments and at pasture.

Following initial infection, animals will, over a period of several months, develop life-long immunity and protection against further disease, although they may continue to harbour subclinical infections and shed small numbers of oocysts. Where infectious burdens and ongoing exposure remain light to moderate, this immunity can be obtained without clinical disease manifesting. Lambs are typically most susceptible to infection at around 4–8 weeks of age once their maternally derived immunity has waned. Older animals may also show signs of clinical disease where very high levels of environmental contamination with oocysts exist or

John Graham-Brown

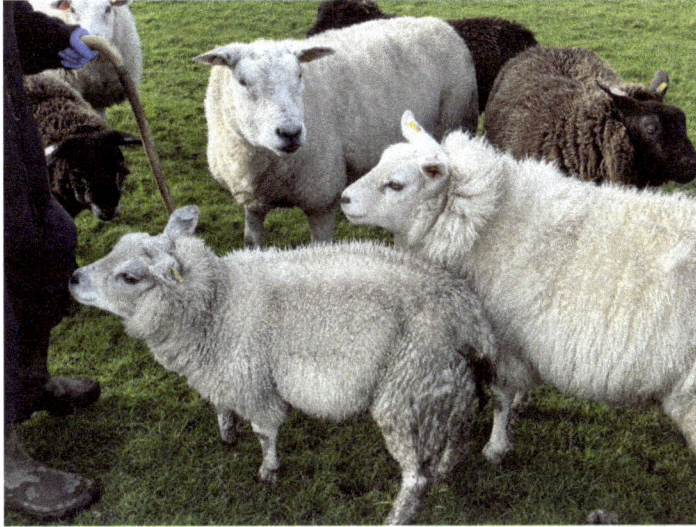

Fig. 9.2. This poorly grown lamb may be suffering the long-term effects of parasitic disease (photo Agnes Winter).

where there is another underlying issue such as poor nutrition or a stressor event (e.g. transportation, tail docking, castration, inclement weather etc.). The degree and rate of environmental contamination is heavily influenced by on-farm management and husbandry practices. In particular, higher stocking rates inevitably lead to higher levels of oocyst accumulation in the environment. Even lambs that have initially acquired light infections can shed oocysts in very high numbers. Where animals are maintained within the same environment (pens, sheds, paddocks etc.) continuously, risk will increase substantially after around 2–3 weeks once these initial infections become patent. Furthermore, where successive groups of lambs are moved through the same environment, oocysts produced by a previous older group of animals will pose an immediate disease risk to subsequent groups of younger, immunologically naïve animals.

Diagnosis

Oocysts are easily observed in faecal samples via microscopy following a standard salt flotation method as small refractile structures measuring 10–40 μm in diameter, often in large numbers (100,000+ oocysts per gram). However, their detection within a sample should not be relied on to diagnose coccidiosis since clinical disease can occur within the pre-patent period of infection, yielding false negative results, whilst the presence of non-pathogenic *Eimeria* oocysts (which can be present in very high numbers) in samples may yield false positive results. Fortunately, clinical signs and history of disease on-farm are often sufficient to make a correct diagnosis, with oocyst counts serving as a useful way to monitor the progress of infection and recovery. Identification of *Eimeria* to the species level can be performed by specialists through morphology of sporulated oocysts and/or molecular techniques. This additional step may be valuable for farms where large numbers of oocysts are routinely observed within growing lambs but the significance of these is unclear. For example, where infected lambs are already out at grass, co-infection with coccidia and *Nematodirus battus* is not uncommon since both infections occur in animals of a similar age. It has been shown that concurrent infection with *E. ovinoidalis*, *E. crandallis* and *N. battus* causes a more severe disease than any of these parasites would by themselves, meaning determining whether any coccidia present are pathogenic may influence subsequent treatment and control.

Treatment and control

Animals with severe clinical disease should be treated immediately with diclazuril (1 mg/kg p.o.) or toltrazuril (20 mg/kg p.o.) and removed to a clean environment free from oocysts. Where severe diarrhoea and dehydration are present, supportive fluid therapy and hospitalization may be indicated. As previously discussed, clinical signs often persist even after successful treatment as a result of residual gut damage.

Where farms routinely experience issues with coccidiosis, a review of their facilities and management may help to identify high-risk areas and practices and inform practical changes. In general, avoiding excessively high stocking rates and good hygiene management reduces disease risk substantially. This includes ensuring objects that lambs interact with regularly, such as milk and creep feeders, water buckets, troughs and mangers, remain clean and free of faecal contamination. In housed animals, ensuring good ventilation and drainage along with regular provision of fresh bedding will help to limit oocyst build-up in the environment. Similarly, thorough cleaning and disinfection of sheds and pens between groups of animals will reduce environmental contamination for the incoming animals. This is particularly important where the new occupants are younger and more susceptible compared with the previous group. It should be noted that very few disinfectants are truly effective at killing oocysts in the environment making the physical act of cleaning the more important aspect of this practice for coccidiosis control. For animals at pasture, initial infectious challenge can be reduced by turnout onto 'clean' grazing (fields not used by young lambs in the previous or current season) and moving creep feeders to a new location every 2–3 days to prevent build-up of oocysts and transmission potential in one specific place.

Whilst management practices can limit the degree of exposure and infection, in many instances these alone are insufficient to prevent clinical disease. Decoquinate is a commonly used feed additive available under prescription which helps to limit the severity of infection and degree of oocyst shedding into the environment at peak risk periods. Formulation is recommended at 100 mg per kg of feed, meaning lambs must be eating a minimum of 100 g creep feed per day to achieve the prophylactic dose of 1 mg/kg. Alternatively, the anti-coccidials diclazuril and toltrazuril are licensed and available for use in sheep as oral drenches. Both are principally intended for use in the prevention of clinical disease as opposed to infection. Consequently, timing of their administration is generally recommended in advance of peak risk periods for disease. Practically speaking, this can usually be assumed to be 1–2 weeks after initial exposure, whilst infections are still pre-patent. Such treatment regimens are intended to allow natural exposure and acquisition of immunity whilst reducing the impact of resulting parasite burdens, subsequent oocyst shedding and build-up in the environment. Whilst a single well-timed dose is often sufficient to prevent clinical disease, in the face of heavy environmental contamination a follow-up treatment after 3 weeks may be indicated, particularly when using diclazuril since this has no residual activity.

Parasitic Gastroenteritis (PGE)

PGE is a major cause of thin, scouring lambs globally. The distribution and prevalence of gastrointestinal nematode parasites in sheep is essentially ubiquitous. Disease normally occurs in lambs aged 2 months up to a year old as they are exposed and become infected over the course of their first grazing season. Following this initial exposure, a strong immunity typically develops meaning that clinical signs are rarely, if ever, seen in ewes. One notable exception to this rule is the Barber's pole worm (*Haemonchus contortus*), which can infect and cause clinical disease in animals of all ages. The clinically important nematode species for lambs in the UK and northern Europe are *Teladorsagia circumcincta*, *Trichostryongylus axei* and *Haemonchus contortus*, found in the abomasum, and *Nematodirus battus*, *Cooperia* and other *Trichostrongylus* species in the small intestine.

Clinical signs

The classically defined presentation of PGE in sheep is caused principally by *Teladorsagia circumcincta* alongside co-infecting *Trichostrongylus* and *Cooperia* species (*T. circumcincta* is generally considered the most pathogenic of these). It is characterized by chronic scours and unthriftiness and/or subclinical parasitism with non-specific signs of reduced weight gain and poor body condition. Whilst mortality is often not a major feature, the widespread and chronic nature of this type of PGE is of major significance from both a welfare and economic perspective. The relative contribution of the different parasite species to infection and disease varies through the year, with risk peaking in early to mid-summer (July) but continuing into the late winter.

In many aspects of its epidemiology and life cycle, *N. battus* differs significantly from the standard model for PGE and consequently should be considered separately in terms of its management, treatment and control. PGE caused by *N. battus* (nematodirosis) is characterized by sudden onset and severe scours, loss of bloom, dehydration, loss of condition and death in young lambs (usually aged 6–12 weeks) early in the grazing season, typically between May and June, with a further potential risk period in the autumn.

Haemonchus also differs significantly from the other PGE-causing nematode species in a number of ways, not least its blood-feeding behaviour. This parasite is discussed in detail elsewhere in the context of its wider impact on flock health (see Chapter 4).

Life cycles and epidemiology

All nematode species named in this section are from the superfamily Trichostrongyloidea and share the same direct route of transmission and basic life cycle. Sheep become infected through the ingestion of infective third-stage larvae (L3) present on pastures. Upon reaching their specific predilection site within the gastrointestinal tract (abomasum or small intestine depending on species) these L3 moult to L4 and begin to feed and develop, moulting once more to emerge as pre-adult L5s. Once sexually mature, adult male and female worms will copulate to produce fertile eggs which are then produced more or less continually by patent females to be shed in the faeces. Eggs develop on pasture first to L1 and undergo a further two moults to L2 and, finally, infective L3.

The pre-patent periods for *T. circumcincta*, *Trichostrongylus* and *Cooperia* species are all around 2–3 weeks. In certain extraneous circumstances, for which the mechanisms are poorly understood, larvae may arrest their development and undergo a quiescent period, or hypobiosis, within the gut mucosa (or gastric gland in the case of *T. circumcincta*). This normally occurs in the latter stages of the grazing season and is believed to be an evolutionary mechanism that allows these parasites to survive more effectively over winter. Hypobiosed larvae will then recommence their development and emerge to become patent adult burdens the following spring. Again, the specific mechanism that facilitates this is poorly understood, but in younger animals (store lambs) the triggered mass emergence of large numbers of encysted

L4 of *T. circumcincta* in spring will occasionally precipitate an acute onset scour referred to as 'type 2' disease (type 1 being the classical presentation of PGE). In older animals, hypobiosed populations are generally smaller, and whilst their recrudescence is not normally associated with clinical disease, a significant increase in worm egg counts can occur. This is particularly apparent in pregnant ewes around lambing, often referred to as the peri-parturient rise. Newborn lambs going out to pasture for the first time in spring do not consume large quantities of grass initially, and consequently do not acquire significant worm burdens in the early part of the grazing season. However, due to their lack of immunity, once infected, spring lambs will shed eggs onto pastures in large numbers over the ensuing weeks and months. The subsequent development from eggs through to infective L3s is largely temperature-dependent and can occur within 2 weeks under optimal conditions. As temperatures rise moving into the summer months, a set of circumstances can arise where substantial numbers of infective L3 are developing and emerging on pastures leading to high levels of infection and clinical disease in lambs.

Outbreaks of PGE at this time can be devastating economically in a commercial flock as the majority of animals will normally be destined for sale imminently. Whilst the early summer is considered to be the 'peak' risk period for PGE, infective L3 can remain viable on pastures for weeks and months. In particular, the L3 of *Trichostrongylus* species (*T. axei* and *T. colubriformis*) can survive and develop in a range of temperatures and conditions, meaning they will persist and continue to emerge on pastures late into the grazing season. These parasites are often associated with black 'winter scours' in store lambs being kept on pastures over winter.

Nematodirus battus is believed to have evolved as an arctic/sub-arctic parasite and has subsequently adopted a different strategy to maintain transmission from one grazing season to the next. This is largely dependent on its survival on pastures over winter as a larvated egg. Unlike other trichostrongylids, *N. battus* L1 do not hatch immediately, instead developing and moulting through to L3 within their eggs, which are highly resilient and can survive for extended periods of time (up to 2 years in some instances). Lambs typically acquire a strong and life-long protective immunity in the months following initial exposure and infection, meaning that they only shed significant numbers of eggs and contribute to pasture burdens in their first grazing season. Ewes do not appear to have any meaningful role in the ongoing transmission of *N. battus* whatsoever. In general, *N. battus* can therefore be considered an infection and disease (nematodirosis) of young lambs, with direct transmission from one crop to the next over consecutive years. The pre-patent period of *N. battus* is 14–16 days.

The development and hatching of larvated *N. battus* eggs is a key epidemiological aspect in terms of disease risk. The majority of this hatching occurs in the spring once ambient temperatures begin to rise above 11°C consistently. Following the prolonged chill period of winter, eggs require a cumulative period of time equivalent to 7 days within an 11.5–17°C temperature range before they will hatch. On an individual farm, clearly the majority of overwintered eggs present on pasture are subject to the same environmental conditions meaning they all tend to develop and hatch at the same time. The consequence of this is a 'spring hatch' event resulting in the mass emergence of infective L3 on pasture. Where susceptible lambs, typically 6–12 weeks old, are grazing pastures at a time such hatch events occur, the overwhelming infectious burdens they acquire as a consequence can precipitate widespread and severe clinical disease.

Due to the close relationship between egg development and temperature it is possible to use local weather data to calculate the likely timing of spring for a geographic region. This technique is employed by a nematodirus risk forecast published annually through SCOPS (www.scops.org.uk) to give an indication of the likely timing of disease risk and allow planning of grazing and treatments of susceptible animals appropriately. When using climate-based risk models it is important to acknowledge the apocryphal view that 'all models are wrong, but some are useful'. A number of factors affect temperature (and therefore timing of hatch) even within a discrete area. For example, higher than average temperatures are experienced at lower altitudes and on south-facing slopes. Where a model predicts a specific hatch date for a given location, clinicians and farmers should therefore consider this as a guide and approximation rather than an absolute prediction and factor in local conditions on-farm, and how the forecast has corresponded to on-farm risk previously; if hatch is known historically to have occurred on a specific farm earlier than the forecast predicted, this can be factored in its interpretation in future years.

Whilst the classical pattern of transmission of *N. battus* in the UK is spring to spring, it has been shown that the chilling effect on eggs over winter is not an absolute requirement for their development and hatching; some eggs may instead larvate and hatch in the autumn months of the same season. Where this coincides with groups of lambs grazing pastures late in the season that missed initial exposure to the spring hatch, clinical disease may also occur. It is suspected that autumn hatching is becoming more common, especially in southern UK, and could indicate parasite adaption to climate change.

Diagnosis

A tentative diagnosis of PGE can usually be made based on clinical signs, seasonality, groups of animals affected and grazing history. Where severe outbreaks occur, the timely submission of fallen stock for PME can allow identification and enumeration of adult parasite burdens and/or associated pathology, the compartments of the GI tract affected and the species responsible. Otherwise, in most cases diagnosis can be confirmed by faecal worm egg counts (FWECs) following a standard salt flotation method of sample preparation. The majority of strongylid nematodes (including the Trichostrongyloidea) produce very similar eggs, making distinction of species presence and abundance on morphological appearance alone difficult. The exception to this is the genus *Nematodirus* (including *N. battus*), which produce much larger eggs, typically ~150 μm in length compared with the ~90 μm of other strongyle eggs. It is important to note, however, in cases of acute nematodirosis, that clinical signs may manifest in the pre-patent period. Recent advances in molecular techniques including PCR and 'nemabiome' sequencing allow for greater levels of insight into species presence and abundance, although at the time of writing, slow speed of turnaround makes its use as a tool for real-time decision making impractical. Specialist techniques can be used for the diagnosis of *Haemonchus* specifically where this is of concern (see Chapter 4).

In general, FWECs remain a central tool for the diagnosis and control of PGE in sheep using both individual or pooled faecal samples (for the latter this is usually a composite of 10× healthy individual animals). Egg counts per gram of faeces are largely speaking proportional to adult worm burdens, meaning thresholds can be established; as a rule of thumb for individual FWECs <250 e.p.g. is generally considered indicative of light infections, 250–750 e.p.g. moderate and 750+ e.p.g. heavy. FWECs are most effective when deployed as an ongoing regular (typically monthly) testing regimen. This allows farmers, veterinarians and/or registered animal medicines advisors (RAMAs) to monitor burdens and take timely and informed interventions as appropriate. Additionally, FWECs can be deployed in the targeted selective treatment (TST) of animals to reduce use of anthelmintics and selection for resistance, and to test treatment efficacy through egg count reduction tests where treatment failures due to anthelmintic resistance is a concern. For the latter, healthy animals with no recent history of prior treatment with anthelmintics should be randomly selected and assigned to a treatment or control group (15–20 animals per group). Individual faecal samples are taken ahead of treatment, with subsequent counts performed at 7–14 days post-treatment depending on the treatment used (7 days for group 2-LVs, 14 days for group 1-BZs and group 3-MLs). Anthelmintic resistance is indicated where reduction in FWEC observed in the test cohort is <95% when compared to the control group. Ideally, pre-treatment FWECs should be >200 e.p.g. to allow unambiguous interpretation of results. A simplified protocol where only post-treatment FWECs are performed may be useful as an initial investigation. In either instance, dosing should be performed under veterinary supervision to rule out treatment failures for other reasons such as under-dosing, incorrect administration etc.

Performing FWECs is a relatively straightforward process and can be conducted in-house by the majority of veterinary practices with minimal investment in additional equipment and consumables. In addition to conventional microscopy approaches, newer technologies are becoming available that aim to streamline sample preparation and automate the screening process through digital image capture and web-based diagnostic platforms, making more direct sample processing and submission by farmers and RAMAs possible, thereby increasing uptake and timeliness of diagnostic information for informed treatments.

Treatment and control

With appropriate treatment and control measures in place, outbreaks of clinical PGE should be largely avoidable. The early recognition of clinical signs and use of FWECs will allow the timely treatment of lambs before severe lesions of villous atrophy develop.

In the face of an outbreak of clinical disease, affected animals should be treated without delay. It may be advisable to remove severely affected animals to a housed environment for supportive therapy and a period of convalescence, and to move the remainder of the affected group to a safe, clean pasture 2–3 days after treatment (discussed further below).

Planning grazing strategy ahead of the grazing season can reduce risk considerably; pastures grazed by lambs in the mid- to late grazing season should ideally be avoided in the early part of the next grazing season, as these will almost certainly be the most heavily contaminated pastures with overwintered eggs and larvae. Later into the grazing season these pastures will become safer as overwintered L3 populations die off and the spring lamb crop becomes more resilient. Where possible, making use of hay and silage aftermaths in the late summer/autumn can also provide a good option for clean grazing, whilst pastures predominantly grazed by cattle in the summer months can provide useful grazing opportunities for ewes and store lambs over the winter period. Further grazing management strategies are discussed below in the context of anthelmintic stewardship and sustainability.

It is also important to consider genetics and selective breeding in the context of host resilience and immunity. It is possible to select breeding rams to produce lambs which develop immunity to worms more rapidly. Estimated breeding values for genetic resistance to worms are becoming available for rams in terms of expected FWECs, clinical disease risk etc. Such considerations have become a central aspect of breeding programmes in places like Australia where anthelmintic resistance is a particular concern (www.sheepgenetics.org.au - accessed 5/11/24).

Although there are an enormous number of proprietary anthelmintic drugs available to farmers for the treatment of gastrointestinal nematodes, the vast majority fall into one of five main chemical groups:

- Group 1-BZs (benzimidazoles)
- Group 2-LVs (imidazothiazoles)
- Group 3-MLs (macrocyclic lactones)
- Group 4-ADs (amino-acetonitrile derivatives)
- Group 5-SLs (spiroindoles)

Broadly speaking, actives within these groups have common characteristics. However, it is also important to consider that drugs within the same class will carry different licences of efficacy, pharmacokinetic properties, routes of administration etc. meaning it is always necessary to check the data sheet for efficacy, range of activity, residual action and withdrawal periods prior to prescription and administration. Groups 1–3 are considered conventional wormers, having been available for decades, whilst groups 4 and 5 are much more recent additions.

Group 1-BZs are by far the oldest group, first introduced in 1961. Widely known as 'white drenches', all benzimidazoles (except the flukicide triclabendazole) are effective against all active stages of the nematode life cycle, including eggs in most instances. Many also carry a licence of efficacy against hypobiosed larvae (specifically albendazole and fenbendazole products), lungworms, *Moniezia* tapeworms and adult-stage fluke infections. All preparations currently available come in the form of oral drenches, some of which are fortified with cobalt and selenium to support growing lambs. None of the group 1-BZs has residual activity.

Of the group 2-LVs, levamisole is the only active molecule currently licensed in the UK. These 'yellow drenches' are presently only available as oral treatments in combination with flukicides. Levamisole is effective against all active stages of GI nematodes and lungworms.

The group 3-MLs (macrocyclic lactones or 'clear drenches') are by far the most diverse group of wormers, available as injectable, pour-on and oral drench formulations. Group 3-MLs are considered broad-spectrum wormers with claims of efficacy against a wide range of gastrointestinal nematodes and lungworms, including hypobiosed larvae, as well as ectoparasites including sheep scab mites (*Psoroptes ovis*) and ticks (see Chapters 12 and 16). It is important to check the data sheets carefully when using these products as advice and withdrawal periods can vary considerably. It is also important to note that whilst many of the active ingredients within this group are considered to be long-acting with persistent activity against re-infection, this claim is not presently made on the majority of product data sheets for sheep parasites. One exception to this is moxidectin, which (at the time of writing) has oral and injectable formulations with claims of persistent efficacy against a broad range of sheep endo- and ectoparasites, including PGE-causing nematodes, lasting 2–5 weeks depending on the particular species.

The groups 4-AD and 5-SI are each represented by a single active compound at present; monepantel and derquantel, respectively. Both are available as oral drenches with broad spectrum activity against GI nematodes. Monepantel also carries a claim of efficacy against hypobiosed larvae, whilst derquantel is effective against lungworms. Derquantel is only licensed and available as a combination wormer with a group 3-ML (abamectin). This approach has been taken with the explicit aim of minimizing risk of selection for resistance against the group 5-SI component. Given the relative newness of these drugs and their introduction after anthelmintic stewardship and responsible use became mainstream thinking, it is generally accepted that these products should be reserved for specific tasks such as break-drenching and quarantine treatments as opposed to more routine use.

When discussing anthelmintics and their use in the context of PGE in sheep it is important to acknowledge and consider the risk posed by anthelmintic resistance. Historically, over-use through blanket prophylactic treatments has selected heavily for resistance within parasite populations. Anthelmintic resistance, including resistance to multiple groups, e.g. to groups 1-BZ and 3-ML, is widely reported worldwide making long-term sustainable control a major challenge, particularly since resistance status is irreversible once established. In the UK, resistance has been confirmed against group 1–4 products. It should also be noted that resistance against one wormer within a group will mean resistance or reduced efficacy of all other wormers within the same group. This is particularly true for group 1-BZs. This situation has necessitated a substantial change in approach to parasite control.

Considerable effort is now directed towards developing adjunctive and supportive control measures alongside use of anthelmintics with a view to reducing selection pressure for resistance and preserving their remaining efficacy long-term. To this end, the UK's Sustainable Control of Parasites in Sheep (SCOPS) steering group was formed in 2004 largely to focus on responsible use of anthelmintics and produce evidence-based, practical guidelines for industry stakeholders (www.scops.org.uk). Much of this advice is based on the principle of parasite populations *in refugia*–parasites not exposed to anthelmintics and, therefore, not subject to selection

John Graham-Brown

for resistance. Maximizing this *in refugia* population helps to dilute resistance genes where they are selected for throrough anthelmintic treatments, thereby preserving efficacy within the population as a whole. *In refugia* populations can be considered as parasites within the environment (on pasture) and within untreated animals. For the former, thought should be given to the timing and administration of anthelmintics relative to larval pasture burdens. For this reason the blanket treatment of ewes at or soon after lambing ahead of spring turn-out to counter the peri-parturient rise in their FWECs, and again at pre-tupping, is no longer recommended since this leads to ewes contaminating spring pastures with only resistant parasites whilst having little to no direct health benefit for the ewes themselves. Similarly, advice has moved away from the conventional 'dose and move' strategy of sending animals to clean pasture immediately after treatments (much to the frustration and in some cases anger of farmers who were previously informed this was best practice). Instead, a modified policy of 'dose, wait and move' is now recommended, where animals are left on contaminated pastures for a period of 2–3 days ahead of moving. The rationale behind this is that it allows animals to become lightly re-infected with susceptible parasites (assuming the product used has no residual activity). Therefore, when moved to clean grazing they will contaminate this with a mixed population of resistant and susceptible parasites rather than exclusively resistant parasites if moved immediately after treatment. Co-grazing of goats with sheep is not recommended, given their ability to rapidly metabolize most anthelmintics and subsequently expose parasites to sublethal doses.

With respect to maximizing the *in refugia* population within animals, quite simply this is achieved through administration of fewer treatments. There is evidence demonstrating that robust monitoring of PGE in lambs by routine (monthly) FWEC and/or production performance (typically weight gain) can reduce the overall frequency of flock treatments and the proportion of animals requiring treatments without compromising animal welfare and productivity. The aim is generally to leave at least 10% of animals untreated. Such targeted selective treatments (TSTs) are now recommended by most sheep specialists, although it should be acknowledged that these can only be implemented successfully by individuals that are engaged and committed to the process – knowledge exchange

and understanding of the rationale behind such approaches is essential, as is the keeping of thorough and accurate records (diagnostics and performance monitoring) to inform decisions.

Choice of wormer is clearly important. As a general rule it is advised to use specific wormers only when indicated. This equates to use of single actives and narrower-spectrum wormers where possible unless there is a specific indication for broader treatments. For this reason, group 1-BZs are typically recommended earlier in the season when nematodirosis is the principal concern, with the timing of administration informed by likely risk period (e.g. nematodirus forecast). It should be noted, however, that group 1-BZ resistance is reported in *N. battus*. Otherwise, treatments should largely be informed by the presence or absence of resistance. Where resistance is suspected, or status is unknown, testing should be performed as described previously. It is important to note that conclusions should not be jumped to without first gathering the necessary evidence. Treatment failures with anthelmintics can and have been attributed to a range of factors including improper dosing, administration and storage of products. Similarly, where products with no residual activity are used and pasture management is not considered, animals may immediately become re-infected with significant parasite burdens whilst still recovering from the intestinal damage caused by the burden that was treated. In the instance of a farm struggling with resistance and control of PGE within the grazing season resulting from ineffective or partially effective treatments, a one-off 'break-drench' later into the season with a group 4-AD or 5-SI may be indicated. Assuming these two classes are normally held in reserve, it is expected that their deployment under such circumstances will effectively clear any parasite burdens irrespective of their resistance to other worming groups. Ideally, break-drenching should not be a regular occurrence. Where they are necessary, a review of on-farm parasite control practices should be undertaken ahead of the following grazing season.

Routine use of moxidectin (particularly injectable) is not recommended due to its importance as an ectoparasiticide (specifically for treatment of Sheep Scab; see Chapter 12) and because of the complications its long persistent activity has for resistance selection against group 3-MLs. Current guidance dictates this should not be used within a flock more than once in a season, either as a break-drench for PGE, or treatment of scab. Where it is used for one of these purposes, alternative treatments should be sought for the other if indicated.

In addition to implementing sustainable practices to reduce resistance selection on-farm, minimizing the risk of introducing resistance should also be considered and mitigated through adequate quarantine procedures. It should be assumed that any bought-in stock will be carrying some degree of parasite burden, and that these could include resistant strains. Current guidelines therefore recommend treating with a group 4-AD and group 5-SI product on arrival and housing for 48 h. These animals should then be turned out separately onto pastures grazed previously by the home flock for 3–4 weeks to pick up parasite burdens native to the farm, after which mixing can occur. Faecal egg counts at 14 days post-quarantine treatment may be useful to check these treatments have been effective. Clearly, where animals are being bought in for breeding purposes (rams and replacement ewes), this should be planned well in advance of the start of breeding.

Cestode Infections

Adult tapeworms of the genus *Moniezia* are extremely common intestinal parasites of young lambs. Strings of white segments are frequently observed in the faeces by farmers and blamed for any clinical signs which may be present at the same time. There is little evidence to suggest that these parasites exert any adverse effect on production, although intestinal impactions are occasionally reported with very heavy infections. Similarly, this species of tapeworm poses no risk to humans or any other species. Most group 1-BZ drugs (e.g. albendazole) are licensed and very effective against adult *Moniezia* infections, although their use for this specific purpose alone is questionable from the perspective of sustainability.

Whilst not a specific issue of growing lambs, it is worth noting here that sheep also act as an intermediate host for several species of taeniid cestodes. Infection occurs through the ingestion of onchospheres in the faeces of an infected definitive host – usually a dog (Fig. 9.3) or wild canid (e.g. red fox). Upon reaching the intestines, larval tapeworms hatch and migrate to a species-dependent predilection site where they establish and develop into metacestodes, the infective stage for the definitive host by ingestion through feeding on infected tissues/

carcasses. The most important of these in sheep from a clinical perspective is *Taenia multiceps*, which forms a coenurus type metacestode in the cranial cavity and causes neurological signs (see Chapter 14). Most other species have little to no impact on the health and welfare of their sheep intermediate host but are of significance in terms of ongoing transmission to definitive hosts. Such infections can also be economically important as their identification at slaughter may lead to the rejection of organs and carcasses.

Taenia hydatigena, a common tapeworm of sheepdogs (and foxes), forms fluid-filled cysticerci (metacestodes) on the serosal surface of the liver and within the peritoneum. Very occasionally heavy infections occur in young, usually pet, lambs kept in close proximity to dogs (and their faeces). The mass migration of larval tapeworms through the liver can result in acute haemorrhage and death. *Taenia ovis*, a tapeworm of dogs and foxes, forms smaller cyst-like cysticerci in striated muscle, with a particular predilection for cardiac muscle. In heavy infections, this 'cysticercosis' may be generalized, resulting in whole-carcass condemnation.

Echinococcus granulosus forms large, fluid-filled hydatid cysts in the liver and lungs resulting in condemnation of offal. Whilst clinical signs are not normally seen in sheep, hydatid disease is a potentially serious and fatal anthropozoonosis. Whilst hydatid cysts themselves do not pose a direct infectious risk to humans, their observation in sheep carcasses indicate on-farm transmission and, therefore, a potential public health risk. Historically seen in the major sheep-rearing regions (particularly central Wales), human cases are now few and far between in the UK due to improved control of tapeworm infections in dogs. Eradication schemes have been successfully carried out in a number of regions including Tasmania, New Zealand, Uruguay and Cyprus, but this parasite and its cousin *Echinococcus multilocularis* remains a public health issue in many parts of the world.

No licensed, efficacious products exist for treating metacestode infections in sheep, meaning control is almost entirely dependent on the regular treatment of farm dogs for adult tapeworms, which should feature as part of a sheep health programme (see Chapter 18), preventing direct access of other (pet) dogs to sheep where practical, and prompt removal and correct disposal of fallen stock to prevent onwards transmission.

John Graham-Brown

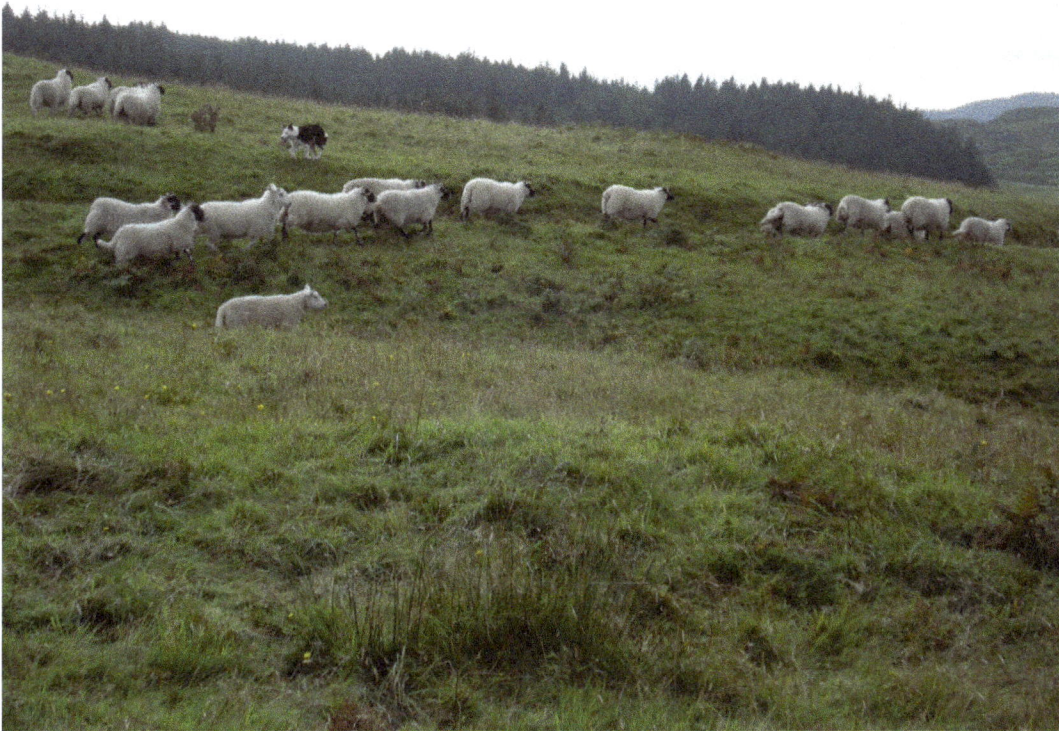

Fig. 9.3. Dogs can host several species of tapeworms which can infect sheep so should not have access to sheep carcasses and should be wormed regularly (photo Agnes Winter).

Cobalt Deficiency

Cobalt deficiency is the cause of 'pine' or 'ill-thrift' in lambs, a condition which is well recognized in all sheep-producing countries of the world. The incidence is highest in areas where soils are derived from acid igneous rocks and where there are coarse, sandy soils. In Scotland, cobalt deficiency is widely distributed but in England, the localities most likely to be deficient are in the limestone areas of the Pennines, the old red sandstone areas of Hereford, Shropshire and Worcester, Dartmoor and the Greensands at the edge of the chalk in south-east England. As well as these areas where cobalt deficiency is endemic, other areas became cobalt-deficient as a result of farming practices, such as liming and reseeding which have improved pastures and, in so doing, lowered the available cobalt. A constant intake of cobalt is needed to allow rumen organisms to produce vitamin B_{12}, and the disease caused by cobalt deficiency is thus an induced vitamin B_{12} deficiency.

Clinical signs

The typical disease is characterized by:

- loss of appetite
- reduced weight gains proceeding to weight loss and extreme emaciation;
- lambs have a dry coat and a tight skin; and
- severe anaemia and lachrymation in the terminal stages

Subclinically, a marginal deficiency of cobalt may be of considerable economic importance since typical signs may not be present but weight gains may be reduced. PGE is often also present and its clinical effects are more serious, whilst copper deficiency may be a further complicating factor in some countries including Australia, New Zealand, South Africa and the USA but rarely in the UK. However, farmers tend to suspect deficiency states with little evidence so care should be taken over diagnosis.

The adult ewe may show signs of cobalt deficiency in late pregnancy due to fatty liver, leading to perinatal mortality.

Diagnosis

- History of farm and geographical area.
- Clinical findings.
- Response to treatment – this is often very marked after cobalt administration, but it should be noted that lambs with reduced appetite due to other causes may also show a response to dosing with cobalt.
- Laboratory confirmation
  - in the animal, by serum and liver vitamin B_{12} concentration;
  - in the food, by herbage and soil cobalt concentration.

Treatment and prevention

There is no placental transfer of vitamin B_{12} and only low concentrations in milk; lambs require colostrum for their first supply.

Possible methods of treatment and prevention include:

- Cobalt boluses – the most effective treatment is to give each lamb, at about 8 weeks of age (not before, because they are too small to dose, and the rumen is not fully developed) a cobalt pellet or bolus. There are a number of different boluses containing various combinations of minerals, so these need to be matched to particular demands on individual farms. Beware of giving products containing copper unless there is a proven need for it.
- Oral dosing with cobalt – a drench of cobalt sulfate can be given to affected lambs which will need to be repeated every 3 weeks.
- Cobalt supplementation in mineral mixture – it is unlikely that lambs will be on concentrates but, if so, the mineral mixture should contain sufficient cobalt to raise the whole feed to 0.11 mg Co/kg DM.
- Injection of vitamin B_{12} – this will deal rapidly with an immediate problem, but cost and the need for injections every 3 weeks precludes this as a preventative measure.
- Application of cobalt sulfate to grazing land – cobalt sulfate may be applied as a spray or as a granular top dressing at 2.0 kg/ha. Dressing need only be repeated every 3 years (or 6 years if the deficiency is only marginal) and only one-third of the grazing need be treated (at 6 kg/ha), since the sheep graze the treated strip selectively. The pasture should not be treated soon after liming.

10 Sudden Death and Found Dead

AGNES WINTER

Department of Livestock and One Health, Institute of Infection, Veterinary and Ecological Sciences, University of Liverpool, UK

Abstract
This chapter addresses the most common causes of sheep of all ages being found dead. It emphasizes the value of post-mortem examination (PME) in any investigation. The various clostridial diseases and pasteurellosis are the most common causes of death if a full vaccination schedule has not been followed. Parasitic diseases such as acute fasciolosis and haemonchosis should also be considered.

Sudden death or, more accurately, 'found dead' is a common problem in sheep-keeping. Since the sheep flock is usually not as carefully observed as other animal enterprises – at best twice a day in lowland flocks and infrequently in the case of high hill flocks – the actual death is rarely observed and may have taken place at any time since the last inspection, so making an estimate of how recently death occurred is important (freshness, appearance of eyes, smell, autolysis). The age of the sheep affected and whether few or many are involved will help in the diagnostic process. The rest of the group or flock should be observed carefully to see if any more sheep are showing early clinical signs of disease.

PME is an important diagnostic tool but it should be remembered that autolytic changes occur rapidly due to the insulating qualities of the fleece so carcasses need to be as fresh as possible. If illness is observed in in-contact animals, consideration should be given to sacrificing a sheep for PME. If this is done, it is advisable that the PME be performed by a Veterinary Investigation Officer (VIO) from APHA, SRUC, AFBI or other specialist providers. PMEs performed by such agencies are subsidized as part of the UK government's scanning surveillance activities.

Some of the diseases which must be considered in the differential diagnosis of sudden death are described in other parts of this book and will only be briefly mentioned here.

AHDB produces an excellent guide on to how to get the most out of an on-farm PME (https://project-blue.blob.core.windows.net/media/Default/Beef%20&%20Lamb/GettingTheMostOutOfPostMortems2731_191120_WEB.pdf accessed 21/2/24). However, if multiple deaths are occurring or if you suspect losses may be associated with, for example, commercial feed formulation or adverse reactions to a medicinal product, it is advisable to consult a VIO through whom detailed investigations can be undertaken.

Common Causes of Sudden Death or Found Dead by Age Group

Young lambs

In young lambs up to about 4 weeks old, a small number of deaths may be caused by:

- accidents;
- starvation/exposure (e.g. where a ewe develops unobserved mastitis or a lamb becomes mismothered);
- watery mouth where colostrum intake is delayed or absent;
- abdominal catastrophes such as gastric torsion; and
- lamb dysentery associated with faults in vaccination technique, individual ewes being missed or lack of colostrum intake.

*Email: a.winter@liverpool.ac.uk

If many lambs are involved, the most likely causes are:

- hypothermia as a result of extreme weather conditions;
- lamb dysentery in a non-vaccinated flock; and
- septicaemia associated with *M. haemolytica*.

Growing lambs

Up to about 6 months old, a small number of deaths may be due to:

- redgut (torsion of the mesentery) particularly if being artificially reared or on *ad libitum* creep feed; and
- dosing-gun injuries if drenching is carried out by an unskilled person.

If many growing lambs are involved (Fig. 10.1) the main possibilities are:

- pulpy kidney disease;
- braxy;
- acute abomasitis (*Paeniclostridium (formerly Clostridium) sordellii*);
- acute pneumonia due to *M. haemolytica*;
- septicaemia due to *Bibersteinia trehalosi*;
- massive parasitic infections, particularly of *Nematodirus, Haemonchus*, coccidiosis or acute fasciolosis, but in these cases others in the flock will be showing less acute signs aiding diagnosis. Specific diagnostic testing of live animals, e.g. faecal examination, serology may be of value in arriving at a diagnosis;
- rumen acidosis can occur in lambs receiving creep feed especially if it is introduced too quickly. Lambs may be found dead although it is likely flock-mates will be showing clinical signs of scour, dullness, ataxia etc.

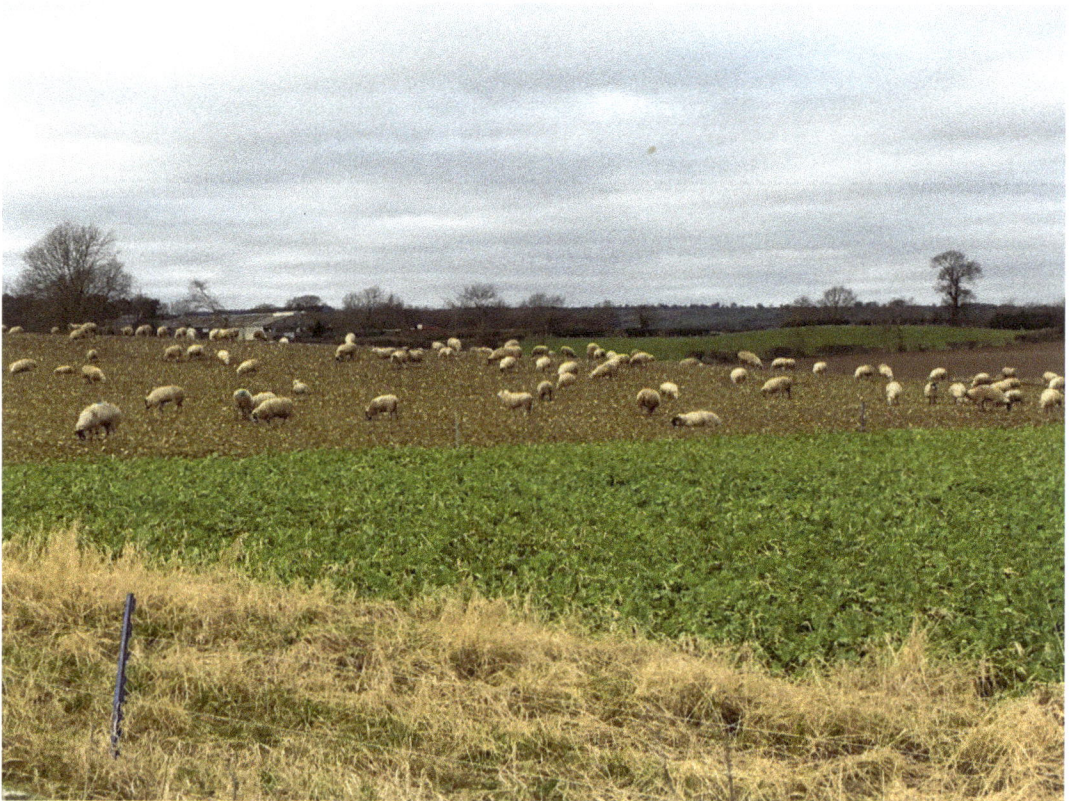

Fig. 10.1. These fattening lambs grazing stubble turnips are vulnerable to clostridial diseases and systemic pasteurellosis if not fully vaccinated (photo Agnes Winter).

Adult sheep

In adult sheep, single or a few deaths may be associated with:

- accidents such as newly introduced rams fighting and fracturing the occipital process of the axis;
- sheep in fat condition becoming cast on their backs (common);
- periparturient problems in lambing ewes; and
- ruminal acidosis associated with either feeding an excessive amount of concentrates or a too sudden introduction of concentrate feed.

If many sheep are involved, the most likely causes are:

- metabolic disorders, particularly hypocalcaemia or hypomagnesaemia (see Chapter 6);
- clostridial diseases, especially black disease, struck, blackleg or acute abomasitis;
- acute pneumonia associated with *M. haemolytica*;
- acute haemonchosis or fasciolosis; and
- toxicity associated with, e.g., copper, yew, rhododendron or nitrites.

Clostridial Diseases

Clostridial diseases have already been discussed in Chapter 3 so refer to that chapter too.

Clostridia are ubiquitous in the environment, especially as very resistant spores in soil, so sheep are potentially always exposed to infection. Furthermore, many species, e.g. *Clostridium perfringens*, are normal gut commensals. Today's farmers tend to be unaware of the catastrophic losses from these diseases which occurred in the era before vaccines were available. The majority of these diseases (apart from tetanus and botulism) cause rapid collapse and death so sheep are usually found dead with few or no clinical signs having been observed. Clinical signs, if seen, and death are associated with the production of powerful toxins by different species or types of clostridia which multiply in a number of different sites in the body.

Diagnosis

This needs to be speedy if control is to be effective. It is usually dependent upon obtaining, from the farmer, accurate and relevant historical information (a trigger factor or other reason for the disease) supported, where possible, by a PME of fresh carcasses and laboratory demonstration of relevant toxins. It is important not to rely on PME alone, not least because the material is often too decomposed for useful interpretation.

The information you need includes:

- Did the sheep die 'suddenly' or was it 'found dead'? (Time since last inspection?)
- Has clostridial disease occurred on the farm before?
- What has the farmer done to control clostridial diseases? Have vaccines been used? (If so, closely check what and when and if individuals could have been missed or colostrum not provided to affected lambs.)
- Were there any obvious abnormal signs (scouring, convulsions, stiffness)?
- Is a particular age group affected? (note the age ranges for the different clostridial diseases).
- Has the farmer done anything to precipitate or introduce the disease (e.g. change to better pasture or more concentrate fed; injected with dirty needles or irritant material; used rubber rings)?
- What season is it? (Spring grass predisposes to pulpy kidney and struck, fluke in winter links with black disease, frost in autumn precipitates braxy.)
- Are the affected sheep in good condition? (Clostridial diseases often affect the greedy, fatter animals.)

Treatment

This is rarely an option and is usually unrewarding even if the animal is seen alive.

Control

Clostridial vaccines are cheap and effective (though no vaccine is ever guaranteed 100% effective) so that it is not unreasonable to expect very few losses from these diseases. In recent years, though, problems with production and availability of some vaccines have led to shortages. Laboratory reports continue to show that serious losses due to these diseases still occur and are usually due to mistakes in vaccine application, for example: (i) choosing the wrong vaccine combination; (ii) injecting at the wrong times; (iii) 'dirty' injections (slick and clean SC injection technique and use of guarded needles are needed to avoid abscess formation); or (iv) just not vaccinating at all. The vet has a significant part to play in promoting a suitable vaccination schedule as part of a planned flock health programme.

The recipe for control contains three ingredients:

1. Avoid the predisposing factors: in practice, this really means the control of fasciolosis, the use of sterile instruments and working in clean, dry conditions with dry, clean sheep.
2. Antibodies derived via vaccination for all age groups and adequate colostrum provision for lambs. Antisera for lambs from unvaccinated ewes are no longer available.
3. Antibiotic cover (LA antibiotic) following trauma (e.g. assisted lambing, dog bites).

Main clostridial diseases

These can be grouped into diseases:

(i) causing enterotoxaemia affecting the digestive system, liver or kidneys (lamb dysentery, pulpy kidney, braxy, struck, abomasitis, black disease and bacilliary haemoglobinuria);
(ii) causing muscle or soft tissue necrosis (blackleg, big head); and
(iii) affecting nerve function (tetanus, botulism).

Lamb dysentery

This is seen in young lambs, up to about 3 weeks old, caused by *C. perfringens* type B. A few lambs are found dead, often only a few days old, with older lambs being affected later in the outbreak. A few lambs may be seen with signs of abdominal pain before death, with a hunched-up appearance. Dysentery is not necessarily present but PME usually shows haemorrhages in the intestinal walls and haemorrhagic gut contents. As with many clostridial diseases, the largest, best-fed lambs are often affected. Up to 25% of the lambs in the batch may die.

Pulpy kidney

This is the most common clostridial disease and is caused by *C. perfringens* type D. It is seen especially in the best growing lambs of around 4–10 weeks old and in store lambs being finished in the autumn on good grass or in the winter, often being fed concentrates. Rams may be affected, especially those on supplementary feed prior to mating. Most affected lambs are found dead as the disease is usually peracute, but some may show ataxia and convulsions before death. PME shows typical softening of one or both kidneys and yellowish fluid in the pericardium. A quick test is to check the urine for glucose.

Braxy

This is seen in autumn and winter in lambs or shearlings, often after eating frosty grass, and is caused by *C. septicum*. Affected sheep are found dead or may show abdominal pain or recumbency prior to death. PME shows acute abomasitis.

Struck

This is seen most commonly in the UK in adult sheep in spring, caused by *C. perfringens* type C. The disease often follows a change in diet and feeding of concentrates. Signs are the classic 'found dead' with others showing dullness and recumbency. Losses are usually low. PME shows haemorrhagic enteritis and excess fluid in body cavities.

Acute abomasitis

Abomasitis caused by *P. (formerly C.) sordellii* is seen in growing lambs of 4–10 weeks old, almost always in housed creep-fed lambs. These bacteria also cause toxaemia in older lambs and adults.

Black disease

Infectious necrotic hepatitis, or black disease, caused by *C. novyi* type B is seen in adult sheep during the winter and is associated with migrating immature liver flukes. These damage the liver and give rise to the conditions which allow the bacteria to multiply. The classic dark haemorrhagic appearance of the liver gives the disease its name.

Bacillary haemoglobinuria

This disease is caused by *C. haemolyticum* (*novyi* type D) and affects the liver and kidneys. The disease is sporadic and uncommon, occurring in adults in winter, also often associated with migrating liver flukes. Haemorrhage in the kidneys colours the urine dark red which may cause staining of the wool in the perineal area. Affected animals may live long enough for jaundice to develop.

Blackleg and big head

These diseases are caused by *C. chauvoei* and *C. novyi* type A, respectively (malignant oedema is similar but caused by other clostridia). These diseases are associated with injuries and wounds which allow the multiplication of clostridia in the damaged tissues and are often called gas gangrene because of the typical necrosis and gas formation which quickly develop in the affected area. The sites affected most commonly are the muscles of the hindlimbs, shearing wounds, uterus, pelvic and perineal areas in recently lambed ewes and the heads of fighting rams.

Tetanus

Affected animals are usually seen alive and show rigidity of muscles including those of the jaws and limbs. It is usually unrewarding to treat. For more details see Chapter 14.

Botulism

This is occasionally seen in sheep which have come into contact with manure from poultry sheds. The bacteria multiply in decaying carcasses, producing toxins which, when ingested, cause progressive muscle paralysis. So, unlike the other clostridial diseases in which toxins are produced from bacteria within the body, in this case the toxin is preformed. Signs include salivation and increasing flaccidity of muscles. It is usually fatal.

Systemic Pasteurellosis

This disease caused by *B. trehalosi* is a major killer of fattening lambs in autumn, particularly following weaning, transport or movement on to richer pasture and should always be at the top of the list of possible diagnoses, along with pulpy kidney, when losses are experienced in this age group. For further details see Chapter 13.

Toxicity

A variety of poisons, both organic and inorganic, cause severe illness and death. The most common are: (i) copper (usually a result of feeding concentrates or minerals formulated for cattle); (ii) plants such as yew and rhododendron (often in sudden wintry weather when grazing is inaccessible, or from garden waste thoughtlessly thrown into fields); nitrite poisoning from too-rapid introduction to turnip tops or grazing after late fertilizer application; rape and kale containing S-methylcysteine sulfoxide (SMCO) which after bacterial fermentation in the rumen is converted to dimethyl disulfide, which causes haemolysis. Obvious indicators may be present – jaundice and dark-coloured urine in the case of copper toxicity, SMCO or nitrite poisoning, or the presence of plant material in the mouth or rumen in cases of other plant poisoning. Laboratory assistance may be necessary to confirm diagnosis.

Acute fasciolosis

Sudden deaths, with others in the group showing weakness, abdominal pain and severe anaemia, can result from mass migration of immature flukes through the liver parenchyma. These can cause massive damage to the liver with severe haemorrhage. Lambs are most commonly affected but any age group is potentially at risk. For details of epidemiology, treatment and control see Chapter 4.

Acute haemonchosis

This disease, caused by the roundworm *Haemonchus contortus*, can occur in explosive outbreaks in suitable weather conditions leading to collapse or sudden death due to anaemia as a result of these blood-sucking parasites. For more information see Chapter 4.

11 Lameness

JENNIFER DUNCAN* AND JOSEPH ANGELL

Department of Livestock and One Health, Institute of Infection, Veterinary and Ecological Sciences, University of Liverpool, UK

Abstract

Lameness in sheep is a very common and important problem which can have severe implications on welfare and production in many flocks. Interdigital dermatitis, footrot and contagious ovine digital dermatitis are the most important causes. Correct diagnosis is a key starting point in any investigation.

Lameness is so common in most flocks of sheep that many farmers regard it as a 'fact of life' and give it only irregular attention. Apart from the discomfort to the sheep, the loss in production can be considerable and inadequate food intake by pregnant and lactating ewes contributes to reduced scanning results, pregnancy toxaemia, and neonatal diseases. It is therefore one of the major welfare concerns in sheep farming in the UK and worldwide (Fig.11.1). The prevalence of lameness in a flock varies with: (i) climate; (ii) pasture moisture; (iii) age; and (iv) stocking rates. For example, over 50% of lowland lambs can be lame with scald or footrot (FR) or contagious ovine digital dermatitis (CODD) if the weather and pasture conditions are suitable.

Causes of Lameness

The main causes of lameness are:

- interdigital dermatitis (ID, scald)–inflammation of the interdigital skin;
- footrot (FR) – classic separation and under-running of the sole and often the wall with a characteristic foul smell; and
- contagious ovine digital dermatitis (CODD) – separation and detachment of the hoof capsule starting at the coronary band.

Other common causes are:

- soil and grass accumulating between the claws (soil balling);
- interdigital hyperplasia (sometimes called a 'fibroma');
- granuloma caused by over-trimming or other injury, or associated with FR;
- white-line problems:
  - localized tracks in the white line with pus formation; or
  - generalized white-line separation with impaction of soil and debris (shelly hoof);
- Infection and sepsis in the pedal joint;
- non-infectious and infectious arthritis;
- myopathies (most commonly white muscle disease of lambs);
- fractures; and
- neurological diseases associated with lameness/ataxia;

Therefore, it is necessary to examine the whole limb/animal not just the foot.

Common Foot Conditions

See Fig. 11.2 for the main diagnostic features.

Interdigital dermatitis (ID, scald)

Dichelobacter nodosus can initiate ID lesions following damage to the skin of the interdigital space. If not treated, it may progress to FR, depending on the bacterial load, virulence and host immunity. The main features of ID are:

---

*Email: jsduncan@liverpool.ac.uk

© CAB International 2025. *A Handbook for the Sheep Clinician, 8th Edition*
(A.C. Winter and D. Grove-White eds)
DOI: 10.1079/9781800626355.0011

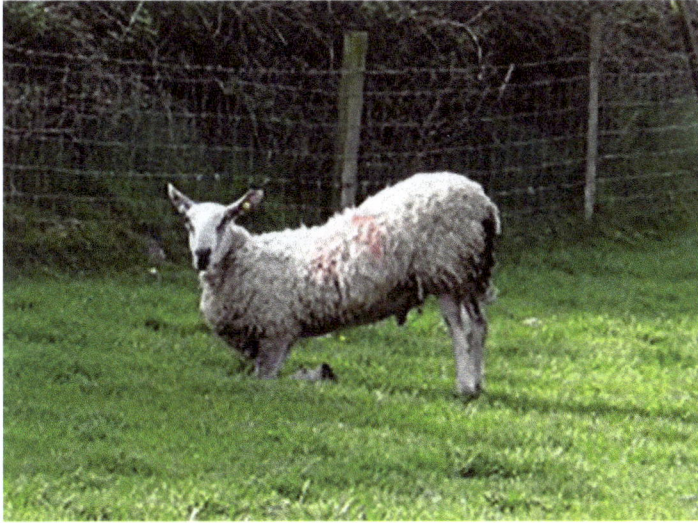

Fig. 11.1. Lame sheep should be treated as soon as possible (photo Joseph Angell).

- the lesion is limited to the skin between the claws;
- this looks moist and reddened, or greyish white, often with loss of hair;
- it is common in growing lambs;
- it is often associated with long, wet grass, in warm weather;
- it can affect a large number of animals and develops quickly (overnight);
- it may affect more than one foot;
- it may progress to FR.

Most flocks are vulnerable, and it is difficult or impossible to eradicate in the UK.

Footrot

This is a result of the primary action of *D. nodosus* with *F. necrophorum* as a complicating factor. These are both anaerobes. *D. nodosus* invades the horn resulting in separation of the sole beginning at the interdigital skin/horn junction near the heel (Fig. 11.3). The degree of horn separation and severity of FR depends upon the strain of *D. nodosus* involved (there are at least 11 strains varying from benign types which cause little under-running, to virulent very aggressive forms) and may be further aggravated by other secondary organisms such as spirochaetes and corynebacteria.

The main features of the disease and the causal organism are:

- separation and under-running of the horn of the sole, starting from the interdigital space, often spreading across the sole to affect the wall (degree depends on virulence);
- a characteristic necrotic smell with dirty greyish cheese-like debris under the horn;
- it often affects both claws and may affect more than one foot;
- most of the horn of affected claws may become detached, often remaining only attached near the toe;
- *D. nodosus* only lives in sheep's feet – survival on pasture is less than 2 weeks;
- it may also be spread by deer and cattle, but these are not thought to be important vectors and infected sheep are the usual source of infection;
- it only spreads in warm, damp weather, therefore spread is much reduced in hot dry summers and in cold dry winters; and
- it can spread rapidly in housing, especially if pens are damp and inadequately bedded.

There is little naturally induced immunity, reinfection is common, and feet may show more than one stage of the disease. As the main causal organism only lives in sheep's feet, it is possible to eradicate the

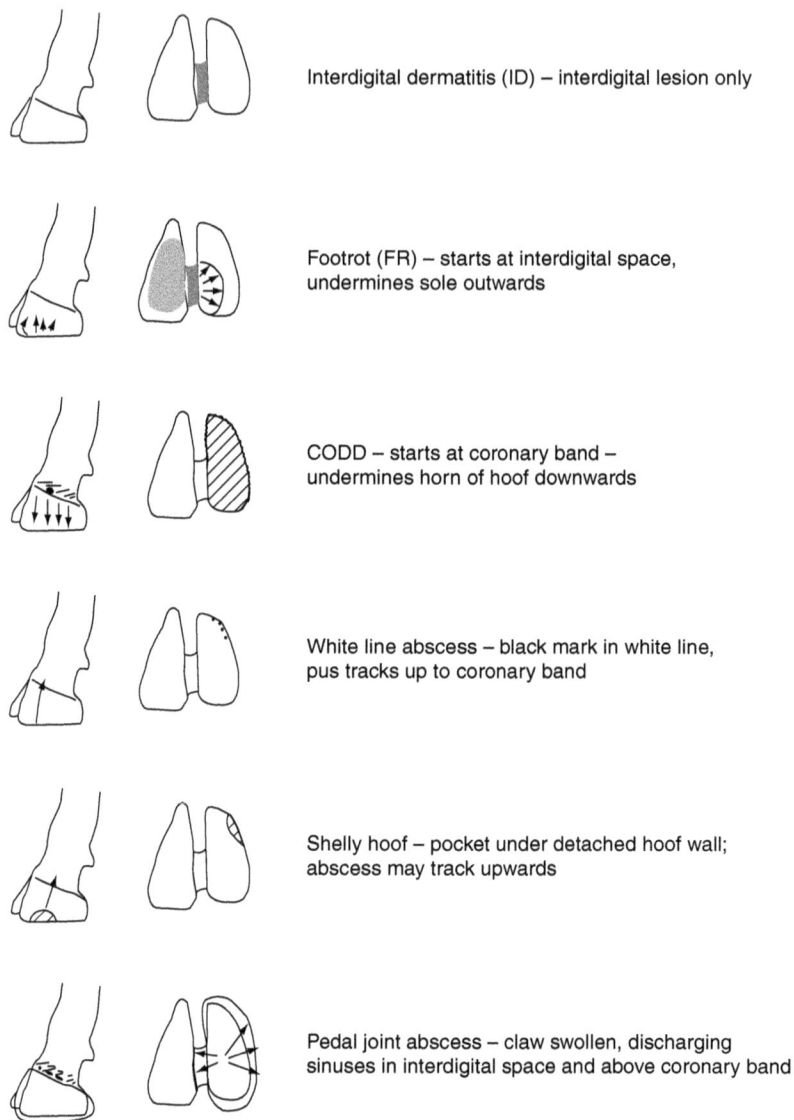

Interdigital dermatitis (ID) – interdigital lesion only

Footrot (FR) – starts at interdigital space, undermines sole outwards

CODD – starts at coronary band – undermines horn of hoof downwards

White line abscess – black mark in white line, pus tracks up to coronary band

Shelly hoof – pocket under detached hoof wall; abscess may track upwards

Pedal joint abscess – claw swollen, discharging sinuses in interdigital space and above coronary band

Fig. 11.2. Diagnostic features of foot lesions

disease and have a FR-free flock. This can be difficult to achieve as carrier animals are common.

Contagious ovine digital dermatitis (CODD)

This disease, which is distinct in appearance from ID and FR, was first reported in 1997 in the UK and initially called 'new virulent footrot'. However, it soon became clear that it was a different clinical entity and subsequent work implicated spirochaetes similar to those found in digital dermatitis in cattle (*Treponema* spp.) as causal agents, hence the name given to the novel condition (Fig. 11.4).

Jennifer Duncan and Joseph Angell

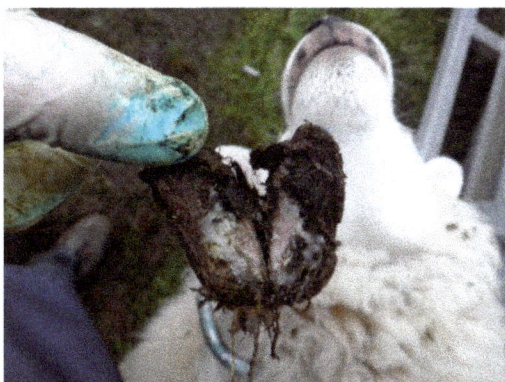

Fig. 11.3. Typical appearance of footrot with separation of horn from interdigital space across sole (photo Joseph Angell).

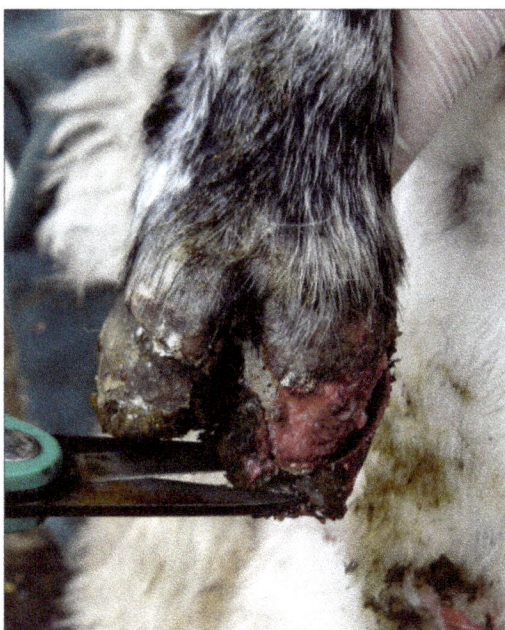

Fig. 11.4. Typical appearance of CODD with separation of horn starting at coronary band (photo Joseph Angell).

It is a severe disease with the main features being:

- the lesion starts at the coronary band and is often bloody in appearance;
- it spreads down from the coronary band rapidly detaching the horn capsule;

- there is loss of hair above the coronary band; and
- if not treated, the foot may sustain permanent damage.

Dealing with Flock Lameness

Diagnosis

It is essential to examine a representative sample of the group or flock to establish which conditions are present. It is common to have cases of ID and FR, and CODD occurring together. Treatment(s) should be based upon a thorough understanding of the diseases present and it is likely that a combination of measures will be required. Picking out and treating only obviously lame individual animals will never get on top of a flock problem.

Methods of treatment of infectious foot diseases (ID, FR, CODD)

A selection of treatments will be required in most flocks, the choice depending on: (i) the type of flock; (ii) management; (iii) the main problems present; and (iv) farm resources.

Vaccination

An effective vaccine is available for FR and may be used as a treatment as well as for prevention so is worth considering as part of a treatment package. An overall improvement is usually seen following the first injection. Timing and frequency of subsequent injections depends on the individual flock situation and identification of main risk periods. Antibodies generated by the vaccine last approximately 6 months, so considering this alongside any risk periods can influence the timing of any booster vaccination.

Topical sprays

Various brands of antibiotic spray are available which are effective for treating ID and should be used in addition to injectables in treating FR and CODD. Treated sheep should not be immediately released into wet grass, which will wash off the spray.

Parenteral antibiotics

Injectable antibiotics are now the method of choice for treating FR and CODD. These should be administered to all lame sheep and any others with lesions. LA oxytetracycline is effective against FR and is currently the treatment of choice, with an expected cure rate of about 75% from a single injection. LA amoxycillin has had satisfactory results; however, it is necessary to repeat the treatment every 48 hours until the foot has healed, and the sheep is sound. Macrolide antibiotics such as tulathromycin and gamithromycin, which have a longer duration of activity than oxytetracycline or amoxycillin, are also used for FR and CODD in sheep under the cascade.

Footbaths

Foot bathing is appropriate for treating outbreaks of ID, as a precaution after gathering for any procedures in handling pens, and before housing. However, facilities must be clean, and the bathing must be carried out correctly. Poor foot-bathing technique is likely to worsen lameness problems. The trend is to build larger, wider footbaths in which a group of sheep can be held for the required length of time. After leaving the bath, keep the sheep in a concrete drying pen for at least 30 minutes.

- Formalin is cheap but unpleasant to the shepherd and sheep and very painful to sheep with severe foot lesions. In some countries its use is not allowed. The strength used should never be more than 5% and 2–3% is adequate and effective for treating ID. 'Walk-through' formalin is effective but be careful of rushing animals through as the solution can be splashed into eyes. Formalin 'goes off' quite quickly especially when contaminated by organic matter so fresh solutions are needed after a few days. Formalin hardens the horn and is associated with the development of granulomas so it should not be used excessively.
- Zinc sulfate (10%) can be highly effective for FR. Stand-in times vary according to the formulation of the product. For ID treatment, a stand-in time of 2 minutes is usually adequate. For prevention, a 30 second walk-through has been shown to be effective. For FR, up to 15 minutes or even longer may be necessary, usually repeated weekly, though daily treatment will speed up the cure rate. Zinc sulfate does not deteriorate and is still effective when it appears contaminated. It has no adverse effect on horn. In a single UK study, 10% zinc sulphate foot bathing with a 15-minute stand-in time, and repeated daily for five days, was reported to be highly effective in treating ID, FR and CODD.
- Various proprietary preparations are available (often containing organic acids) through agricultural merchants, and these are favoured by some farmers.

Check that data are available on efficacy before recommending their use.

Trimming

Foot trimming has been shown to be detrimental in treating sheep with ID and footrot but has not been studied directly with regard to CODD. Its use is no longer recommended, unless absolutely necessary to improve welfare in isolated individual clinical cases. With regard to managing foot abscesses, careful paring may be necessary to relieve the pressure of the abscess. Trimming infected sheep feet can easily result in damage to the underlying soft tissues resulting in bleeding, a slower healing response, the development of granulomas, and increases the risk of transmission of infective bacteria from one foot to another.

Control of Infectious Foot Diseases (ID, FR, CODD)

In the UK, the Five Point Plan is recommended as the basis of lameness control in flocks. However, it is important that its application should be tailored by the veterinarian to each individual flock. Factors to consider are: (i) which diseases are present; (ii) what is the prevalence of lameness at its worst; (iii) what are the risk factors for disease in the flock; (iv) what is the buying-in policy; and (v) what resources are available in terms of facilities and labour.

1) Prompt identification and treatment of lame sheep

Identifying, treating and isolating lame sheep early is key. This will improve sheep welfare, reduce bacterial spread, reduce medicine use, and accelerate return to production. The vet and farmer need to work together to develop effective, practical treatment protocols for each flock. An appropriate duration of treatment is key here; the sheep should be isolated and treated until the foot is healed and they are no longer lame.

2) Vaccination

The footrot vaccine in the UK covers all ten strains of *D. nodosus* and is licensed to treat and prevent footrot and may also help reduce the development of new CODD cases. The antibodies produced can decline after about 6 months, so repeat vaccination is necessary on some farms every 6 months. It should be used under veterinary direction to help prevent footrot/ID in ewes prior to key risk periods, e.g. lambing time. The vaccine can cause lumps where it has been injected so it is best to avoid using it prior to shearing and users need to be careful in handling it as it can cause severe reactions in people if accidentally injected. In the case of accidental injection, urgent medical attention should be sought without delay.

3) Culling of repeat offenders

Most sheep that develop an infective foot lesion can be successfully treated and recover, provided an appropriate course of treatment is given. However, a few sheep will serve as a reservoir of infection for the rest of the flock. For most commercial flocks two cases of lameness per year should trigger a culling decision. For this to happen successfully, lame sheep should be identified either through EID tags or with a permanent mark (e.g. specific ear tags or zip ties through an ear tag). This will ensure that they can be re-identified for culling at the next opportunity should they become lame again in the future.

Replacement policies should sit alongside culling policies as both are attempting to build a more resilient flock. Keeping replacement ewe lambs that have never been lame and have been reared by ewes that have not been lame has been associated with lower flock lameness.

4) Avoidance of transmission at high traffic areas

Handling pens, 'field furniture', e.g. blocks, licks, troughs, feeders etc., gateways and tracks all allow infected sheep to more easily contact uninfected sheep and transmit bacteria to them increasing the risk of infection. Often these areas can also serve to increase 'trauma' to the foot skin, e.g. poaching around water troughs and feeders, sharp stones in gateways etc. As such, minimizing these areas or improving their surface where possible can help reduce trauma to the feet; however, this is not always possible, but an appreciation of the increased risk provided by these areas is an important part of control. Using lime, improving drainage and limiting contact where possible can reduce the build-up of infective bacteria in these areas and the risk of transmission to other sheep. Frequent use of handling pens may increase the spread; therefore, these should be cleaned frequently and all sheep effectively foot-bathed every time they pass through the pens, even for some other procedure.

5) Quarantine of brought-in stock

Purchased and returning sheep are a risk for introduction of many contagious diseases, including new strains of footrot bacteria, or the CODD-causing treponemes. Farm purchasing policies should include a focus on excellent foot condition, shape, structure and health, alongside preventative quarantine measures.

A simple measure that can be taken by all farmers is to isolate all purchased or returning sheep for three or more weeks. This can allow infections to develop and show up and allow treatments to be used prior to the infection spreading to the rest of the flock. CODD lesions in their early stages tend not to cause lameness until the disease progresses further, so it is advised, ideally, to physically turn over and inspect all four feet of all purchased sheep to ensure a lesion is not missed. Finally, foot bathing of purchased or returning sheep on entry after inspection can disinfect the feet and reduce the risk of infection that may not be visible.

Having got lameness under control, it is then crucial to: (i) carefully monitor the situation; (ii) treat newly lame animals as soon as possible; and (iii) re-impose group or flock treatments if the incidence starts to increase again.

Other Foot Lameness

White-line lesions

There are two common types of white-line lesion: (i) shelly hoof; and (ii) white-line abscess. Shelly hoof occurs when a pocket develops beneath the outer wall of one or more claws. This then becomes impacted with soil and grit. When the loose horn is trimmed away, a characteristic half-moon appearance of the wall results, with the underlying laminae visible. Lameness does not occur until the impacted soil is pushed into the deeper sensitive laminae when pus forms. The sheep then develops acute lameness which is not relieved until the pus is either released by trimming or bursts out after tracking up to the coronary band.

White-line abscesses develop in small discrete tracks in the white line, which again cause acute lameness and can sometimes be very difficult to locate, although the affected digit should be identifiable by pain response and the presence of heat. Careful trimming may release pus.

For both types, if careful trimming does not find pus, application of a poultice covered with a polythene bag and bandaged, left on for a couple of days, will soften the horn and encourage bursting, or at least make re-examination easier. Once the pus has been cleared, healing occurs leaving a loose piece of horn which can be carefully trimmed.

Foot abscess (pedal joint sepsis)

Infection of the pedal joint is a serious condition which needs to be differentiated from white-line lesions. There is severe pain (10/10 lameness) with obvious swelling of the digit and pus bursts out at several sites around the coronary band. One theory is that infection gains access from the interdigital space. Radiography will help to decide if the joint is involved, as will careful examination with a probe. For early cases, irrigating the joint via a cannula inserted either through a lateral coronary band sinus, or by drilling through the lateral hoof wall into the joint has been described and may lead to a satisfactory result. Either of these forms of treatment should be carried out under regional anaesthesia. If recovery is not rapid after this form of treatment, amputation should be considered, and certainly immediately for cases where treatment has been very delayed.

Amputation of a digit

This should be carried out under regional anaesthesia as described here. Clean the lower limb and shave the skin above the coronary band. When anaesthesia has developed, incise through the skin all the way around the affected claw about 0.5 cm above the coronary band. Take great care in the interdigital space that the incision does not damage the opposite claw. Then remove the claw either by sawing through the lower end of P1 using an embryotomy wire or disarticulate the joint between P1 and P2. Place a non-stick dressing over the wound, pack with cotton wool and bandage tightly. Cover with waterproof tape. Then release the tourniquet. The bandage can be removed 2–3 days later. Opinions vary about re-dressing – some people prefer to leave the wound open, others prefer to re-bandage for a bit longer. In any case, the animal should be kept in clean, dry conditions until healing has occurred. This takes about 3 weeks.

Interdigital hyperplasia ('fibromas')

Fibrous outgrowths in the interdigital space (mainly hind feet) are a feature of some breeds. Lameness occurs only when they become ulcerated and infected. Frequent foot bathing maintains some control, but the worst cases require simple surgical removal under local anaesthesia; this is not a job to be done just before tupping time but should be identified and carried out well in advance.

Toe granulomas

Most large flocks have a few sheep with strawberry-like granulomas, usually at the toe, often the result of foot

trimming, but also following injury or FR. Although loose horn will grow over and partly hide the lesion, healing will never occur without radical treatment. Loose horn should be trimmed away (the foot is anaesthetized), the granuloma cut off after application of a tourniquet to the leg, and the base cauterized (a calf disbudding iron is suitable). Alternatively, repeated application of an astringent such as copper sulfate or formalin (5%) may eventually work.

Post-dipping Lameness

This is caused by *Erysipelothrix rhusiopathiae* which can invade broken skin. At the time of dipping, this organism, which is present in soil, can seriously contaminate the dip solution and enter limb wounds sustained in the dipping process. The disease has also been reported without dipping, after sheep passed through muddy pens. Within a day or so, many sheep may be very lame with a local cellulitis of the hairy parts of the limbs. Early treatment with penicillin is essential. In future, ensure that dip and/or handling pens are cleaned before use. Contaminated dip should not be used after standing overnight, especially in warm weather.

Joint Infections
Young lambs up to 1 month

See Chapter 7: Neonatal Lamb Diseases.

Lambs over 2 months – lowland
Stiff lambs/Erysipelas arthritis

On some farms, a significant number of fattening lambs at grass show a stiff, stilted, short-striding walk or hopping run, appearing to be lame on more than one leg. Very careful examination and palpation discloses some synovial swelling, general thickening and pain in some limb joints, particularly the stifle, hock and carpus. Although probably infected soon after birth, the condition is insidious and often irreversible by the time it is recognized. *E. rhusiopathiae* is the most common organism causing this chronic fibrinous synovitis and arthritis. Often the organism cannot be isolated from the joints but a blood ELISA titre ≥ 1/320 is indicative of infection. Badly affected animals should be euthanased on humane grounds, but it is worth treating less severe cases for which penicillin should be effective. Such lame sheep need housing so that

Jennifer Duncan and Joseph Angell

more intensive treatment and feeding can be applied and where they do not have to walk far for food or shelter. Repeated penicillin treatment is advisable. Vaccination is effective (using a vaccine licensed for pigs, under the cascade), but relies on colostral transfer of antibodies; therefore vaccinating ewes in late pregnancy (as for clostridia) is necessary.

In the USA, polyarthritis in lambs has been associated with *Mycoplasma* spp. and, in fattening lambs in feedlots, with *Chlamydophila* infection.

Lambs up to 4 months – hill

Tick-bite pyaemia, following tick bites and staphylococcal septicaemia is the usual cause (see Chapter 16).

Adult sheep

Joint infection as a result of injury may be a problem in individual adult sheep, leading to visible swelling of the affected joint(s). Early treatment with a prolonged course of penicillin is necessary if this is to be successful. Delay leads to irreversible joint damage and welfare issues in affected animals.

A chronic degenerative arthritis of one or more joints, particularly elbows, but sometimes shoulders, hips and stifles, is quite often seen in elderly sheep. Elbows should be carefully examined for characteristic thickening and restricted flexion. Such sheep become progressively more lame and thin and need very careful attention. In pet sheep, welfare improvements can be seen with daily use of NSAIDs. However, should welfare be insufficiently manageable, culling should be advised.

Vitamin E and Selenium Deficiency

Deficiency of either selenium or vitamin E, or both together, can lead to problems affecting muscle function variously known as white muscle disease, stiff lamb disease, nutritional myopathy or nutritional muscular dystrophy. Many areas of the world (e.g. parts of northern Europe, Australia and New Zealand) have soils low in selenium content. Vitamin E content is high in fresh grass but falls in stored forage and grain, so deficiencies can be made worse if home-produced diets are fed.

This is essentially a disease of young lambs which are growing fast. Predisposing factors include: (i) feeding only home-grown foods; (ii) adding preservatives to straw and cereals; and (iii) use of artificial fertilizers with high nitrogen (N) and sulfate (SO_4), promoting rapid grass growth. Selenium-responsive ill-thrift in lambs has been reported in some countries as has early fetal death leading to barren ewes and the increased susceptibility to disease because of reduced phagocytic activity.

Clinical signs

The usual picture is that thriving young lambs (50% occur at 0–30 days old and 25% at 30–60 days old) have just been turned out to fresh spring grass, and within a few hours or days of running around, a few are found down and reluctant to get up; one or two may also be found dead due to cardiac failure. Those that are able to stand, if forced to get up, take a few tottering steps, showing particular stiffness in the shoulders, and lie down again, looking alert and not uncomfortable. Some may show distressed respiration due to failure of respiratory or cardiac muscles, and pneumonia is a secondary risk. This situation is, at first, easily confused with pulpy kidney, pasteurellosis, swayback, polyarthritis, spinal abscess and injury.

Diagnosis

- Suspicion arises if there has been previous evidence of selenium deficiency on the farm and, in particular, if the flock is receiving little concentrate and no vitamin/mineral supplement and also if a lot of root crops and/or poor-quality roughage is being fed.
- The sudden onset in several otherwise healthy-looking lambs (often the fastest growing) should point to this condition and the absence of obvious signs of injury and arthritis should increase the suspicion.
- Necropsy should eliminate pulpy kidney disease and pasteurellosis, but note that the muscle lesions are bilateral and therefore no comparisons are possible within the lamb, and that if there is cardiac involvement, the lungs may look congested. Histopathology of cardiac tissue can be useful.
- If analysis of plasma and whole blood (green tubes) from affected lambs show plasma creatine kinase (CK) levels of over 1000 IU/l, this indicates severe muscle damage, but the blood must be taken very early, as concentrations drop in a few days; and whole blood GSHPx is often <1 unit/ml.

- If analysis of whole blood (green tubes) from ten apparently healthy contacts show suspiciously low levels of GSHPx (i.e. <20 units/ml), inject with vitamin E and selenium and see whether there is a response (it may take a few days).

Treatment

- Inject with vitamin E and selenium, and repeat the next day if there is not much improvement. Usually there is a good (diagnostic) response if caught early.
- Rest the affected lambs – bring inside.
- Consider giving an NSAID injection to affected lambs – this can make them more comfortable and speed recovery.

Prevention

Be careful if recommending products containing several trace elements, particularly those containing copper as accidental copper poisoning may occur in copper-sensitive breeds.

- Ensure there are adequate levels of selenium and vitamin E in the diet of ewes in late pregnancy: avoid low-selenium foods (e.g. turnips) and feeds which reduce vitamin E concentrations (e.g. treated grain, spoilt hay, oil seeds). Ensure a dietary concentration of 0.1 mg/kg DM for selenium and 30–50 mg/kg DM for vitamin E.
- Inject ewes in the third month of pregnancy with a selenium/vitamin E preparation.
- Short-term control in lambs can be achieved by injecting them at strategic times, such as shortly before turnout or folding on roots.
- Some anthelmintics contain added cobalt and selenium. These might be sufficient to help lambs with marginal deficiencies in the short term.
- Long-term control can be provided by supplementing with selenium by various methods including:
  - an annual injection to lambs at weaning and to pregnant ewes, of a LA barium-complex of selenium;
  - dosing at strategic times (tupping, scanning, lambing, weaning) with a proprietary trace-element product containing selenium;
  - dosing weaned lambs and ewes with LA selenium pellets – these give 3 years' protection;
  - if multiple deficiencies of copper, cobalt and selenium, or zinc, cobalt and selenium occur

(particularly on upland farms), it is worth considering use of soluble glass boluses containing these minerals. These give about 6 months' protection.

Techniques
Foot trimming

In general, foot trimming may damage feet and spread infectious bacteria between sheep. Recent work has shown that foot trimming delays the healing of FR lesions and reduces treatment success. The emphasis should be on routine inspection of flocks for lame sheep allowing prompt treatment of cases. Trimming very overgrown horn or trimming loose horn may be a necessary part of diagnosis and (very occasionally) treatment should be done carefully with a good pair of sharp foot clippers. Great care must be taken not to cut into sensitive tissues. It is extremely easy to cut too deeply at the toe causing profuse bleeding. This may lead to the formation of a toe granuloma which will never heal unless treated correctly.

Remember, hoof trimming should never make the feet bleed. If in doubt, don't cut.

Anaesthesia of the foot

For amputation of the digit, removal of granulomas or interdigital fibromas, IV regional anaesthesia is the best technique, though a ring block around the cannon bone is also effective.

Intravenous (IV) regional anaesthesia

Clean and disinfect the distal leg and place a tourniquet around the leg above the knee or hock. Identify a suitable vein distal to the tourniquet and inject up to 5 ml of local anaesthetic. Anaesthesia develops in about 10 minutes. The tourniquet should not be released for 15–20 minutes to avoid potential toxicity problems.

Ring block

The cannon bone of the affected leg is cleaned and prepared. Then 8–10 ml local anaesthetic is injected at sites around the leg. Following this procedure, the leg sometimes swells at the site of injection, so it may be worth putting a firm bandage on for a day or two.

Jennifer Duncan and Joseph Angell

12 Skin and Wool

EMMA FISHBOURNE* AND JOHN GRAHAM-BROWN

Department of Livestock and One Health, Institute of Infection, Veterinary and Ecological Sciences, University of Liverpool, UK

Abstract

Problems affecting the skin and wool of sheep are common. The most important are infestation with external parasites (mites and lice) which often affect a large number in a flock or group. Accurate diagnosis is essential in order that appropriate treatment and control measures can be applied.

Although a number of specific conditions affect the skin and wool of sheep (see Table 12.1), it must be remembered that because the production of wool is an active process, many systemic diseases or stress will result in local or generalized loss of wool (Fig.12.1). In addition, primitive sheep shed the fleece in early summer, a feature which is still seen to a limited degree in some breeds and crosses. However, this characteristic has been selected for in certain breeds such as the EasyCare in order to obviate the need for annual shearing.

Disorders Associated with Pruritus

Pruritus is a very obvious, but non-specific, clinical sign characterized in sheep typically by restlessness, stamping of feet, rubbing against fencing and posts and nibbling or biting at areas of the body (Fig. 12.2). Correct diagnosis of the underlying condition is clearly very important, particularly given the implications of some differentials (Table 12.1). Incorrect treatments based on farmer diagnosis and/or assumptions without diagnostic confirmation may be ineffective, delay and potentially reduce likelihood of resolution and, in the case of the parasitic diseases, contribute to the development of drug resistance.

Where pruritus is apparent, it is essential to establish the proportion of animals showing signs; to examine individuals to determine the areas affected; to establish the nature of the underlying lesions (including involvement of the skin); and include taking samples for further confirmatory diagnostics, particularly identification of parasites.

Parasitic conditions

Sheep scab (psoroptic mange)

Sheep scab occurs in most sheep-keeping countries, although Australasia is considered disease-free having pursued a successful eradication programme in the 1800s. It was eradicated in Great Britain in 1952 by compulsory dipping but, unfortunately, reintroduced through importation of infested sheep from Ireland in 1973. Due to its severity and highly contagious nature, it became a criminal offence in the UK to keep, move and/or leave visibly affected animals untreated under the Animal Health Act (1981). At the time of writing (2024), its status and significance varies by region. It is presently a notifiable disease in Northern Ireland and Scotland. In England and Wales responsibility for treatment and control lies with the farmer, but local authorities have power under the Sheep Scab Order (1997) to restrict movements and enforce treatments of visibly affected animals under the guidance of a DEFRA-appointed Official Veterinarian. In Scotland, the Sheep Scab (Scotland) Order 2010 requires notification to APHA on suspicion of the disease and puts in place automatic movement restrictions until sheep are either treated/slaughtered or disease is ruled out.

*Email: emma.fishbourne@liverpool.ac.uk

Table 12.1. Summary of conditions affecting skin and wool.

Condition	Cause	Pruritus	Area affected
Non-infectious			
Natural shedding	Genetic	No	Neck, back, belly
Wool break	Illness, debility	No	Body
Wool slip	Winter shearing	No	Flanks
Sunburn	Lack of pigment	No	Ears
Photosensitization	Photodynamic plant, liver damage	Yes when healing	Face, ears
Parasitic			
Sheep scab	*Psoroptes ovis*	Intense	Body
Ear mites	*Psoroptes cuniculi*	Head shaking	Ears
Foot and scrotal mange	*Chorioptes bovis*	Medium	Lower legs, scrotum
Lice	*Bovicola ovis*	Medium	Body
	Linognathus ovillus	Slight	Head
	Linognathus pedalis	Medium-severe	Legs
Keds	*Melophagus ovinus*	Little	Body
Blowfly strike	*Lucilia sericata*	Intense	Breech, shoulder
	Phormia terrae-novae		
Headfly	*Hydrotaea irritans*	Intense	Head, base of horns
Infectious			
Mycotic dermatitis	*Dermatophilus congolensis*	Little	Back, ears, nose
Staphylococcal dermatitis	*Staphylococcus aureus*	Little	Periorbital, nose, legs, teats
Caseous lymphadenitis	*Corynebacterium pseudotuberculosis*	No	Abscesses in lymph nodes esp. parotid
Actinobacillosis	*Actinobacillus lignieresi*	No	Head and neck abscesses
Fleece rot	*Pseudomonas aeruginosa*	No	Body
Orf	Parapox virus	No	Lips
Strawberry footrot	*D. congolensis* and orf	No	Lower leg
Ringworm	*Trichophyton verrucosum*	No	Head
Ulcerative balanoposthitis/vulvitis	*Streptococcus zooepidemicus?*	No	Prepuce, vulva
Scrapie	Spongiform encephalopathy	Usually intense	Tail, flanks, head

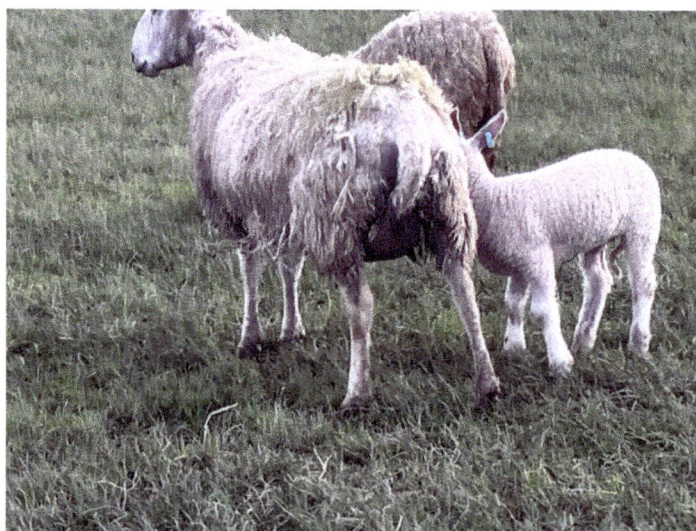

Fig. 12.1. This ewe is losing some of its fleece (woolbreak) (photo Agnes Winter).

Emma Fishbourne and John Graham-Brown

Recent advances in diagnostics, specifically the development of a serum antibody ELISA, and evidence of its successful implementation in reducing transmission has led to a renewed discussion of treatment, control and eradication prospects in the UK with expert opinion suggesting a re-unification of policies across the devolved nations is essential to avoid inconsistencies and loopholes.

Clinical signs

Sheep scab is a highly infectious, severe and debilitating disease caused by infestation with the non-burrowing mite *Psoroptes ovis*. These mites live, reproduce and 'graze' on the skin surface, feeding on secretions. Their presence, in particular their faeces, elicit a strong immune response characterized by local inflammation, erythema and serous exudate, thus establishing an ideal environment for mites to continue feeding and cycles of reproduction.

The predominant initial sign of scab infestation within a flock is intense, unrelenting pruritus as a consequence of this allergic-type immune reaction, with classical foot stamping and lip-smacking behaviours. Pruritus and discomfort can be so intense that the reactive behaviours elicited may occasionally resemble neurological disorders and/or lameness. Animals show signs of wool drop and fleece tags, and are observed continually nibbling at accessible areas (shoulders and lower back) and/or rubbing themselves on any available surface, including fence posts, wire etc. Upon physical restraint and clinical examination affected areas of skin have shed their fleece and appear thickened, inflamed and ulcerated with classic 'scab' lesions of crust formed by dried serous ooze covering the skin surface. Such lesions are initially discrete, measuring a few centimetres, but will expand concentrically outwards as the disease progresses to cover a significant proportion of the body surface in the latter stages. Active mite populations are present at the leading edge of these expanding lesions, setting up further inflammatory responses and lesion expansion. Extensive and severe skin damage can leave affected animals susceptible to secondary skin infections which, accompanied by ongoing inflammatory responses to the mites and serous discharge, can lead to weakness, loss of body condition, systemic illness, and death in the absence of timely and appropriate interventions.

Epidemiology

Psoroptes ovis is both sheep-specific and highly contagious. It is normally transmitted through direct contact between animals, although mites can also survive and remain infective within the environment in cool, humid conditions for up to 18 days. Clinical disease is most apparent over the winter months when increased stocking rates associated with housing and thick-fleeced animals make conditions for its transmission favourable. After initial infestation, clinical signs are slow to appear, with 'scab' lesions starting initially as microscopic foci, expanding into visible lesions as successive generations of mites emerge and reproduce *in situ*. Due to its initially slow disease progression and highly infectious nature, a large proportion of the exposed group may be affected once clinical signs become apparent. The life cycle of *P. ovis* takes around 10–14 days to complete, with a single adult female expected to produce 40–50 eggs over its approximately 16-day lifespan. Mite burdens double roughly every 6 days, with peak burdens typically occurring at 6–12 weeks post-infection. Strain variation exists which can affect both virulence and susceptibility to treatment.

Where *P. ovis* is present within a flock, clinical signs will develop and necessitate treatment. Outbreaks of disease are therefore typically the result of its introduction onto the farm from an external source, although subclinical carriage by lightly infested animals can facilitate continuation of transmission and subsequent outbreaks of clinical disease where treatments are unsuccessful. For most flocks, risk mainly lies with the purchase of subclinically infested animals and ineffective quarantine measures. Where it is practised, common grazing has also been identified as a significant risk factor for disease, with transmission occurring either through direct contact with infested flocks, or use of contaminated areas immediately after infested flocks, with indirect transmission via fomites (e.g. live mites residing on fence posts, fleece tags etc.). Maintenance of farm boundaries is important to provide adequate separation from neighbouring sheep flocks with adjoining pastures. Consideration should also be given to external contractors (e.g. scanners and shearers) and their own biosecurity measures for decontamination and disinfection of equipment and PPE between flocks.

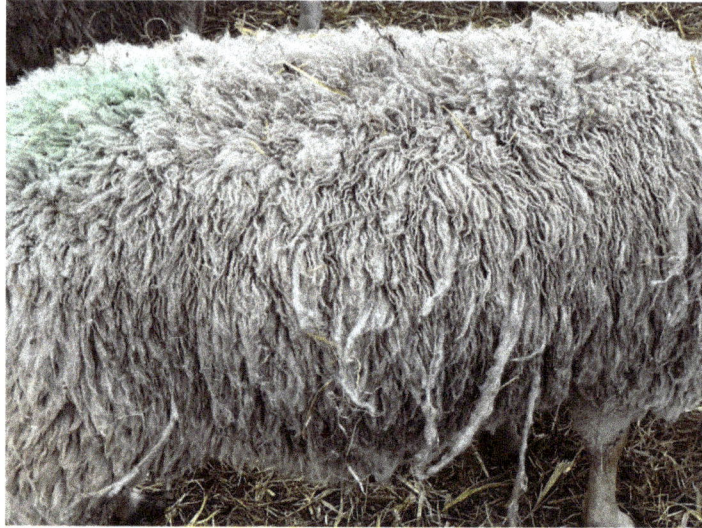

Fig. 12.2. This sheep has wool tags which may indicate pruritus (photo Agnes Winter).

Diagnosis

In outbreaks of clinical sheep scab the high proportion of the flock affected combined with the characteristic scab lesions make tentative diagnosis relatively straightforward. With heavy burdens, mites may be just visible with the naked eye. Confirmation is achieved through microscopic examination of superficial skin scrapings. These should be taken from the edge of the lesion where the majority of active mites are present and examined either directly to observe live mites or following boiling with 10% KOH to clear skin debris. *Psoroptes ovis* can be distinguished from *Chorioptes bovis* based on their pointed mouthparts and jointed, funnel-shaped pedicels on the ends of their front legs (Fig. 12.3).

Recently, a serum antibody, ELISA, has been developed that allows detection of pre-/subclinical *P. ovis* infestations from as early as 2 weeks post-infestation with reported test sensitivity and specificities exceeding 90%. The advent of this ELISA has created new opportunities for screening of flocks and bought-in animals. In the case of the latter, it is now recommended that the sheep scab ELISA is employed as part of routine quarantine measures for purchased stock, with animals isolated on arrival away from the rest of the home flock and tested after 2 weeks, by which time any subclinically infested animals should have seroconverted, with treatments as deemed necessary.

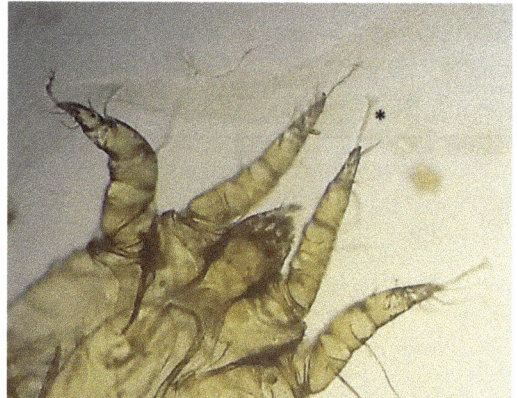

Fig. 12.3. Wet preparation of *Psoroptes ovis* from a skin scraping by boiling in 10% KOH solution (40x magnification). *Psoroptic* mites are identifiable based upon the jointed, trumpet-shaped pedicels on the ends of their legs(*) (photo Joseph Angell)

Further research into the effective implementation of this new diagnostic assay in effective disease control measures is ongoing.

Treatment and control

Where infestations are identified, treatments should be administered at the earliest opportunity with the

Emma Fishbourne and John Graham-Brown

aim of eliminating disease. It should be assumed, unless there is a strong case to the contrary, that all animals within the flock have been exposed and, therefore, require treatment. Handling and management of animals within their environment is important whilst treatment and elimination is ongoing; some products have long periods of residual activity against *P. ovis* but, since mites can persist within the environment for 2+ weeks, it is generally advisable to avoid placing animals back into areas and environments (e.g. paddocks, sheds, handling facilities) they occupied pre-treatment for at least 3 weeks. The same is clearly true for any animals left untreated.

Presently, two active groups are licensed and available in the UK for the treatment of *P. ovis* infestation, organophosphates and macrocyclic lactones.

ORGANOPHOSPHATES Diazinon is licensed for use in plunge dips and is effective against sheep scab and most other ectoparasites of clinical significance (lice, keds and ticks) with residual protection up to 60 days. Whilst highly effective, its use is not a simple matter. Formulation is dependent on factors including numbers of sheep and dip container volume, with regular replenishments required over the course of whole flock treatments to ensure efficacy. Animals' bodies must be fully immersed for a period of not less than one minute, with the head fully submerged (but not held) at least once during this process. Additional factors to consider include safety precautions for dip operators and handlers such as PPE and adequate ventilation, whilst subsequent storage and disposal of dip is also not straightforward. It is generally recommended that farmers employ a professional sheep dipper. There are a number of such individuals in the UK with mobile dipping apparatus, trained and licensed to use and dispose of diazinon correctly. Due to historic misuse and concerns over ineffective treatments and/or selection for resistance, the use of diazinon via other means such as jetters or showers is now illegal and should be reported. There are presently no reports of resistance to diazinon within *P. ovis* populations in the UK. As such, this is generally considered the gold standard treatment for sheep scab, and preferred option for quarantine treatments. Whilst highly effective against various other ectoparasites, its prescription should be reserved specifically for outbreaks of scab. It should also be noted that

treatments with the anthelmintic levamisole and diazinon should not be administered within 14 days of one another.

MACROCYCLIC LACTONES (GROUP 3-MLS) Discussed elsewhere as anthelmintics, group 3-MLs are also potent ectoparasiticides. Of these, injectable preparations containing ivermectin, doramectin and moxidectin carry licences of efficacy against *P. ovis*. Pour-on and oral formulations of group 3-MLs are **not** suitable or licensed for this purpose. In general, for products with a claim of efficacy against *P. ovis*, the following regimens and stipulations typically apply (check the data sheets of specific products for claims of efficacy):

- Ivermectin-based products will typically require two separate injections (200 µg/kg) at 7-day intervals with no ongoing protection against re-infestation.
- Doramectin 1% (w/v) can be administered via intramuscular injection as a single dose (300 µg/kg) with no protection against re-infestation.
- Moxidectin-base preparations may require 1 or 2 doses via subcutaneous injection depending upon their formulation; 1% (w/v) formulations required two doses (200 µg/kg) at a 10-day interval with subsequent protection against re-infestation for up to 28 days, whilst 2% (w/v) formulations require a single dose (1 mg/kg) with subsequent protection against re-infection for up to 60 days post-treatment.

Whilst several such group 3-ML products with claims of efficacy are available, it is important to note that drug resistance (including multiple drug resistance) has been confirmed in the UK. Follow-up diagnostics and close monitoring of flocks pursuing such treatment options are therefore critical to prevent further disease outbreaks and onward transmission. Given the concerns over drug resistance, widespread reports of treatment failures and lack of any residual activity in the face of re-infection from the environment, it is the opinion of a number of experts that, despite carrying licences of efficacy, use of injectable ivermectin- and doramectin-based products for the treatment and control of sheep scab is questionable. Of the group 3-ML products mentioned, due to their higher dosage and longer period of protection, moxidectin 2% formulations are considered a viable alternative to diazinon for use as a quarantine dose. It is also important to acknowledge (as discussed in Chapter 9), that moxidectin 2% should be used sparingly for general and whole-flock treatments due to its importance as a potent endectocide. Where it has been used previously for roundworms, its use for control of sheep scab in the same year should be avoided to reduce selection for resistance.

Whilst effective and useful for control of other ectoparasites (discussed below), no formulations of synthetic pyrethroids or other actives should be used to treat sheep scab.

Other mange mites

Aside from *P. ovis*, a number of other mites are found on sheep. *Chorioptes bovis* are most commonly found on the scrotum of rams and the udder of ewes as well as the lower legs and brisket. Affected animals show itching of the legs (e.g. rubbing against troughs or on fence wire). Affected rams show thickening of the skin of the scrotum which may decrease fertility. The mites are surface dwelling and are relatively easily picked up using a tape strip, rather than a skin scraping, and can be differentiated from *Psoroptes* due to their rounded mouth parts and unjointed, cup-shaped pedicels. As surface dwellers and feeders, injectable MLs are generally not effective, whilst synthetic pyrethroids do not carry a licence of efficacy. Diazinon dips are effective.

Sarcoptes scabiei is not considered a problem of sheep in the UK or northern Europe, but is prevalent in the Middle East, Asia and Africa. This likely relates to breed preferences in these regions (specifically haired versus wool breeds) since *Sarcoptes* prefers parasitizing non-fleeced skin. These burrowing mites live in the dermal layer and require diagnosis by deep skin scrapes. *Sarcoptes scabiei* is also an anthropozoonosis.

Lice and keds

There are two types of lice: (i) chewing, *Bovicola ovis*; and (ii) sucking (blood feeding), *Linognathus ovillus* and *Linognathus pedalis*. The sheep ked, *Melophagus ovinus*, is a blood-feeding wingless species of fly. All of these species are host-specific and obligate parasites (all life stages are present on the sheep) with direct sheep-to-sheep transmission occurring particularly in overwinter housing in heavily fleeced animals.

Both sucking and chewing lice are a major problem in Australia and New Zealand where they affect wool growth and hide quality. In the UK, chewing lice (*Bovicola*) are the species most commonly encountered. In many instances, *Bovicola* infestations are light and will not require specific treatment. In heavy infestations there may be an underlying cause (e.g. malnutrition) that warrants further investigation. In this context, pediculosis is mainly of significance because animals present with pruritus and irritation involving a high proportion of the flock with result rubbing, nibbling and damage to fleece similar to sheep scab; thus, differentiation is an important point for disease control. Collection/submission of wool samples from affected sheep alongside skin scrapes to allow identification of lice are therefore an important step in determining the likely cause of pruritus and, therefore, what treatment is appropriate. Adult keds are large brown insects with flattened bodies and are easily visible upon clinical examination, as are their pupae, which remain glued to the fleece of infested animals, with heavy infestations potentially causing anaemia and ill-thrift.

Both lice and keds are susceptible to most insecticidal drugs including diazinon (dips) and topical synthetic pyrethroids (SP), although resistance to the latter is recorded in lice and is of major concern in Australia. Due to their blood-feeding behaviour, sucking lice and keds (but not chewing lice) are also susceptible to systemic endectocides (e.g. injectable group 3-MLs). Where indicated, treatments are usually more effective if administered after shearing, which in and of itself helps to reduce burdens, clinical signs and onward transmission.

Blowfly myiasis (flystrike)

Strike is a common condition worldwide. In the UK it is predominantly seen throughout the summer months but can occur earlier if the weather is unseasonally warm. Adult female *Lucilia* (greenbottle flies) and *Calliphora* (bluebottle flies) are important primary agents of fly strike, attracted to soiled fleece, skin wounds etc. to lay their eggs. L1 larvae will hatch within 12 hours to invade skin and wounds, feed on living tissue and cause extensive damage, expansion of lesions and underrunning of the skin. Once this primary myiasis is established, other secondary species (*Phormia, Calliphora* etc.) may then also colonize struck animals. Adults flies are attracted to foul-smelling necrotic tissues, and their maggots subsequently feed on these. The resulting tissue damage combined with accumulation of

Emma Fishbourne and John Graham-Brown

toxins produced by large maggot populations lead to extreme discomfort, systemic illness and death (Fig.12.4). Mature L3 maggots will drop off the host to pupate in the soil. Under optimal conditions of high temperatures and humidity, this life cycle may complete in as little as 2 weeks, with animals at risk of becoming struck and severely diseased in a very short space of time. The most commonly affected areas are: (i) around the breech associated with soiling due to scouring, particularly in lambs affected by PGE; (ii) footrot lesions, and along the side of the body where fleece becomes contaminated when sheep lie down; (iii) various sites associated with wounds including shearing injuries and primary infections such as dermatophilosis. Affected animals are restless, show vigorous wagging of the tail when the breech is affected, or biting and nibble at affected areas which often appear damp and discoloured. Struck animals are often separated away from the flock.

Treatment and control

Treatment and control are principally dependent upon good husbandry and prophylaxis. Ensuring good foot health and control of PGE limits opportunities for strike to establish initially, including trimming (dagging) of soiled fleece from around the back ends of animals with clinical PGE. Regular (daily) inspection of animals for early signs of disease and pre-emptive treatments are necessary during high-risk periods. In the UK, a temperature-driven regional blowfly alert is published annually and updated every 2 weeks over the course of the grazing season to help farmers be aware of risk in their area (www.nadis.org.uk). Where animals with established strike are identified, treatment may be attempted, but the extent of lesions (which is not always immediately apparent due to under-running) should first be established–euthanasia on welfare grounds may be a more appropriate treatment in some advanced instances. Otherwise, affected areas should be clipped and visible maggots removed and animals treated with a topical SP. NSAIDs may help with discomfort and inflammation, and since secondary bacterial infections are common, antibiotics may also be indicated.

Due to the severity and rapid onset of disease, in addition to practical management, prophylactic treatments are also recommended during peak risk periods. SPs (cypermethrin and deltamethrin) as pour-ons and spot-ons will treat and protect for up to 10 weeks depending on the specific product used. The insect growth regulator dicyclanil is also available in topical formulations for the control (but not treatment) of blowfly larvae, and similarly provides residual protection for up to 19 weeks (check the data sheets of specific products). It is

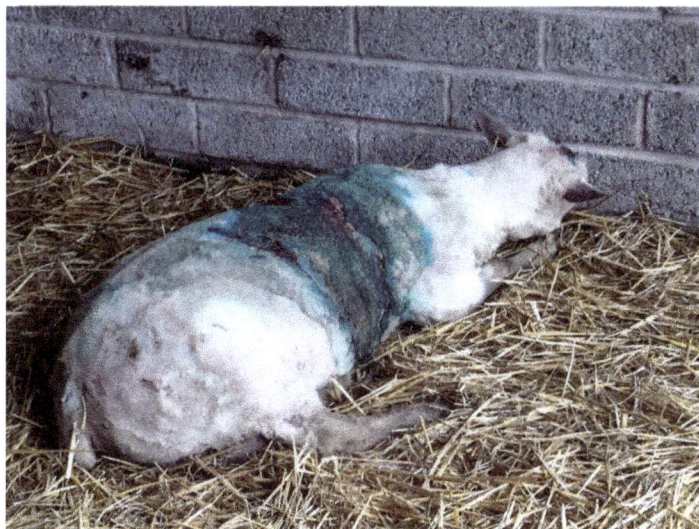

Fig. 12.4. This sick-looking sheep has had a large area behind the shoulder affected by fly strike (photo Joseph Angell).

important to note that for long-lasting protection these topical treatments must be applied correctly following the manufacturer's recommendations. This includes keeping animals dry immediately after application, meaning they should not be applied when rainfall is forecast. Whilst it is not recommended, diazinon is prescribed for this use; where dipping is conducted for scab, this will also effectively treat blowfly and provide further protection for up to 60 days.

Headflies

The non-biting muscid fly, *Hydrotaea irritans*, may be seen swarming around the heads of sheep (and cattle) in the summer months, causing rubbing which leads to self-trauma. These flies then feed on the exudate of blood and lymph leading to further attacks. The base of the horns is a common site for small breaks in the skin to form, making this a particularly important issue in horned breeds. In reality, any open wound is liable to attack. These wounds do not heal while the flies are active and extensive lesions involving much of the skin of the head can result, leading to loss in condition and disfigurement.

These flies are typically most active over the summer and into the autumn months on still, warm humid days, with a single generation of flies each year. Non-feeding females rest in trees and can fly up to 0.5 km/day. Each female produces one or two batches of about 30 eggs which hatch to larvae in pasture soil (not dung) from September to May especially near woodland.

Many methods of control have been tried; none is entirely successful. Of the current products available, topical SPs can help but may require multiple applications over the season.

Ticks

See Chapter 16.

Midge hypersensitivity

In addition to their important role as vectors for viral pathogens such as BTV and Schmallenberg, hypersensitivity to midge bites has been observed in certain breeds, particularly those with black wool (Black Welsh Mountain, Zwarbles) or black belly wool (Torddu) resembling sweet itch in horses. This condition may be seen at any time when midges are active. Affected animals show severe itching and discomfort with thickened, scabby, often bleeding lesions on the hairy parts of the body, especially face, ears, ventral abdomen, udder and perineum. Realistically, effective control is a challenge, but improved habitat that is less attractive and conducive to midges (mowing overgrown grass) and regular application of topical SPs prior to and during active midge periods may reduce severity and make the condition more manageable.

Non-parasitic Conditions

Scrapie

Scrapie should be suspected when an individual adult sheep begins to rub, nibble or suck its fleece for no obvious reason, leading to bilateral semi-bald patches on its flanks, hind legs, bridge of the nose and top of the head. The skin and fleece appear normal except for self-inflicted healing scabs. The irritation is increased by firm finger rubbing of the back and itchy areas. Other neurological signs are often present (and sometimes on their own) and there is a worsening over days/weeks. Scrapie is notifiable. For details see Chapter 14.

Disorders with Usually Little or No Pruritus

Infectious

Orf (contagious pustular dermatitis, scabby mouth)

This disease, which occurs worldwide, is a constant worry to sheep farmers as shown by the priority they give it for further research. If it occurs around lambing, it threatens to develop into an outbreak and spread to the teats of ewes, which in turn can lead to difficulty for lambs to suck and mastitis developing in the ewe. Later in the year, it can disrupt sales of fat or breeding animals. Occasional cases also inexplicably develop extensive and persistent lesions. **It is a zoonosis so there is a risk of spread to anyone handling infected animals**, particularly those caring for orphan lambs; lesions on the fingers, face or neck are, at best, irritating and painful, and at worst there is a very marked reaction with local lymphatic involvement. Doctors are often unfamiliar with this infection – sometimes the vet diagnoses it first!

Emma Fishbourne and John Graham-Brown

Control measures are difficult and the epidemiology of the condition remains unclear. However, while the appearance and site of the lesions in and around the mouth suggest a lot of discomfort and interference with sucking and grazing, many lambs survive without problems; most cases self-cure in a few weeks and the incidence in most flocks remains low.

Orf is caused by a parapox virus which survives in dry scabs, from year to year indoors, but for shorter periods outside; small scabby lesions on the hairy areas of the face and limbs are also persistent sources of the virus; it is susceptible to iodophor disinfectants. It has a distinct shape and size and is easily recognized by electron microscopy (EM), although it is morphologically indistinguishable from the paravaccinia (pseudo-cow pox) virus found in teat lesions of cattle. It has an affinity for hairy areas, particularly at the weak junctions between skin and mucosae (e.g. commissure of lips) but it requires some surface damage to allow invasion (e.g. splitting of lips, eruption of incisors, rough grazing and teat sores following vigorous sucking and incisor injury by hungry lambs).

The lesions are characteristic and diagnostic, although when in doubt, unpreserved scabs should be sent to the lab for EM examination. They start as raised red papules which coalesce and, in a few days, proceed through vesicles and pustules to thick scab formations which are firmly attached to what looks like exuberant granulation, and removal causes haemorrhage. Secondary mixed bacterial infection is common and exaggerates the local response. The lesions are often confined to the outside of the lips and are sometimes barely noticeable, but in young lambs, granulomatous lesions may occur within the mouth, involving the gums and sometimes the tongue. Despite their appearance, the lesions do not appear to cause much distress unless particularly exuberant and extensive, and while there may be some lambs that fail to thrive, most will self-cure within 3–6 weeks. The situation becomes much more serious, however, if and the lesions secondarily arise on the teats of ewes (see Chapter 8).

TREATMENT Individual severe cases should be separated to ensure proper nursing with daily application of topical antibiotic to tackle secondary bacterial infection. Ewes should be inspected for teat lesions and these should be treated with antibiotic. Ointments containing local anaesthetic may allow lambs to carry on sucking until healing

occurs; in extreme cases it may be necessary to wean and hand rear their lambs (easier said than done as lambs will often refuse a bottle, plus the risk of frequent handling) and to dry off the ewe following infusion of LA antibiotic. Where necessary, sheep should also be removed from pastures that appear to be causing face or limb abrasions (e.g. thistles). Where possible, contaminated pens should be cleaned out and disinfected before reuse, and again at the end of housing.

PREVENTION Immunity following primary infection is incomplete and short-lived, lasting only a few months, although subsequent infections are likely to produce milder lesions which heal more rapidly. Immunity is largely cell-mediated, and although humoral antibodies are produced, they are not protective, and therefore neither is colostrum.

A vaccine is available which consists of live virus. It is applied by skin scarification, usually on the hairless area of the inner thigh. Its efficacy and timing is debatable but it probably shortens the recovery time if not preventing infection. It is commonly applied to ewes in early or mid-pregnancy, especially to those which will be housed at lambing, in an attempt to reduce the weight of infection in carriers, and to protect the teats. It is sometimes applied to lambs in the summer a few weeks before sale, in an attempt to avoid lip lesions and subsequent refusal at markets. It is also sometimes applied to young lambs in contact with infections, or where there has been a previous history of disease, and even to those with lesions, in an attempt to prevent or control an outbreak; the consensus seems to be that this should be a last rather than a first resort. It certainly should not be used on ewes within 7 weeks of lambing nor in flocks that have no history of the disease, as the induced scabs are a source of further infection. The vaccine, like the natural infection, needs to be handled with care. **It should never be used in a flock without a previous history of the disease.** Sometimes altering the lambing pattern can help with disease control, especially on farms where lambs get abrasions from rough grazing. Anecdotally, control of thistles in the summer months can be helpful in controlling orf, presumably by reducing abrasions and scratches etc.

Strawberry footrot

Occasionally, lambs at pasture, often in wet, muddy and abrasive conditions, develop orf-like granulomatous lesions on the skin of the lower limbs particularly around the coronary bands, making the lambs obviously lame. The condition does not involve the foot and has no resemblance to FR, but the granulation tissue is likened to a strawberry. Orf virus particles can usually be isolated from the scabs, but so also can *Dermatophilus congolensis*, the organism more commonly associated with lumpy wool; it is uncertain which gets there first! Treatment should be for both, which means local dressing and systemic antibiotic. The lambs need to be removed to dry pasture or housed. Some cases are particularly persistent and extensive, like other forms of orf, and these require euthanasia.

Ulcerative balanoposthitis (pizzle rot) and ulcerative vulvitis

It is quite common to find a scabby ulcerative lesion at the junction of the skin and mucosa of the prepuce in rams and vulva in ewes. Raw, bleeding tissue is exposed if the scabs are removed, rather like orf, but the lesion is ulcerative rather than proliferative and it is unusual to find orf virus particles. In some cases in rams, the ulceration is confined to the glans penis and therefore goes unnoticed. The incidence can be quite high and is sometimes associated with tupping time, suggesting venereal transmission.

Most cases self-cure or remain as minor lesions and there is no interference with breeding or fertility. However, occasionally, the lesions are extensive with swelling, superficial sepsis and necrosis; in rams, this may mean the involvement of both the glans penis and the mucosa of the sheath which becomes noticeably pendulous; subsequent scar tissue may interfere with breeding.

The cause is still uncertain, although ureaplasms or *Streptococcus zooepidemicus* have been found in some outbreaks. Antibiotic aerosol spray is adequate for mild cases, but the more severe ones require systemic antibiotic and frequent local dressing and irrigation.

Staphylococcal folliculitis

Small discrete pustules are often seen around the lips, muzzles and under the tails of very young lambs, and on the udders of ewes (mammary impetigo). The surrounding skin is hyperaemic but not proliferative, as is orf, and a crater is left when the pustules rupture, which heals quickly leaving a white patch if the skin is pigmented. Treatment is rarely necessary although local dressing and antibiotics directed at the causal organism, haemolytic coagulase positive *Staph. aureus*, may occasionally be justified.

Staphylococcal dermatitis (facial or periorbital dermatitis or eczema)

This is another variant of the skin lesions associated with *Staph. aureus*. Extensive, suppurating scabby lesions, which bleed easily and have a deep ulcerated centre surrounded by a zone of hair loss, are seen over bony prominences such as the orbit, nose and lower legs. Sheep feeding at crowded sites are usually affected, typically late-pregnant ewes being fed concentrates with insufficient trough space, where they both injure themselves and each other, and transmit the infection to one another. Removal from the source of the problems and treatment with local dressing and antibiotics usually leads to rapid improvement, although serious and disfiguring complications can arise from eye involvement and from scar tissue. In future, adequate trough space must be provided (at least 45 cm per ewe) and the food spread evenly and quickly to minimize aggression or adopt floor feeding if this is practical.

Mycotic dermatitis (lumpy wool)

This condition occurs in many countries and in many if not most flocks, but generally as a low-grade self-limiting infection, and is of little consequence in the UK other than some downgrading of the fleece. However, occasional outbreaks occur where the infection becomes more active and extensive, and secondary problems arise such as flystrike; treatment is then necessary.

The disease picture is an exudative dermatitis passing rapidly through the stages of hyperaemia, exudate and scab formation. It is caused by an actinomycete *D. congolensis*, which also infects other species (e.g. horses, cattle and occasionally humans) and can remain viable in dry scabs for many months. It induces only weak local immunity, all of which means that successive 'attacks' are common and eradication is not an option.

The condition is often only noticed when a sheep is handled (e.g. being condition-scored) and on parting the fleece, bundles of wool fibres are seen matted together by rough scabs. These scabs originate from the skin and are carried up in the growing fleece, eventually working to the tips and

Emma Fishbourne and John Graham-Brown

breaking off. The back and top sides of sheep are most commonly affected as these are the sites which get soaked following heavy rain or dipping; fat, flat-backed, close-wooled sheep are the most susceptible, where the fleece acts as a sponge. Other areas do get infected, appearing as scabs on the ears, head, limbs, udder of ewes and scrotum of rams, and these are constant sources of re-infection elsewhere.

The distribution of the scabs and the general lack of pruritus are usually sufficiently diagnostic but if there is doubt, impression smears should be made of skin exudate or scabs taken, preferably those close to an active lesion, for laboratory examination.

Significant outbreaks usually follow wet weather or dipping, but it can also follow shearing when skin wounds may admit infection.

Sheep that need treatment should be housed and given suitable systemic antibiotic treatment; topical dressing with aluminium or zinc sulfate may be justified to prevent further surface spread. Combined insecticidal and antimycotic dips are no longer available.

Other fleece problems

- Fleece rot is caused by *Pseudomonas aeruginosa* leading to discolouration (green, brown or blue) of the wool.
- *Pseudomonas* infection has also been associated with severe fatal necrotic dermatitis, probably induced as a result of bad dipping practice.
- Canary stain is a permanent yellow colouration of the wool.

Ringworm

This is not particularly common in sheep, perhaps because of lack of contact with other hosts such as cattle or because of the protective fleece, but housed, shorn ewes occasionally develop the condition, particularly if housed in buildings also used by cattle. It has also been seen on the heads of rams. It is caused by the fungus *Trichophyton verrucosum*. On the hairy areas of head and face it looks just like the condition in cattle, but the infection in the woolly areas often produces more obvious circular raised plaques which eventually lift off, leaving the more typical crusty skin beneath.

The condition usually has to run its course, waiting for immunity and turnout; topical iodine sprays may be useful but **handle with care as the disease is a zoonosis.**

Caseous lymphadenitis (CLA, cheesy gland)

This disease, seen in many sheep-keeping countries including Australasia, was first identified in the UK in 1990 in imported goats. It spread to sheep and is present in some pedigree flocks producing terminal sires and is being seen increasingly in commercial flocks, usually introduced by infected rams. There is also a real possibility of spread via contaminated shears and shearing equipment if these are not adequately disinfected between flocks.

The disease is caused by *Corynebacterium pseudotuberculosis* and is seen as chronic abscesses in superficial lymph nodes (Fig. 12.5). These often burst producing greenish cheesy or putty-like pus. Abscesses repeatedly wall off, producing a characteristic 'onion-ring' appearance. Abscesses may also form in internal organs especially the lung and mediastinum, causing chronic wasting, or signs resulting from pressure on vital structures from large internal abscesses. Confirmation of diagnosis is by identification of the organism from samples of pus.

An important differential diagnosis is bovine tuberculosis (TB) which is widespread in cattle in parts of the UK. Fortunately, sheep seem to be relatively resistant to TB although a small number of flock outbreaks have been reported.

EPIDEMIOLOGY In the UK, the mode of spread and the lymph nodes most commonly affected are rather different from those in Australia where the disease is common. In both countries, discharging lymph nodes in the lung form a common source of infection.

- In Australia, the disease spreads at major gathering times such as shearing and jetting or dipping. Entry of the disease is via skin abrasions; hence, body lymph nodes such as the prefemoral and popliteal are commonly affected.
- In the UK, spread appears to take place more commonly via the oral route – trough feeding facilitates the spread from discharging lung abscesses, thus head lymph nodes, especially the parotids, are commonly infected. These are situated just below the ears (see Fig. 12.5) and should always be carefully examined during any ram examination, as well as the main superficial nodes (submandibular, prescapular, prefemoral, popliteal, supramammary). Infection also spreads directly from sheep to sheep from discharging abscesses.

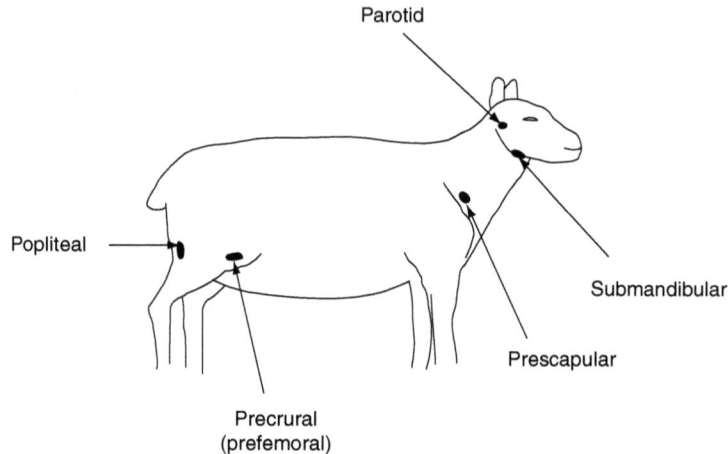

Fig. 12.5. Important superficial lymph nodes.

TREATMENT Although the organism is susceptible to antibiotics, the nature of the abscesses means successful treatment is unlikely. Treatment of superficial abscesses is of little use since inevitably other lymph nodes become infected and infected internal nodes cannot be detected.

CONTROL Vaccination is widely used in Australia and other countries (usually in combination with clostridial vaccine) and seems to be quite effective. The vaccine is prepared from the bacterial toxins. This vaccine is not generally available in the UK, but in certain circumstances can be imported under special licence from the VMD. Autogenous vaccines made from killed bacteria have been used in the UK and recent information is that they may provide more protection than the Australian vaccine. It is possible that a new vaccine may become available in the UK in the reasonably near future.

It is best to try to avoid introducing infection into a flock by careful selection of purchased animals and quarantine. An ELISA test is available offered by SRUC.

If infection gets into a flock, measures to reduce spread include: (i) floor feeding rather than trough feeding; (ii) weaning of lambs as early as possible ('snatching' lambs at birth and artificial rearing in extreme cases); and (iii) keeping age groups separate, and when shearing, shear from the youngest to the oldest. Ram breeders may sell ram lambs rather than keeping them to shearlings and risk infection. Blood testing using the ELISA test with culling of positive animals has had some success in eradicating the disease from some flocks, but is expensive.

Actinobacillosis

The main differential diagnosis for CLA is sporadic cases of actinobacillosis ('cruels') where abscesses occur along the lymphatics in the head and neck region. These are responsive to appropriate antibiotic treatment.

Non-infectious

Wool break

A wool break (thinning or breaking of the fibres) usually follows any severe illness or prolonged debilitating condition including inadequate nutrition. It is most marked during pregnancy and lactation, particularly following pregnancy toxaemia, difficult lambing or acute mastitis. It is common to see ewes, often in poor condition, in late winter or spring patchily shedding their complete fleece and in the process looking very 'moth-eaten'. Underneath, the skin is normal and providing the precipitating factors are reversed, normal wool regrows.

Emma Fishbourne and John Graham-Brown

Wool slip

This is an allied but specific condition sometimes seen in housed, winter-shorn ewes. Here, there is patchy loss of wool mainly confined to the hind quarters and back, developing within a few weeks of shearing. It is thought to be related to the stress of housing, shearing and cold, resulting in raised blood cortisol concentrations. The ewes are not obviously adversely affected but it can lead to delay in turnout.

Sunburn

Occasional cases of sunburn follow exposure to bright sunlight, particularly in recently shorn white-faced breeds. Marked skin erythema and oedema develop in exposed surfaces such as the ears, back and udder and necrosis with extensive scabs may develop. Affected sheep need housing and if secondary infection is suspected (e.g. *Dermatophilus*) antibiotic therapy is indicated. Shade will be required in future.

Photosensitization (yellowses)

Bright sunlight can also induce photosensitization if the white sheep have previously been eating a photodynamic agent as found, for example, in St John's wort (*Hypericum perforatum*), or they have raised circulating concentrations of the photodynamic agent phytoporphyrin (a breakdown product of chlorophyll), which arises when liver function is impaired. This impaired liver function can be caused by a variety of factors including copper toxicity, toxic plants and fungi, and some drugs, so the precise factor is rarely discovered, particularly if only one or two sheep in a flock are involved. In northern Europe, the plant bog asphodel (*Narthecium ossifragum*), found growing on natural hill or mountain pasture, is widely associated with the problem. In New Zealand, the condition, known as facial eczema, is caused by ingestion of sporidesmin fungal spores.

The most noticeable feature is the marked oedema of the head and face including the eyelids and ears, which makes the sheep look very 'droopy' and miserable; other non-pigmented areas may also be affected and, if severe enough, there is necrosis and eventual sloughing, particularly of the tips of the ears which then look 'cropped'.

Cases should be housed and carefully nursed. Blood samples for liver enzyme estimations may help to decide the prognosis. If cases continue in a flock, look at copper blood concentrations, check for toxic plants and investigate recent treatments.

13 Respiratory Diseases

PEERS DAVIES* AND JOHN GRAHAM-BROWN

Department of Livestock and One Health, Institute of Infection, Veterinary and Ecological Sciences, University of Liverpool, UK

Abstract

Respiratory diseases are common in all age groups of sheep. Causes can be bacterial, viral or parasitic and can be responsible for significant losses ranging from acute with sudden death through typical pneumonic disease to chronic conditions often responsible for thin ewe problems. Accurate diagnosis is very important on which to base suitable control measures and post-mortem examination is usually an important part of this process.

Several respiratory diseases (see Table 13.1) are involved in two important areas of loss: (i) sudden death; and (ii) thin adult sheep. In both cases PME is going to be an important part of the diagnostic process in addition to clinical examination of any live animals. Recently, ultrasound examination of the chest has been developed as an aid to diagnosis of lung lesions, although some experience is required in obtaining and interpreting images.

Pasteurellosis

Although microbiologists have periodically reclassified various *Pasteurella* spp., the livestock diseases they cause are still predominantly referred to by clinicians and farmers as **Pasteurellosis**. The bacterium *Pasteurella haemolytica*, which used to be divided into two biotypes, was then split into two separate species, *Mannheimia haemolytica* and *Pasteurella trehalosi*. The latter has more recently been reclassified as *Bibersteinia trehalosi*; however, in this book we will continue to refer to the diseases by the term 'pasteurellosis'. This group of bacteria is a common and an important cause of pneumonia and rapid or sudden death in sheep.

As most sheep carry *M. haemolytica* in the nasopharynx or tonsils, the mere isolation of this organism in nasal swabs or at PME does not establish the diagnosis; it is generally held that it requires some stress factor or intercurrent disease to precipate pasteurellosis.

There are three different manifestations of disease:

1. Septicaemia and rapid death in young lambs (a few days to 3 months old) caused by *M. haemolytica* – affected lambs are usually simply found dead or profoundly depressed with a high temperature and a PME is required to confirm diagnosis.
2. Pneumonia in older lambs and adults, also caused by *M. haemolytica*, most commonly in late spring and early summer (May–July) but also in store and fattening lambs in the autumn and winter. Affected animals are febrile and depressed with nasal discharge, coughing and laboured respiration. Some may survive but go on to develop chronic disease with weight loss.
3. Septicaemia and rapid death in the fattening and store lamb (6–9 months old) in the autumn and winter caused by *B. trehalosi* (systemic pasteurellosis). The most common first sign is one or two sheep found dead. A few others may appear very ill and separated from the rest and unwilling to be driven; they are usually febrile (over 40°C) and show increased respiratory rates. Some may have crusted eyelids and nostrils and usually there is some coughing in the group. About 10% may become affected in an outbreak.

Diagnosis

● Necropsy of fresh carcasses, if available. In the septicaemic and systemic forms, widespread

*Email: Peers.Davies@liverpool.ac.uk

© CAB International 2025. *A Handbook for the Sheep Clinician, 8th Edition*
(A.C. Winter and D. Grove-White eds)
DOI: 10.1079/9781800626355.0013

Table 13.1. Summary of main respiratory diseases.

Organism	Disease	Main age group affected
Bacteria		
Mannheimia haemolytica	Septicaemia	Young lambs
	Pneumonia (acute and chronic)	Growing lambs, adults
Bibersteinia trehalosi	Systemic pasteurellosis	Growing lambs in autumn
Mycoplasma ovipneumoniae	Atypical pneumonia	Growing lambs
Trueperella pyogenes	Laryngeal chondritis	Adults, especially heavily muscled terminal sire breeds
Internal parasites		
Dictyocaulus filaria	Parasitic bronchitis, husk	Growing lambs
Viruses		
Retrovirus	Ovine pulmonary adenocarcinoma (OPA, Jaagsiekte)	Adults over 2 years (occasionally in growing lambs)
Lentivirus	Maedi	Adults over 2 years

petechiae and ecchymoses are usually present with varying degrees of pleurisy and lung pathology present in all forms. *Mannheimia/Bibersteinia* need to be isolated in large numbers to confirm diagnosis and ask the laboratory for serotyping to check against the vaccine serotypes.

- Try to find a predisposing reason for the deaths or illness; in particular, with systemic pasteurellosis, enquire if the group has been moved or handled in the last day or so, or if the weather has been noticeably different, for example wet and windy (rain/wind-chill factor) or warm and still. Other intercurrent infections such as parainfluenza virus type 3 (PI3), Jaagsiekte and tick-borne fever may also predispose to clinical outbreaks of the pneumonic form.
- Consider clostridial diseases as the main differential, in particular pulpy kidney and braxy, and check on the vaccination history and dates.

Treatment and control

- For young lambs, control is by vaccination of ewes (for colostral antibodies) and early vaccination of lambs – remember, colostral protection is short, only 2–4 weeks. Also improve the ventilation of lambing sheds. Administer antibiotics such as oxytetracycline or tilmycosin (not if under 15 kg) if animals are seen alive.
- For older lambs and adults, control is by vaccination before the risk period, and improving ventilation if poor housing is a trigger (Fig. 13.1 and Fig. 13.2). Administer antibiotics as above

in acute cases. Chronic cases may not respond unless the course is very prolonged and this may not be economical.

- Systemic pasteurellosis can be difficult to deal with and control:
  - Sometimes the group is large and inaccessible, which means the incidence is unsure, PME is delayed and there is a very real difficulty in deciding when to do something, that is whether to gather (which may make matters worse) and treat (all?). Often a number of deaths occur over a period of days or weeks and then unaccountably cease.
  - Remove and isolate affected sheep – treat these and as many contacts as seem worthwhile. Tilmycosin is very good for pneumonia but is vet-only administration, so if you as the vet are going to treat sick animals yourself this might be the drug of choice. If the farmer has to treat, other drugs will have to be used, for example LA oxytetracycline given twice at a 4-day interval.
  - Recommend vaccination – a dead vaccine is available, containing most of the serotypes known to cause the disease, and requires two doses at approximately a 4-week interval to provide useful protection. If given to ewes in late pregnancy it not only affords protection to the ewes that spring, when the incidence of *Mannheimia* pneumonia is highest, but also to the lambs via colostrum for the first 2–4 weeks of life and so helps to cover the first major risk period for this type of septicaemia (contrast with passive clostridial protection

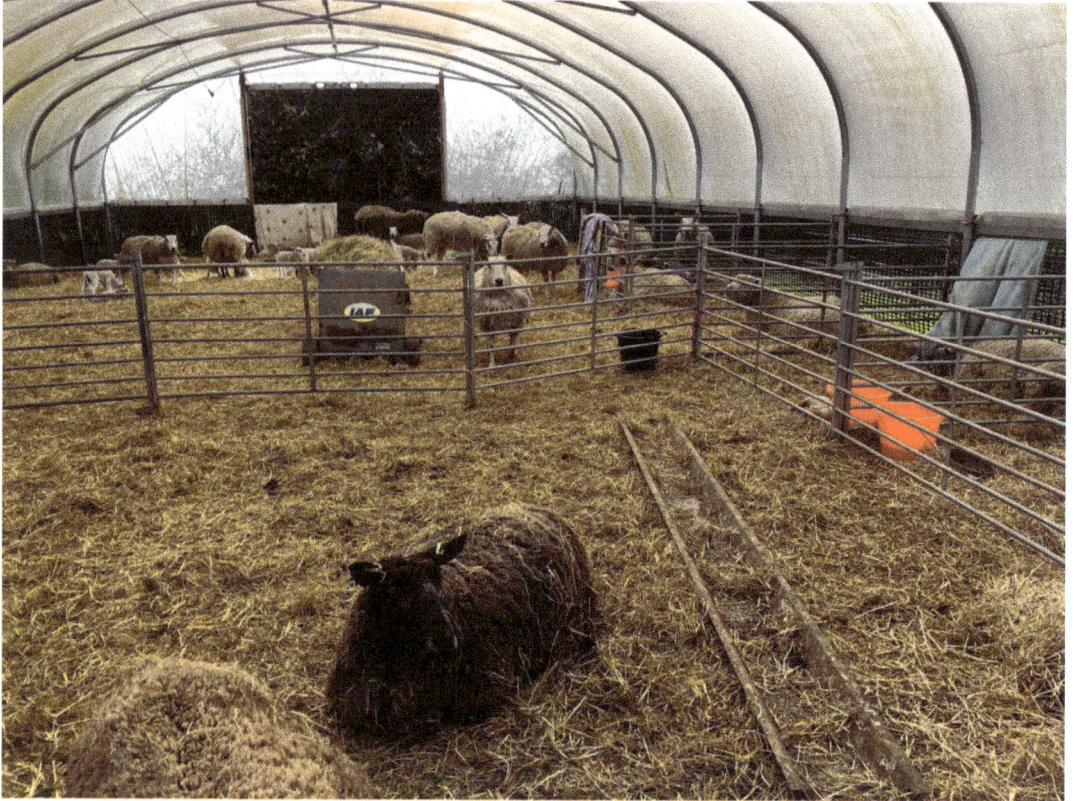

Fig. 13.1. This polytunnel provides shelter with good ventilation (photo Agnes Winter).

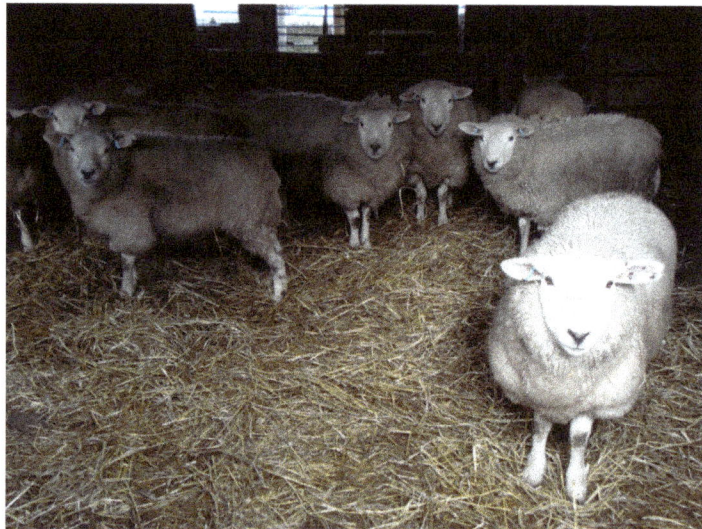

Fig. 13.2. Poor ventilation in this shed predisposes these fattening lambs to pneumonia (photo Agnes Winter).

Peers Davies and John Graham-Brown

which lasts 12–16 weeks). To cover adequately the next few weeks and months, lambs need to be given two doses of vaccine at a 4-week interval, starting 3 weeks after birth; there is evidence that any colostrum-derived antibody does not interfere with the response to this early vaccination.

- Look at the environmental conditions (e.g. wet, exposed, overcrowded, lush food) and consider providing plenty of shelter or moving the group, although the moving could make matters worse.
- In the long term, avoid, if possible, very exposed wet and windy sites which induce stress and encourage the flock to crowd into small sheltered sites which, in turn, intensify the aerial spread of pathogens. Also, avoid putting store lambs on lush grass in the autumn without considering vaccination first.

The position regarding vaccination is complicated by combining this vaccine with a clostridial vaccine to form a very popular product which is considerably more expensive than clostridial vaccines alone. While such a combination is ideal for the vaccination of ewes, it matches the needs of lambs less well because of the disparate length of protection by colostral antibodies for the two categories of disease. In practice, if this combination is to be used in flocks where there is a significant incidence of septicaemia and sudden deaths in young lambs which is diagnosed as pasteurellosis, the normal lamb clostridial vaccination schedule needs to be brought forward to 1 and 2 months rather than the usual 3 and 4 months; alternatively *Pasteurella* and clostridial vaccines can be given separately at appropriate times.

The pasteurellosis vaccine was improved a few years ago and is now more effective in the control of disease in the later store and fattening lamb. Antigenicity of some serotypes involved in this form of the disease was improved by growing the bacteria in a very iron-depleted medium which increased the expression of some important antigens on the surface of the bacteria.

Parasitic Pneumonia (Parasitic Bronchitis)

The most common species of lungworm associated with clinical disease in sheep is *Dictyocaulus filaria*. Oviparous adult worms reside in the trachea and bronchi, producing larvated eggs that are coughed up, swallowed and shed in the faeces as L1, or aspirated into the alveoli and small airways. It is the combination of adult and pre-adult worms in the airways and aspiration of eggs and L1 larvae that causes clinical disease characterized by coughing, ill-thrift and, occasionally, tachypnoea and dyspnoea. Disease risk typically peaks in the later part of the grazing season (September–November) with increasing pasture infectivity, although signs of coughing may be seen at any time. Lambs are at greatest risk due to a lack of prior exposure. Animals generally develop a strong immunity after their first season, although older animals can still act as subclinically infected carriers.

Parasitic pneumonia in sheep is not considered to be as common or important compared with 'husk' in cattle. Modern TST-based approaches for PGE may leave a greater opportunity for lungworm infections to manifest and, anecdotally, appear to be becoming more commonly diagnosed in some parts of the UK. In many instances lambs will be sent to slaughter before peak pasture infectivity occurs. Where clinical disease outbreaks occur, these are commonly found accompanying high PGE worm burdens and, consequently, are often not considered the primary clinical concern. Onward transmission of *D. filaria* is achieved through survival of infective larvae on pastures over winter and renewed shedding by carrier animals.

Diagnosis, treatment and control

Diagnosis is based on clinical signs and seasonal incidence and can be confirmed by examination of fresh faecal samples for first-stage larvae by the Baermann apparatus. In addition to *D. filaria*, *Protostrongylus rufescens* and *Muellerius capillaris* may be found infecting the small airways and lung parenchyma, respectively. Neither is considered particularly pathogenic; both are oviparous. *Dictyocaulus filaria* L1 can be distinguished from these other species in that they: (i) are long (500 µm); (ii) have a blunt tail; (iii) have a cephalic knob; and (iv) contain refractile food granules.

Where clinical disease is identified, group 1-BZ, 2-LV, 3-ML and 5-SI products all carry licences of efficacy against *D. filaria*. Monepantel (group 4-AD) does not carry a licence of efficacy against lungworms.

Atypical Pneumonia

This is an unsatisfactory name given to the type of pneumonia which closely resembles that which is so commonly found in the fattening pig and housed calf. It is associated with a variety of agents such as *Mycoplasma ovipneumoniae*, PI3 and adenovirus. It is principally a disease problem in housed or densely stocked fattening or store lambs (3–12 months old), although *M. ovipneumoniae* has been found in extensively kept sheep and wild sheep in some countries. It is particularly common following the mixing of lambs introduced from the market in autumn and winter.

Clinical signs

The disease is characterized by chronic coughing, ocular and nasal discharges, and is usually afebrile, although the occasional acute pneumonic lamb arises which is febrile, off-food, listless, and with obvious respiratory distress; these cases are associated with secondary *M. haemolytica* infection. Affected lambs take several weeks longer to reach slaughter weight and consume more food to do so.

Diagnosis

This is based on the clinical signs, environmental conditions and pathology of lungs, which show collapsed areas in the lower parts of the lung lobes at PME or slaughter.

Control

For pigs and calves:

- supply more fresh air;
- reduce numbers under one roof, and in any one group;
- split groups according to age, size and origin;
- treat sick animals with appropriate antibiotic (Mycoplasmas are not susceptible to penicillins); and
- consider pasteurellosis vaccination to protect against additional disease caused by these pathogens.

Slow Viral Pneumonias

Ovine pulmonary adenocarcinoma (OPA, sheep pulmonary adenomatosis, SPA, driving sickness, Jaagsiekte)

Although this condition has caused worrying losses in some flocks, particularly of Scottish origin where the incidence can be up to 10%, it usually only causes sporadic deaths, but its potential danger is illustrated by the losses that occurred when introduced into Iceland where sheep are housed for long periods. It is a contagious adenomatous tumour of the lungs of sheep and possibly goats, and caused by a retrovirus, with an incubation period of up to 3 years.

Clinical signs

The signs are of loss of condition and severe respiratory distress, but without much coughing, in an individual adult sheep when driven. This respiratory embarrassment, which sounds like 'bubbly porridge' on auscultation, increases over several weeks. Characteristically, if the ewe is held with its head lowered (the 'wheelbarrow' test), relatively large volumes (30–300 ml) of clear mucous exudate flow from the nostrils; this fluid contains virus so is infectious. There is no fever and the animal feeds up to the terminal stages when there is often fulminating pasteurellosis.

Diagnosis

Diagnosis is based on clinical signs (including the 'wheelbarrow' test) and PME – which is the preferred method of diagnosis; the lungs may weigh up to 4 kg (1.5 kg is normal) and show areas of grey tumour tissue with frothy white fluid in the trachea and bronchi. Ultrasound scanning of the lungs can be a useful supportive diagnostic test in sheep showing clinical signs. Unfortunately, the sensitivity and specificity is too poor for it to be a suitable screening test in whole flocks where the prevalence of the disease is low and thus the risk of a large number of costly false positive misdiagnosis is high. Although the virus can be detected in laboratory tests, no commercial test is yet available for either antibodies or antigens. Pasteurellosis may mask the presence of OPA, so where significant losses of older sheep occur from pasteurellosis, lungs should be checked histologically for OPA.

Control

There should be prompt slaughter of the obviously affected animals. Active surveillance of all on-farm deaths by PME is strongly recommended, followed by culling of all dam, progeny and siblings of infected cases where linkages between individuals are known. This is in order to reduce the number of animals in the flock at high risk of being infected and thus reduce the risk of further onward horizontal transmission. The disease has been eliminated from a few flocks by removing lambs at birth and rearing them artificially in the same way as used to produce maedi-free animals from infected flocks (see below).

Maedi visna (MV, ovine progressive pneumonia)

Maedi means 'air hunger', visna means 'wasting'. Maedi is seen as a chronic progressive pneumonia affecting sheep over 3 years old and visna is the nervous form of the disease, again affecting older sheep. Both diseases are caused by a lentivirus, similar but not identical to that causing caprine arthritis encephalitis in goats. The virus causes lesions in the lungs, CNS, joints and udder. Maedi was first recognized in the UK in 1978, having probably been introduced from the continent, where it was common, with imported stock. It does not occur in Australia and New Zealand.

A number of flocks have had clinical cases. Because of the insidious nature of the disease which takes 3–4 years for clinical signs to develop, it is likely that many more flocks have subclinical infection. In 1993, a random check on blood samples showed a seroprevalence of 0.4%, which extrapolated to at least 70,000 seropositive sheep at that time. Another survey in 2013 showed the number of infected flocks had doubled as had the number of infected sheep per flock. Doubtless the disease has continued to spread since then. Economic losses occur from premature culling of infected ewes, from reduced lamb growth rates and reduced conception rates. Unless sheep farmers take the threat from this disease seriously, it could have a major impact on the health of the national flock in the foreseeable future.

Unlike OPA, diagnostic serological tests can be used to identify MV-free flocks and this is applied in the SRUC Premium Sheep and Goat Health Scheme (https://www.sruc.ac.uk/media/wbobswkd/mv_insert_2020-1.pdf accessed). This has particular application for the pedigree breeder, especially those wishing to export sheep, but should be taken up more widely by commercial breeders. A monitoring scheme aimed at commercial flocks is available with less rigorous rules than the accreditation scheme and a screening package is also available for finding out if the disease is present in a flock.

The disease is spread in various ways:

1. by coughing or sneezing infective droplets, which is important in housed sheep;
2. by multiple use of contaminated needles, ear punches etc; and
3. most importantly, by colostrum and milk from infected ewes, which contains the virus.

Clinical signs

Maedi is seen as a chronic progressive pneumonia affecting sheep over 3 years old and is invariably fatal. Affected sheep lose condition and lag behind when driven, with characteristic difficulty in breathing which becomes progressively worse over a period of months.

Visna is the nervous form of the disease, again affecting older sheep, in which weight loss and vague, slowly progressive neurological signs occur. One recognizable feature may be the development of a unilateral conscious proprioceptive deficit of one hindlimb, with dragging and scuffing of the toe progressing to paralysis of the hind legs.

The virus also affects the udder causing an indurative lymphocytic mastitis with reduced milk yield which is not always recognized because milk remains normal in appearance, but lambs from affected ewes have been shown to weigh 3 kg less at weaning than those from healthy ewes. Arthritis and vasculitis are other possible components of the clinical picture.

Diagnosis

In the individual, this is based on clinical signs and PME. Serological tests such as the agar gel immunodiffusion test (AGID) and, particularly, ELISA are useful at the flock level (see above), but false negative results, due to delay in antibody production or immunosuppression, do occur, which makes them less useful in the individual animal.

Control

- Slaughter affected animals.
- Do not breed from the offspring of affected ewes.
- Be careful about the source of ewe colostrum fed to lambs.

- Keep a young flock and only keep replacements from the young ewes.
- Purchase from accredited flocks only.
- Join the Premium Sheep and Goat Health Scheme and eradicate by test and slaughter.

Because the infection is not passed to the lamb before birth, it is possible (though demanding) to obtain uninfected lambs from an infected flock by supervising lambing and immediately removing lambs, certainly before sucking the ewe. Lambs are then given colostrum substitute and reared artificially.

Laryngeal Chondritis

This acute obstructive upper respiratory condition, seen most commonly in 'short-necked' breeds, the Texel being the most numerous, is characterized by severe dyspnoea with laryngeal stridor and is often fatal if not treated quickly. The laryngeal occlusion results from chronic suppurative lesions within the arytenoid cartilages. Rams, ewes and growing lambs are all known to have been affected. Initial studies comparing the dimensions of the larynx of Texels with Bluefaced Leicesters have shown a shorter, narrower airway compounded by increased muscle mass in the neck which probably predisposes to the condition.

Treatment

These cases are often presented as emergencies.

- Treat with a large dose of steroid, intravenously if possible, and broad-spectrum antibiotic. Carry on with reduced doses for 5–7 days. This regimen alone may be adequate for less severe cases.
- If dyspnoea is severe, an emergency tracheostomy is necessary under local infiltration anaesthesia. This usually gives immediate relief, but good aftercare is needed with the tube changed twice daily, initially, reducing to once daily if the tube remains clear of discharges. After the tracheostomy tube has been in for 2–3 weeks, infection may have subsided, so try leaving the tube out. If dyspnoea is still present, the only remaining option, rarely worthwhile, is surgery to try to remove the necrotic tissue from the larynx.

The prognosis should always be extremely guarded as recovered cases very commonly relapse, sometimes just being found dead. It is probably unwise to use recovered animals for future breeding or semen collection, even if they are said to be valuable and it is worth considering changing to genetically unrelated stock in future breeding policy.

Peers Davies and John Graham-Brown

14 Neurological Diseases

NIALL CONNOLLY* AND HELEN WILLIAMS

Department of Livestock and One Health, Institute of Infection, Veterinary and Ecological Sciences, University of Liverpool, UK

Abstract

Neurological diseases are common in sheep and are a particular challenge for the clinician to make a firm diagnosis. Performing a full neurological examination, together with obtaining a full history including number of animals affected (individual or group), speed of onset of clinical signs, age, husbandry, recent management changes etc. are a starting point to arrive at a presumptive diagnosis. Response to therapy following a presumptive diagnosis may offer valuable clues as to true disease status.

A full clinical and neurological examination will help determine whether disease is generalized or has a specific neuroanatomic location (see Appendix 2 'Neurological Examination of Sheep'). Distinguishing between severe systemic disease and neurological disease is not easy, as diseases such as pneumonia, acute fascioliosis, severe emaciation, septicaemia or toxaemia, e.g. clostridial disease, will all be differential diagnoses in a collapsed sheep. In addition, multiple limb lameness, muscle weakness or stiffness, e.g. vitamin E and selenium deficiency, can be confused with gait and proprioception deficits. Due to the diagnostic challenges in the live animal, post-mortem examination including brain histopathology is often required to arrive at a final diagnosis. This is particularly the case where, as with many sheep diseases, the key finding may be collapse or sudden death.

The main neuroanatomic syndromes which should be identifiable following neurological examination are:

- **Cerebral** – depression, blindness, circling, proprioceptive deficits, head turn.
- **Cerebellar** – wide-based stance, high head carriage, ataxia, dysmetria, intention tremors, nystagmus.
- **Vestibular** – head tilt, circling, stumbling, nystagmus, sometimes facial paralysis;

- **Ponto-medullary (brainstem)** – depression, multiple cranial nerve deficits especially V, VII and VIII.
- **Spinal cord** – varying degrees of ataxia, paresis or spasticity depending on location of lesion.

Table 14.1 shows the main neurological differential diagnoses for each of these neuroanatomic syndromes.

Metabolic Diseases of Ewes (Pregnancy Toxaemia [PT], Hypocalcaemia, Hypomagnesaemia)

See Chapter 6.

Space-occupying Lesions: Gid (*Coenurosis*), Abscess, Tumour

Space-occupying lesions of the sheep brain, which may produce clinical signs, include gid cysts, abscesses and tumours. A variety of signs may be present depending on the location (see Table 14.2). CT or MRI can be used to give a definitive location in the live animal, however this is only viable in animals of high economic or sentimental value. In reality, gid cyst is the only treatable space-occupying lesion.

---

*Email: conno11y@liverpool.ac.uk

DOI: 10.1079/9781800626355.0014

Table 14.1 Neurological diseases in the sheep by anatomical location, with information regarding history.

Location of lesion	Disease	Typical onset/progression	Age affected	Flock Problem	Individual Problem	Further Information
Cerebral (generalized)	Cerebro-Cortical Necrosis (CCN)	Acute – 24 hrs	Usually weaned lambs but sometimes adults	+	+	
	Bacterial meningitis	Acute – 24 hrs	Usually young lambs within 1 week of age	+	+	Chapter 7
	Pregnancy toxaemia	Sub-acute – 2–4 days	Ewes	++	+	Chapter 6
	Scrapie	Chronic – months	2–5 years old	+	+++	
	Lead poisoning	Acute – 24 hrs Sub-acute – over several days	Any but usually not pre-weaned lambs	+	+	
	Vitamin A deficiency	Chronic but seizures can be acute	Any age but usually only in sheep which have been housed for long periods	++		
Cerebral (focal)	Schmallenberg disease	Congenital disease	Newborn lambs	+	++	Chapter 7
	Ram fighting injury	Acute – instantaneous	Adult rams		+++	
	Gid	Acute – 2–4 weeks Chronic 3–8 months	Weaned lambs and adults up to 2 years old (occasionally up to 3 years old)		+++	
	Brain abscess	Sub-acute – over 7 days	Any		+++	
	Brain tumour	Chronic – weeks/months/years	Adults		+++	
	Listeria	Acute – 1–3 days	Mostly adults		++	
Cerebellar	Gid	Chronic – months	Weaned lambs and adults		+++	
	Border disease	Congenital disease	Newborn lambs but they can survive so can be first noticed when older	+	++	Chapter 7
	Scrapie	Chronic – months	Adults 2–5 years old		+++	
	Louping-ill	Sub-acute – days	Usually less than 2 years old but most young lambs are protected by maternal antibodies	+++	+ (if endemic)	Chapter 16

Niall Connolly and Helen Williams

Location	Condition	Onset	Details			Chapter
Brainstem	Listeriosis	Acute – 1–3 days	Most frequent in sheep 18–24 months but other ages can be affected		++	
	Louping-ill	Sub-acute – days	Usually less than 2 years old but most young lambs are protected by maternal antibodies	+++	+ (if endemic)	Chapter 16
	Pituitary abscess syndrome	Can be acute or develop over weeks	Any age but often adult rams		+++	
Spinal cord	Injury	Acute – instantaneous	Any age		+++	
	Spinal cord abscess	Sub-acute – 1–7 days	Most common in young lambs as part of the joint ill complex of diseases however can occur occasionally in older sheep. May be caused by damage to neck with dosing gun.		++	Chapter 7
	Cervical Myelopathy "wobblers syndrome"	Chronic - months	Young Rams (usually Texel or Beltex) approx. 15–18month old	+++		
	Swayback (Copper Deficiency)	Acute for congenital form, or chronic for delayed form	Either newborn with acute congenital form or 4–12 weeks for the delayed form	++		Chapter 7
Vestibular disease	Middle or inner ear infection	Sub-acute – days to weeks	Can be any age but typically adults or older lambs		++	Chapter 15
Peripheral neuropathies	e.g. radial nerve damage	Acute – instantaneous	Any age		+++	Chapter 11

Table 14.2. Clinical signs associated with space-occupying lesions and the likely lesion location.

Indicator sign		Possible location
Behaviour	Depression	Cerebrum (rostral)
	Excitability	Cerebrum (temporal)
Head position	Tilt	Cerebellum or vestibular
	Aversion (turn)	Cerebrum
	Raised	Cerebellum
	Head tremor	Cerebellum
Movement	Circling – wide	Cerebrum (ipsilateral, superficial)
	Circling – tight	Cerebrum (contralateral, lateral ventricle or basal nucleus)
	Dysmetria (hypermetria)	Cerebellum
Posture	Wide-based stance	Cerebellum
Wheelbarrow and hemi-walking tests	Unilateral deficit	Cerebrum (contralateral)
	Bilateral deficit	Cerebellum
Vision	Unilateral blindness	Cerebrum (contralateral caudal)
	Bilateral blindness	Cerebellum
Eye movement	Nystagmus	Cerebellum or vestibular nuclei
Eye position	Strabismus	Brainstem nuclei of CNs III, IV and VI

Note:

- Head tilt is the head rotated but the nose pointing forward. The cyst or lesion is usually on the side of the lower ear.
- Head aversion is the head rotated and turned to the side and usually down. The direction is not a good indicator to the side affected.
- Circling may be indicated by a plait of straw wound round the leg on the inside of the circle. The diameter of the circle may indicate whether it is in the right or left side of the brain and depth of the lesion or cyst.
- Unilateral menace deficit indicates that the lesion or cyst is in the opposite cerebrum because approximately 90% optic axons cross over; residual vision could be from the 10% that are in the nasal field which do not cross over.
- Spontaneous nystagmus indicates vestibular involvement. Cerebellar nystagmus is induced by eye movement and is an intention tremor of the eye muscles.

Coenurosis (Gid, Sturdy, Bendro)

Coenurosis is now an uncommon disease of sheep in the UK due to the availability of effective anthelmintic drugs for dogs and more strictly enforced legislation on carcass disposal. The causative agent is the metacestode (larval) stage of the life cycle of *Taenia multiceps* (*Coenurus cerebralis*), a tapeworm which dogs can acquire through scavenging dead sheep. The adult cestode also occurs in the fox but the worms seldom reach maturity and become gravid, so foxes should not be blamed until every possible dog source of infection has been considered. The metacestode is also recorded in cattle, goats, horses and deer, but at a much lower incidence than in sheep, and, very rarely, in humans.

Once a sheep or lamb (pet lambs are often most vulnerable as they may be kept in close contact with dogs) has ingested the tapeworm eggs the larvae hatch and migrate in the bloodstream throughout the body but can only continue their development within the CNS. Over a period of 2–8 months, the *Coenurus* grows into a fluid-filled cyst containing around 100 scoleces (Fig. 14.1). Multiple cysts have been thought to only occur occasionally in natural infections, possibly because an established cyst inhibits the development of further cysts, but recent magnetic resonance imaging (MRI) investigation has shown some animals with multiple cysts.

Clinical signs

Acute coenurosis is uncommon and usually goes unnoticed. Some 2–4 weeks after a sheep has ingested a large number of tapeworm eggs, nervous signs such as ataxia, blindness, muscle tremors, nystagmus, excitability and collapse may be seen.

Niall Connolly and Helen Williams

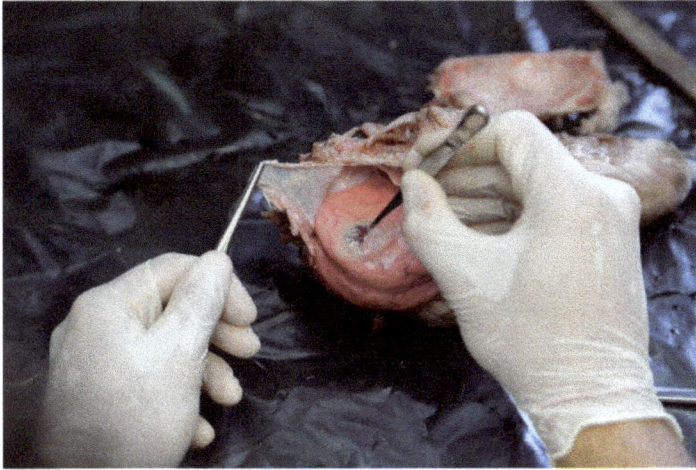

Fig. 14.1. *Coenurus cerebralis* (Gid cyst) in a sheep's cerebrum (photo John Graham-Brown).

Diagnosis is extremely difficult and is usually at PME where haemorrhagic tracts and migrating parasites are found in the brain.

The chronic form of the disease is more frequently seen. The onset of clinical signs is usually 3–8 months after infection. The affected animal shows a variety of neurological deficits, usually correlating closely with the location of the cyst within the CNS. About 80% of cysts are in the cerebrum, 10% in the cerebellum, 5% are multiple cysts in several locations and the remainder are in the brainstem and spinal cord. Differentials for diagnosis include other space-occupying lesions such as abscesses or tumour.

Affected sheep are usually identified initially by the farmer because of abnormal behaviour such as standing apart or failing to respond to the dog. As the cyst develops, the clinical signs gradually increase in extent and severity, progressing to recumbency and death (over days or weeks) if the cyst is not removed surgically. In diagnosis, it is important to perform a full neurological examination to identify the full combinations of signs rather than relying too heavily on any one deficit, e.g. unilateral blindness. This will allow better spatial identification of the cyst. Locating the cyst and subsequent surgical removal is an interesting clinical challenge, though rarely financially viable.

Diagnosis

The disease usually occurs sporadically, although occasional outbreaks are seen. It is characterized by the slowly progressive development of CNS signs in sheep over 4 months old (usually 1–2 years old and very rarely over 3). The chronic nature of the disease and the age of affected animals, together with a known farm incidence, will aid diagnosis. In addition, the presence of skull softening at or near the horn bud site, due to the intracranial pressure, helps with diagnosis but is not a reliable guide to the localization of the cyst.

A differential white blood cell count and CSF analysis may aid in diagnosis including differentiation of a gid cyst from other types of space-occupying lesions. Usually, the white blood cell profile is not altered by coenurosis, thus presence of a neutrophilia will generally indicate another cause of the CNS signs (e.g. listeriosis or abscess). CSF sampling should be carried out with care in cases where a raised intracranial pressure is suspected (e.g. coenurosis); only 0.5 ml should be taken from the lumbar cistern to avoid herniation of the cerebellum. In coenurosis, the CSF does not show any diagnostic changes; surprisingly, there is no eosinophilia.

Treatment

Lambs near killing weight should be sent for slaughter. Surgical removal of the cyst can be attempted in breeding animals or those too small for slaughter. The surgical success rate may be as high as 80% in the case of cerebral cysts, although lower in the case of cysts in other locations.

The operation should be carried out under general anaesthesia. A C-shaped skin incision is made just caudal to the horn bud on the appropriate side (left or right cerebral cortex), or in the midline just rostral to the nuchal line (cerebellum). The skull is trephined (0.5–1.5 cm diameter) and a circular plate of bone removed. Sometimes, the skull is so soft that scissors may be used. However, it is not safe to assume that the site of skull softening indicates the location of the cyst. The bone at the cerebellar site is at least 0.5 cm thick and may bleed. In trephining at the cerebellar site, it is important to avoid the transverse suture line about 1.5 cm rostral to the nuchal line, since this marks the position of the *tentorium cerebelli* and the transverse sinus and serious haemorrhage could follow. The meninges are cut and reflected to expose the cerebrum, which will bulge due to increased intracranial pressure. If the cyst is lying superficially, the translucent pale-grey wall may be visible and should be immediately grasped with artery forceps. If the cyst is not visible, a 14G or 16G needle with cannula (e.g. horse IV catheter) is inserted. When the cyst is punctured, clear cyst fluid wells up the needle. The needle is removed and a 20–50 ml syringe is attached to the cannula and some of the fluid is withdrawn. Cerebral cysts average 35 ml but may contain over 100 ml; cerebellar cysts contain 10–25 ml. Suction is used to trap the pale-grey cyst wall in the end of the cannula which is then elevated to allow the pedicle of the cyst wall to be grasped with artery forceps and can then be removed by applying gentle tension, draining more fluid from the cyst if required. The depth of the trephine hole at the cerebellar site may reduce the angulation of the cannula, making it difficult to grasp a cyst that is laterally situated in the cerebellum. Only the skin incision is sutured, and antibiotic cover is continued for 2 more days; steroids may also be necessary unless cyst removal was straightforward. It is advisable to keep the sheep inside for 7 days in a quiet dark location to avoid excitation. The sutures are removed in 10 days and the skull heals in about 1 month.

The results of surgery can be very rewarding; uncomplicated cases usually make a good recovery within about a week, but excessive probing, haemorrhage and multiple cysts lead to a poor prognosis (better to euthanaze rather than allow to recover from anaesthesia).

Control

- Worm dogs with a drug which is effective against cestodes, for example praziquantel at least as frequently as every 3 months.
- Dispose of sheep carcasses properly, ensuring there is no access to dogs or other scavengers to the carcass whilst awaiting collection by the fallen stock transporter.
- Avoid sheep grazing possibly heavily infected pasture, for example following sheepdog trials or if used by hounds.

Brain Tumours

Brain tumours are an uncommon space-occupying lesion in sheep although a range of types has been reported in the literature. They have been diagnosed in lambs as well as older sheep.

Suppurative brain diseases

In sheep, these include listeriosis, abscesses, pituitary abscess syndrome (Basilar empyema) and bacterial meningitis. Of these, listeria is the most common.

Listeriosis

This is a disease of sheep and cattle caused by the bacterium *Listeria monocytogenes* which is commonly excreted in faeces and milk by apparently normal animals (which can be carriers of the organism for extended periods following exposure) and is found widely in soil. Although many sheep in the flock will be exposed to the organism, clinical disease is usually sporadic. It has been suggested that the level of challenge, immunosuppression, concurrent disease, nutrition or other stressors may all affect the likelihood of clinical disease occurring. It is a zoonotic disease with most human cases being foodborne from ingestion of unpasteurized milk or cheese, contaminated cold meats and fish or soil-contaminated vegetables. It is advisable that pregnant women avoid all potential listeria infection routes. However, cutaneous listeriosis is an occupational hazard for veterinary surgeons and farmers who handle sick animals (usually from contamination during obstetrical procedures when the fetus is infected).

Niall Connolly and Helen Williams

Disease caused by *L. monocytogenes* presents in a number of forms:

- encephalitis – by far the most common and significant form;
- abortion;
- diarrhoea and septicaemia;
- septicaemia and death in young lambs; and
- kerato-conjunctivitis and mastitis have also been reported associated with *Listeria* spp.

Encephalitic listeriosis

Cases of encephalitic listeriosis are most often seen during the winter months particularly when silage is being fed. Poor-quality, badly fermented (i.e. high pH) silage, especially if it is contaminated with soil, and stored where air can get at it, can contain large numbers of *Listeria monocytogenes*.

It is thought that the organism gains entry to the animal via any mouth lesions (e.g. changing teeth) and travels up cranial nerve V (Trigeminal) to involve the nuclei of the V, VII and VIII cranial nerves in the brainstem (pons and medulla). Encephalitic listeriosis appears to have a longer incubation period than other forms of the disease with cases usually occurring 6 weeks after silage feeding starts. This is probably because the bacteria take some time to travel up the nerves to the brain. Thus, it is mainly a winter disease with a peak incidence in February/March when many ewes are heavily pregnant. However, as *L. monocytogenes* is shed in the faeces and has long survival times in the environment, the disease can occur when silage is not being fed and at any time of year, e.g. if sheep are fed concentrates on bare ground they may be exposed to the organism in the soil.

Clinical signs

The signs are variable but classically, the animal is very depressed and there is unilateral V (trigeminal), VII (facial) and sometimes VIII (vestibulocochlear) cranial nerve paralysis. This shows as: (i) drooping ear, eyelid and lip (facial paralysis) (Fig.14.2); (ii) loss of facial sensation; and (iii) paralysis of cheek muscles with consequent dribbling and difficulty in eating and drinking. If the VIII nerve is involved, there is aversion of the head, propulsive circling and falling over onto one side. The animal is unable to respond to the menace test

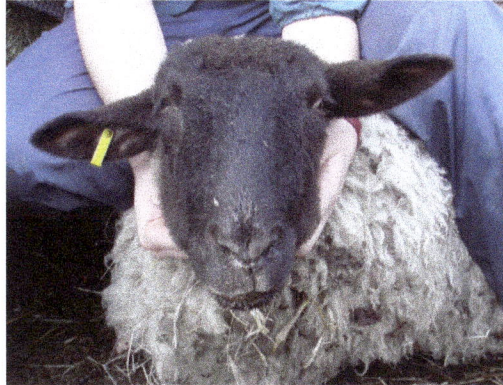

Fig. 14.2. Encephalitic listeriosis causes unilateral facial paralysis (photo Helen Williams and Niall Connolly).

(also palpebral and corneal reflexes may be absent) which may mislead one into thinking that the ewe is blind in that eye as might occur with a space-occupying lesion. Pyrexia may occur early in the course of the disease but is less common as it progresses. Deterioration usually occurs over just a few days, leading to recumbency and death.

Diagnosis

The CNS form requires differentiating clinically from, in particular:

- hypocalcaemia (always check a recumbent ewe for facial paralysis before assuming it is hypocalcaemia);
- middle- and inner-ear infection – confusion may arise because infection spreading from the ear locally to involve the facial nerve will produce classic signs of facial paralysis but without the extreme depression of listeriosis. Such cases usually respond well to antibiotics and probably account for some supposedly 'cured' listeriosis cases; and
- other differential diagnoses such as pregnancy toxaemia, gid, CCN and brain abscess.

Usually, blood haematology and biochemistry are unremarkable and any changes reflect dehydration, anorexia and a stress response whilst serology is unhelpful. Analysis of the CSF can be a useful diagnostic technique with an increased protein concentration and nucleated cell count (often monocytes but sometimes neutrophils) in listeria cases.

However, post-mortem examination, specifically brain histology is necessary to confirm listeriosis.

If, as expected, silage is being fed, or was fed at some time during the previous 6 weeks, examine it for signs of: (i) poor fermentation; (ii) spoilage (mould); and (iii) soil contamination. Most silage contains some *Listeria*, although very rotten silage may be sterile. Take care when handling suspect material, including silage, particularly if you are pregnant or unwell.

Treatment

Therapy for the CNS form can be disappointing and is much less successful than in cattle. The organism is sensitive to a wide range of antibiotics *in vitro*, but despite intensive treatment, many cases fail to respond. Therefore, owners should be warned of the likely poor outcome before embarking on therapy, and euthanasia may be the best option, especially if the sheep is recumbent. Success is more likely if treatment is early and vigorous. Both high doses of penicillin G (44,000 iu/kg per day; roughly 40 mg/kg) and oxytetracycline (10 mg/kg) have been used to treat listeria in ruminants though there is little evidence base regarding comparative efficacy of these treatments. The benefit or risk of corticosteroid use is poorly understood. In humans with meningitis, it is used with a positive effect but since immunosuppression is a risk factor for listeriosis there is a possibility that it may exacerbate the disease. Therefore, a non-steroidal anti-inflammatory drug is often recommended as an alternative. Other supportive therapy that could be indicated include correcting fluid and electrolyte imbalance (metabolic acidosis is common due to loss of bicarbonate in saliva), managing the common unilateral eye complications of corneal ulceration and uveitis, B-vitamins and offering food as a mash.

Control

The main control measure is in reducing contamination of silage. Live attenuated vaccines are available on the continent, but there is argument over their efficacy, and they are not used in the UK. Some argue that they can make matters worse rather than better, since the disease may be an allergic response in a previously sensitized animal.

SILAGE MAKING AND FEEDING Although a few incidents do occur at pasture, particularly when soil is exposed by heavy grazing, most follow silage feeding. It is almost impossible to avoid contamination

by *Listeria*, so one must seek to avoid the conditions in which it multiplies.

- Make high-quality silage with a pH <5 and a D value of >65%, using additives where necessary. Avoid gross soil contamination (e.g. mole hills) by rolling and not cutting grass too short, so that it has an ash content of <100 g/kg DM.
- Compact and completely seal the silage as soon as possible (the same day) and so avoid air getting into the sides and tops of clamps.
- With big-bale silage, ensure wrapping is secure and avoid puncturing wrapping when bales are moved or stored. Increasing the number of layers of plastic wrapping is claimed to improve silage quality and thereby reduce listeria risk.
- If there are persistent problems, try to avoid grazing sheep on fields from which silage will be made later in the season – grass may be contaminated if sheep are passing *Listeria* in faeces.
- Avoid feeding poor-quality silage, as judged on appearance and smell.
- Ideally, do not give more silage than can be cleared in 48 h maximum. However, this is often not possible if big-bale silage is being fed outside.
- It is less risky to feed suspect silage to cattle.

Other forms of listeriosis

The alimentary form often produces diarrhoea and brief general illness although a fatal septicaemia has been reported. If the ewe is pregnant, abortion may follow a week or so later, sometimes with retention of fetal membranes and subsequent systemic illness, but usually not encephalitis. However, others in the flock may show characteristic neurological signs of encephalitic listeriosis. Liveborne lambs from infected ewes may develop septicaemia. For diagnosis, submit faeces, vaginal discharges, fetuses and milk (if any) for culture and paired blood samples for serology.

Pituitary Abscess Syndrome

This is an uncommon disease of individual sheep which is a differential diagnosis for listeriosis. A pituitary abscess can occur following haematogenous spread of bacteria from a chronic infection such as mastitis or pneumonia or by direct extension from a suppurative infection such as sinusitis

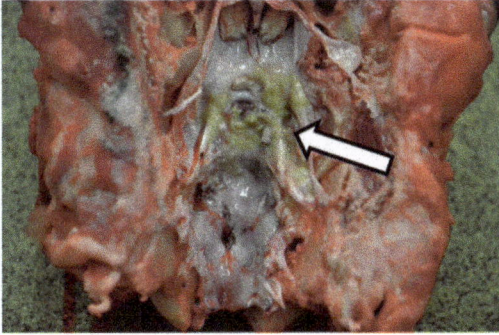

Fig. 14.3. An abscess of the brain base in a 3-year-old ram (photo Helen Williams and Niall Connolly).

or otitis (Fig. 14.3). It is seen more commonly in rams, likely due to damage whilst fighting. The abscess can cause inflammation or compression of the surrounding structures including the hypothalamus, brain stem or retrobulbar region and clinical signs will vary depending on the structures affected. Many cases have similar clinical signs to listeria with depression, anorexia and ataxia and cranial nerve deficits causing unilateral facial paralysis, circling and head tilt. Most affected sheep will have a wide-based stance and extended head. Other clinical signs present in some cases, which may help differentiate the disease from listeria, include bradycardia, exophthalmos and blindness. Treatment is not usually successful, so euthanasia is recommended. Definitive diagnosis is usually made at post-mortem examination.

Non-suppurative Brain Diseases

Cerebrocortical necrosis (CCN, Polioencephalomalacia, 'brain rot')

This is an acute central nervous disease, mainly affecting lambs 2–6 months old (not under 2 months, as it requires a functional rumen), but it may also affect adults. It usually occurs sporadically and 'out of the blue' but there are occasional outbreaks affecting a small number of sheep and lasting a few weeks following a history of a diet (or other) change such as feeding a high level of concentrates, moving to lush pasture or post worm drenching. It is associated with a deficiency of thiamine resultant on both a reduction in thiamine synthesis by the rumen flora, and increased rumen thiamine breakdown due to microbial production of thiaminase in the rumen, e.g. by *Clostridium sporogenes* and *Bacillus thiaminolyticus*. It is postulated that this resulting thiamine deficiency is associated with defects in carbohydrate metabolism in the CNS astrocyte cells such that ATP production by these cells is reduced resulting in cellular damage, leading to cerebral oedema and subsequent pressure necrosis. Diets which are high in sulphur can also induce or exacerbate thiamine-related polioencephalomalacia.

Clinical signs

After a short period (a few hours) of aloofness, dullness and wandering, often 'star gazing' (even circling), the sheep becomes increasingly excitable (over another few hours, even up to 2 days), developing tremors, staggering, bilateral blindness, bilateral strabismus, recumbency, opisthotonus and galloping movements. In some cases, the animal may be found dead. The presence of opisthotonus and bilateral blindness should help to differentiate it from such conditions as pulpy kidney, listeriosis, gid, pregnancy toxaemia and hypomagnesaemia, but it requires some confidence to avoid a 'mass medication' approach at the first examination.

Diagnosis

Diagnosis in the live animal is often made based on clinical signs and response to vitamin B1 treatment. In the dead animal, PME shows bilateral discolouration of cortical gyri and bright white fluorescence under Wood's lamp of the sliced cortex, and the diagnosis can be confirmed histologically.

Treatment

Give 200–500 mg thiamine (vitamin B_1) by slow intravenous injection initially. This should be repeated by intramuscular injection (IM) at 4-hourly intervals up to four times if required. Some veterinarians advise daily IM treatment for a few days. If the case has been 'caught early' (i.e. before much irreversible necrosis), improvement can be expected within hours (not minutes). A sheep showing a positive response to treatment will be quieter and have fewer convulsions, and often there is complete recovery within days, although vision often takes longer to return.

Control

It is reasonable to look at the diet and perhaps suggest changing it; for example, removal from lush grazing or removal/reduction of concentrate feed or lick (e.g. molasses), but such management changes are often speculative in terms of addressing risk factors. There is some suggestion that clinically unaffected group members may appear not to be thriving and may show signs of scouring; thus, it is advisable to inspect the whole at-risk group not just the clinically affected animals identified by the farmer. Some authorities advocate injection of all group members with 500 mg thiamine, but the incidence does not usually justify such intervention.

Lead Toxicity

Subacute lead toxicity may present with similar clinical signs to CCN and listeriosis. Lead competes with calcium, affecting the central nervous system and neuromuscular transmission. This should be considered a differential diagnosis where animals have access to land with a history of lead mining, or contaminated with abandoned lead-acid batteries, bonfire ash, in particular burned building materials, electrical wiring or vehicles, vehicle sump oil, or lead shot from clay pigeon shooting. In the housed environment, lead from old paints and sealants may also cause a problem, particularly when starting to flake. The main clinical signs are extreme dullness, muscle weakness, ataxia, intermittent convulsions and blindness with palpebral reflex absent or reduced, and death. There may be signs of abdominal pain due to ruminal atony and gastroenteritis with constipation progressing to fetid diarrhoea. Diagnosis is often by clinical signs but blood or renal lead concentrations will support diagnosis. A chronic form of lead poisoning associated with access to old lead-mine workings has been described with signs of stiffness and locomotory difficulties, osteoporosis and occasional bone fractures or deformities being observed. If a diagnosis of lead poisoning is confirmed, it is advisable to inform the relevant authorities, namely APHA or Food Standards Scotland (FSS), due to any potential human health implications. Treatment of affected animals is based around chelating available lead using sodium calcium edetate and supportive therapy.

Scrapie

Scrapie is a chronic progressive neurodegenerative disease of adult sheep (and goats). Scrapie is classified as a transmissible spongiform encephalopathy (TSE). There are two forms of this fatal disease, classical and atypical. While atypical scrapie has been identified worldwide, Australia and New Zealand remain free of it.

Scrapie is a notifiable disease in the UK and is actively monitored on an EU-wide basis with the aim of eventual eradication. In the last few years, the number of diagnosed cases in the UK has fallen to a very low level probably due, at least in part, to the genotyping programme which has been in place since 1991.

Classical scrapie

The disease

Scrapie is the result of a misfolding and accumulation of an abnormal form of cellular prion protein (PrP) within various tissues, especially the brain. Although not fully understood, normal PrP functions are thought to include memory, circadian rhythm, calcium homeostasis, myelin maintenance and neuroprotection. Scrapie usually enters a flock through introduction of an infected animal, which is incubating the disease. Once in a flock, it can be spread via vertical transmission from a dam to its genetically susceptible lambs via colostrum and milk. The fetal fluids and membranes are also highly infective and can lead to contamination of the environment and subsequent horizontal transmission. The scrapie agent may persist for several years and is very resistant to heat, formalin and UV light.

Due to its long incubation period the disease most commonly affects sheep between 2 and 5 years of age. True incidence is difficult to assess as there is probably under-reporting and some cases may not be recognized. Usually, just one or two cases occur from year to year in an affected flock; however, outbreaks may occur where there is a high incidence of genetically susceptible individuals born at the same time.

Following the BSE epidemic in the 1990s, European-wide regulations were amended to ensure that controls at the animal level and food chain were in place throughout the UK and EU. Specified offal including brain, eyes, tonsils, spinal cord, ileum and spleen of sheep over 6 months of age were classified as Category 1 materials to be disposed of by incineration, ensuring complete removal from the food chain to prevent possible recycling of infection and to protect human health. Feeding ruminant-derived protein to sheep (and other animals) is banned.

Genetic background and monitoring

It has long been recognized that there is a genetic susceptibility to the disease. Sheep have two copies of the PrP gene, which encode for the production of PrP or prion protein. This protein consists of 256 amino acids and is found in the brain and lymphoid tissues. It is the production of abnormal (misfolded) PrP protein that leads to the development of the disease. There are three sites (codons) on the gene which are significant in determining whether an animal is susceptible or resistant to infection. These are codons 136, 154 and 171. There are five different allele combinations and 15 different genotypes depending on which alleles are inherited from each parent. The genotype is written as ARR/ARR, ARR/AHQ, ARR/VRQ, etc. and sheep are classed in five different categories (Type 1–5) according to susceptibility (see Table 14.3).

In 2001 the National Scrapie Plan was introduced in the UK to promote the breeding of genetically resistant sheep by genotyping. This was largely successful and resulted in a sharp decline in reported cases such that the incidence of scrapie is now

believed to be very low. As a result, this scheme has closed; however, there is an option for flocks to become scrapie-free monitored, which is required for export. There is random testing of deadstock and carcasses and a compulsory scheme for flocks where cases of classical scrapie are confirmed.

Clinical signs

Clinical signs vary and are usually seen in animals over 2 years of age. The most common are shown below and may be present singly or in any combination:

- A change in temperament or behaviour, sometimes the sheep appearing apprehensive, wild and excitable. Some other cases just look dazed and depressed and do not appear to focus properly.
- The most common and obvious sign is irritation, with scratching, rubbing, sucking and nibbling the fleece in an adult sheep. It is often seen at first as restlessness with the sheep darting about from place to place as if it has been bitten, and turning to nibble anywhere it can get at, as well as rubbing on posts and walls, etc. (watching a case one could imagine it feels like 'prickly heat'). The rubbing leads to a loss of fleece or hair over any area which the sheep can get at, including the head and both sides of the flank and hind legs. A fine rough stubble is left, often with scabs. If one rubs the sheep, it responds by standing still and nibbling its lips in apparent pleasure and relief. Note that this test is applicable for all conditions causing pruritus and is not diagnostic of scrapie. If several sheep are affected, remember the possibility of external parasites.
- Change in posture and gait – these usually show incoordination, so that the sheep becomes awkward to catch and to examine. Often, it will not relax sufficiently to allow its head to be held comfortably for a clinical examination. Rams can be quite dangerous and the difficulty in raising the head can suggest a high cervical lesion (e.g. from fighting).

If allowed to live, all these signs worsen over the weeks and sometimes months, and although there is sometimes a temporary stasis or even remission, all animals become progressively thinner and die sooner or later.

Diagnosis

The clinical signs are eventually diagnostic but, obviously, primary skin conditions (e.g. sheep scab) must be ruled out. If in doubt, notify the local

Table 14.3. Alleles[a] involved and their genotypic combinations showing the degree of resistance to classical scrapie.

Codon					
136	154	171	Genotype	Type	Resistance
A	R	R	ARR/ARR	1	+++++
			ARR/AHQ	2	+++
			ARR/ARH		
			ARR/ARQ		
A	H	Q	AHQ/AHQ	3	++
			AHQ/ARH		
			AHQ/ARQ		
A	R	H	ARH/ARH		
			ARH/ARQ		
A	R	Q	ARQ/ARQ		
V	R	Q	ARR/VRQ	4	+
			AHQ/VRQ	5	-
			ARH/VRQ		
			ARQ/VRQ		
			VRQ/VRQ		

[a]A, alanine; R, arginine; H, histidine; Q, glutamine; V, valine.

APHA Office which will arrange examination of the suspect animal, with slaughter and laboratory testing if the disease is suspected. Diagnosis is by immunohistochemistry or rapid immunochemistry, although definitive diagnosis is by brain histology looking for characteristic lesions (these differ between different TSE strains, e.g. the lesion 'profiles' of BSE and classical scrapie are different and distinctive). There is no diagnostic test currently in use in the live animal, although promising results have been achieved by taking biopsy samples of the third eyelid or rectal mucosa immediately adjacent to the anus, which contain lymphoid follicles. These can then be subjected to immunohistochemistry.

If classical scrapie is confirmed, there is a compulsory scheme consisting of genotyping the flock and culling of susceptible genotypes.

Atypical scrapie – a complication

This was first reported in Norway in 1998 and since then a small number of so-called atypical scrapie cases have been identified by surveillance activities in several countries including the UK, where out of over 100,000 random sheep tested, only about 80 were positive. Atypical scrapie appears to differ from classical scrapie and BSE in that there is an absence of vertical transmission in atypical scrapie. The disease only affects one or a small number of animals (usually over 5 years of age) within a flock. Most notably, some cases have had the resistant ARR genotype. The significance of atypical scrapie is unknown but restrictions are not currently placed on flocks if incidence is low. In the case of atypical scrapie, the flock is monitored for 2 years by APHA.

Tetanus

This disease, most commonly seen in young or growing lambs, should not occur if clostridial vaccination has been correctly carried out, since the vaccine is highly effective. It does, however, rely on passive transfer of antibodies via the colostrum, so the disease can occur in vaccinated flocks where colostrum management has been poor. It also needs to be remembered that passive protection only lasts 12–16 weeks, so lambs require active protection after this stage. Most lambs are at risk, since the causal organism, *Clostridium tetani*, is widespread in the environment in the form of very resistant

spores. Routine procedures such as tailing and castration provide perfect sites for the bacteria to multiply and to release the toxins which cause the characteristic clinical signs. Adults are also at risk through injuries or associated with bad lambings.

Clinical signs

These should be easily recognized:

(i) rigidity of muscles, with the affected animal in lateral recumbency with limbs rigidly extended, jaw tightly closed, tail and ears held in a fixed position;
(ii) spasm of the third eyelid; and
(iii) in older animals, bloating of the rumen since they are unable to eructate gas.

Treatment

This is usually unrewarding – consideration should be given to euthanasia on diagnosis. Penicillin is effective against the bacteria and antitoxin can be given to try to 'mop up' free toxins; sedation to help relax muscles and good nursing may help, but the prognosis is always poor.

Prevention

Implementation of a comprehensive clostridial vaccination policy for the flock including vaccination of rams, ewes before lambing and lambs from 6–8 weeks. As for all clostridial diseases, two doses of vaccine 4–6 weeks apart are necessary to provide active immunity. The majority of clostridial vaccines provide tetanus coverage.

Other Neurological Disorders

Focal symmetrical encephalomalacia is associated with *C. perfringens* type D enterotoxaemia, causing vague neurological signs, recumbency and death mainly in growing lambs. However, sheep with classic pulpy kidney disease due to *C. perfringens* type D also exhibit neurological signs including convulsions prior to death and, furthermore, definitive diagnosis is by brain histopathology.

Maedi visna (MV) is an ultimately fatal viral disease of sheep. The disease has a long incubation period, is highly infectious and is difficult to diagnose on clinical signs alone. The symptoms include: pneumonia, progressive weakness leading to paralysis, wasting, arthritis and chronic mastitis. The nervous form of the disease is very rare in sheep. Where nervous signs are suspected, these include hindlimb weakness and ataxia, hypermetria, and paralysis, usually leading to recumbency although affected sheep remain alert and responsive to external stimuli. The main neurological lesions observed are encephalitis or encephalomyelitis usually accompanied by demyelination. See Chapters 13 and 18 for more information about the disease and its control via flock health schemes.

Spinal Disease

Spinal diseases cause sensory and motor defects, which are most obviously seen affecting the limbs in sheep. There is a large range in severity from weakness to paresis and the signs seen vary depending on the level of the lesion. The lesions may be congenital, e.g. swayback (see Chapter 7), or acquired, such as injury or infection. Injury is less common than infection but should be considered when there is an acute onset of clinical signs or a history of trauma.

Vertebral osteomyelitis/spinal abscess

This is most common in lambs 1–4 months old but can affect any age. It is thought that cases develop from haematogenous spread, e.g. from an infected navel or tail post docking. Clinical signs will depend on the location of the abscess. Most are in the thoracolumbar region, which causes paresis of the hind limbs but usually the lamb remains bright. Diagnosis can be aided by CSF examination which will demonstrate increased protein concentrations, if taken caudal to a compressive spinal lesion such as an abscess. If there is sufficient bony change it will be evident on radiography. Prognosis is usually hopeless, despite treatment, so euthanasia is recommended.

Compressive cervical myelopathy (wobbler syndrome)

This is a disease which has been described in young Texel and Beltex rams, causing ataxia and weakness. Although the clinical signs are similar to wobbler disease in horses, which is caused by the presence of bony malformations, in sheep it is caused by a fatty nodule protruding from the dorsolateral intervertebral space at C6-7 compressing the spinal cord at this level. The disease is seen in rams typically around 15–18 months old and is slowly progressive. Clinical signs include a wide-based stance and ataxia of the hind limbs and dysmetria of the forelimbs with exaggerated withdrawal reflexes. As the case progresses the ram may collapse when moved.

Louping-ill

See Chapter 16.

Kangaroo gait

This affects ewes, usually during lactation, and is a neuropathy of the nerves supplying the forelimbs, especially the radial nerve. Affected animals have difficulty using their forelimbs and, as the name suggests, have a strange gait resembling that of a kangaroo. Surprisingly, most cases recover after a few weeks. Weaning may hasten this. Until they recover they need general nursing care to make sure they are able to get sufficient to eat.

Ryegrass Staggers

This is occasionally seen in the UK and more commonly in Australia and New Zealand where it can be a serious flock problem. This is a mycotoxicosis (a toxin produced by an endophyte which is found in ryegrass), causing staggering and tremors. Affected animals may fall into ditches or streams and drown, or are attacked by predators. Recovery usually occurs if removed from the affected pasture.

15 Eyes, Ears and Nose

HELEN WILLIAMS* AND NIALL CONNOLLY

Department of Livestock and One Health, Institute of Infection, Veterinary and Ecological Sciences, University of Liverpool, UK

Abstract

Diseases affecting the structures of the face of sheep are quite common, in particular those involving the eyes which can cause major welfare issues and blindness if neglected. Lesions affecting the skin of the face and ears are also regularly seen and altered ear position may indicate more systemic issues.

Eye Diseases

Eye problems in sheep are common and can have a considerable impact on sheep welfare. Many eye diseases will cause direct ocular pain, with progression potentially leading to permanent damage including blindness. Any loss of vision, either caused by damage to the eye itself or central (brain and optic nerve) blindness, will adversely affect the welfare and the productivity of that animal.

Diagnosis and treating appropriately are important for both individual sheep and protecting the rest of the flock. Initial history taken should include the age and stage of production of the sheep affected, whether it is a single animal or multiple and whether any co-existing systemic illness has been noted.

On a practical level it is useful to consider eye diseases in sheep as two groups for differential diagnoses:

1. Those that present with painful superficial changes affecting the conjunctiva and/or cornea; deeper structures including the iris and anterior chamber may also be involved. Blepharospasm and lacrimation will feature but systemic disease is not usually seen.

The three most common conditions in this category are:

- entropion
- ovine infectious keratoconjunctivitis (Pink eye)
- ovine iritis/uveitis (silage eye).

2. Those that present with blindness and no gross superficial changes. In some cases, abnormalities of the lens or retina may be visible on closer examination; alternatively, the blindness may be neurological in origin and the eye itself remains unaffected. Ocular pain is not always a feature, but in some cases systemic disease may be present. The most common are:

- bright blindness (ptaquiloside toxicity from bracken ingestion);
- closantel toxicity;
- pregnancy toxaemia – See chapter 6;
- lead toxicity – see Chapter 14;
- polioencephalomalacia (cerebrocortical necrosis, CCN) – see Chapter 14; and
- inherited/congenital blindness.

Ocular examination

i. Assess the eyelids for entropion (mainly in lambs) and any abnormalities such as peri-orbital eczema or trauma.

ii. Assess the degree of ocular pain indicated by degree of blepharospasm and lacrimation or discharge.

iii. Assess the conjunctiva for reddening.

iv. Assess the cornea for opacity and ulceration. Application of fluorescein will help determine if an ulcer is present.

v. If possible, use an ophthalmoscope to examine the anterior chamber, iris, lens and retina.

vi. Note whether the pupil responds to light or is constricted suggesting uveitis.

*Email: he1enw@liverpool.ac.uk

© CAB International 2025. *A Handbook for the Sheep Clinician, 8th Edition*
(A.C. Winter and D. Grove-White eds)
DOI: 10.1079/9781800626355.0015

Entropion

Entropion is common in newborn lambs, involving one or both lower eyelids (Fig. 15.1). The in-turned eyelids will quickly cause corneal damage and secondary infection if untreated. The incidence varies between flocks with some evidence of heritability, which is likely to account for the difference. The eyes of any lambs showing ocular discharge should be carefully examined for entropion before assuming it is an eye infection alone. Entropion can also occur less commonly in very thin adult sheep as a result of loss of the fat pad behind the eye.

Treatment and control

In mild entropion cases the eyelid can be easily everted by finger pressure, particularly in newborn lambs. In flocks with an entropion problem, an 'eyelid' check should be routine with correction done as often as necessary and as soon as possible after birth. More severe cases, where the lower eyelid is repeatedly turned in, causing blepharospasm, keratitis and corneal ulceration, require more vigorous attention with options including:

- subcutaneous injection of 0.5–1ml of long-acting penicillin below the margin of the affected lid, after manual correction, sufficient to produce a bleb which everts the lid. This will also treat any infection that may have resulted;
- placing a tuck in the skin below the lid with 14 mm or 16mm Michel clips (Fig.15.2); and
- surgical correction as described for small animals is effective, but this is rarely necessary.

Most cases that have not been corrected immediately after birth merit topical antibiotic eye ointment at the time and for the next day or so to treat any infection which has become established.

On farms where the incidence is high the breeding lines should be considered. If there is a sudden increase, has a new ram been used? It is sensible to mark and record each case so breeding from them can be avoided.

Ovine infectious keratoconjunctivitis (OIKC, contagious ophthalmia, pink eye, New Forest eye, cloudy eye, snow blindness)

This is a very common painful disease affecting sheep's eyes worldwide. The disease can be sporadic, but devastating outbreaks can occur. These often arise in the winter when sheep are gathered close together, e.g. feeding and housing.

There is a wide range of severity of clinical signs. Both eyes are usually affected but not always simultaneously, nor to the same extent. In many cases there is only superficial damage resulting in conjunctivitis, scleral congestion and excessive lacrimation. These

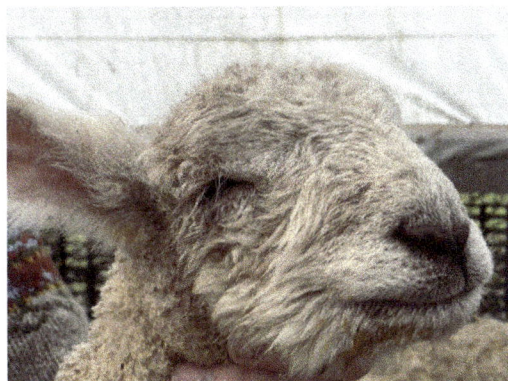

Fig. 15.1. Uncorrected entropion in a lamb of a few days old (photo Agnes Winter).

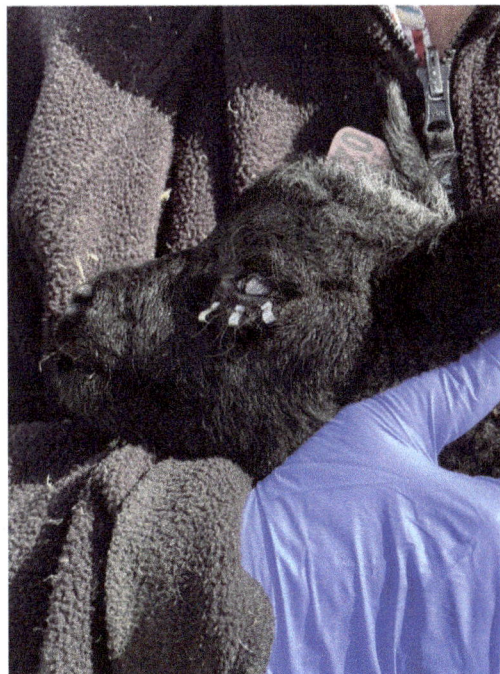

Fig. 15.2. Entropion corrected using Michel clips (photo Agnes Winter).

sheep respond by blinking, progressing to blepharospasm. Keratitis and corneal ulceration occur in more severe cases with neovascularization and pannus spreading from the corneo-scleral margin (Fig. 15.3). This can lead to temporary or even permanent blindness. Severely affected sheep will find it difficult to find food and are accident prone, further compromising their welfare.

Mycoplasma conjunctivae is believed to be the primary organism causing OIKC. However, there is often mixed infection with bacteria including *Moraxella boviculi*, *Staph. aureus*, *Listeria monocytogenes* and *Chlamydia* spp., which may play a role in increasing the severity of the ocular reaction. Even after treatment and apparent recovery, *M. conjunctivae* can be found in the conjunctival sac for long periods resulting in a carrier state, meaning recurrence in individual affected sheep is common and outbreaks are often prolonged. Many outbreaks can be traced back to the purchase of new sheep or rams. It is useful to sample affected sheep to identify the cause – consult the laboratory for type of sample required. Bacterial culture is slow but PCR techniques can produce results within 24 hours.

Treatment

Treatment, especially in the case of outbreaks, is often frustrating as bacterial cure is usually unsuccessful.

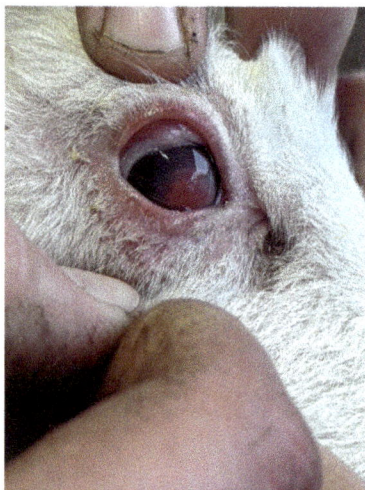

Fig. 15.3. Healing corneal ulcer caused by entropion after correction with penicillin injection into lower eyelid (photo Helen Williams and Niall Connolly).

Despite this, treatment will lessen the severity of disease and reduce time to resolution, improving the welfare of severely affected sheep. There is a lack of evidence base surrounding treatment so often a wide variety of remedies have been tried. It is likely that a flock-level immune response slowly develops to resolve the outbreak rather than any treatment eradicating the disease. There is currently no evidence base regarding whether use of antibiotics will make a carrier state more or less likely than waiting for resolution from an immune response.

In the UK currently the only licensed treatments for ocular disease in sheep are a long-acting preparation of oxytetracycline administered intramuscularly or an eye ointment containing cloxacillin. As *Mycoplasma* spp. are not susceptible to penicillin-based products it is likely that any improvement seen with this treatment is due to reduction in secondary infection or self-cure. Therefore, as a first line treatment a single injection of oxytetracycline is the most practical treatment, particularly if large numbers of animals are affected. Use of other longer acting antibiotics has been tried (e.g. Florfenicol) and subconjunctival injection of antibiotic will increase local concentration of antibiotics which may be beneficial; however, there is no evidence base to support this off-licence use. Administration of a non-steroidal anti-inflammatory drug is indicated in severely affected cases. Separation from the group may be necessary in order to ensure proper care and treatment and may help reduce spread. However, in most cases it is impractical to completely separate cases for long periods of time needed to achieve bacterial cure.

Prevention

The frequent movement and mixing of sheep are obvious hazards and should be kept to a minimum. In order to reduce the risk of importing fresh strains of *M. conjunctivae* into the flock, purchased sheep, e.g. rams, should be quarantined and monitored for eye disease during this time although there is always the risk of these animals being carriers. Antibiotic administration to such animals in an effort to prevent disease introduction is not justified.

Silage eye

Listeria monocytogenes may occasionally be implicated in eye problems as in 'silage eye' in cattle, although this is uveitis/iritis rather than keratoconjunctivitis so should be distinguishable clinically.

Infection probably gains entry to the eye as a result of the sheep burrowing their heads into silage when feeding so it is usually associated with big-bale silage feeding but may also occur if any silage is not cleared away regularly (uncleared silage allows multiplication of the bacteria). Examination of the eye may show folding of the iris with inflammatory changes progressing from the edges of the pupil accompanied by clumps of fibrin underneath the cornea. Unlike in OIKC, corneal ulceration is not a feature. Treatment is by subconjunctival injection of steroid, to alleviate the uveitis. However, due to the risk of secondary infection and immunosuppression from the steroid this should be combined with an antibiotic.

Prevention can be attempted by avoiding contamination of silage with soil, preventing damage to the wrapping of big bales and providing only sufficient silage so that it is eaten within 2 days.

Bright blindness (clear blind, glass-eyed)

This is an irreversible blindness in adult sheep, mainly reported in flocks in the north of England, but occurring in hill flocks in other areas. The condition affects both eyes equally and simultaneously. The retina shows progressive degeneration with atrophy of the rods and cones; the tapetal arteries and veins are narrowed and there is a marked green reflection from the tapetum. Ophthalmoscopic examination of the retina is easy because the pupils are dilated, and the cornea and lens are clear.

It is caused by a toxic factor in bracken (Ptaquiloside) and may require several seasons of bracken consumption before signs become apparent; it is therefore only seen in adult sheep. The prevalence may be over 5% and usually becomes apparent in the autumn following the bracken growth season.

As the condition is slowly progressive, the sheep have time to adapt, and the blindness may only become apparent when the sheep are driven or placed in strange surroundings. They are not unwell, appearing perhaps more alert than usual and are not easy to catch. They are, however, more prone to accidents and to getting lost. They will require culling.

Closantel toxicity

The anthelmintic closantel has a relatively low safety index. Blindness associated with optic neuropathy has been reported at only 1.6 times the recommended dosage. If the overdose is greater, neurological signs such as ataxia and depression are seen, and in severe cases, there is recumbency and death. Onset of clinical signs has been reported to be between 2 and 17 days post overdose, and it is likely that this range is related to the severity of the overdose.

Other genetic defects

Occasionally, lambs, particularly Texels, are born with very small eyes (microphthalmia) or no eyes (anophthalmia). In some breeds with a gene for four horns (e.g. Jacob or Hebridean), sheep may have a defect in the upper eyelid (split eyelid) which, if severe, can predispose to eye infections and subsequent blindness. Inherited night blindness has been described in Wiltshire sheep with the onset of clinical signs being around 2–3 years, where affected sheep struggle to negotiate objects such as gates and fences in low-light conditions due to retinal degeneration. Autosomal recessive gene mutations have given rise to day blindness due to cone destruction in Awassi sheep. As with any inherited disease, certain breeding lines should be investigated and avoided.

Ear Problems

The ear may be involved in a number of different diseases but allowing the ears to droop is usually a general sign that a sheep is unwell. (However, note that normal ear position is very variable between breeds – contrast, for example, Suffolks with Border Leicesters for extremes of normal appearance.)

Specific problems include:

- paralysis of (usually one) ear – listeriosis and middle-ear infection (see Chapter 14);
- rubbing and shaking, with hematoma formation – see *Psoroptes ovis* (*cuniculi*) infection (Chapter 12);
- scabbiness – sunburn, dermatophilus, orf, ringworm (see Chapter 12); and
- swelling of the ears and head – see photosensitization (Chapter 12) and bluetongue (see Chapter 17).

Nose Problems

Nasal discharge

Nasal discharge can be seen in systemic or local disease.

1. Systemic diseases with nasal discharge:

- OPA – affected sheep show weight loss and pass copious clear mucoid discharge, which increases in amount when the sheep's rear end is lifted (the 'wheelbarrow test'; see Chapter 13).
- Pneumonia caused by pasteurellosis or *Mycoplasma ovipneumoniae* causes a serous discharge often accompanied by a cough and, in the case of pasteurellosis, a raised temperature (see Chapter 13).
- Hypocalcaemia – a clear mucoid discharge (saliva) may be seen in a collapsed heavily pregnant or recently lambed ewe (see Chapter 6).
- Regurgitated rumen contents – these may be present in the case of, e.g. rhododendron toxicity, or in advanced cases of hypocalcaemia; this is indicated by green-coloured discharge with a typical smell.

2. Local nasal disease:

- Nasal bots can cause a dirty, possibly bloodstained discharge which can be unilateral and bilateral, accompanied by sneezing.
- Maxillary tooth root abscess will produce a unilateral purulent discharge often with a associated facial swelling.

- Nasal tumour, e.g. adenocarcinoma, is a rare cause of serosanginous discharge often with unilateral airflow disturbance.

Nasal bots

The fly *Oestrus ovis*, which lays larvae inside the nostrils of sheep, is found worldwide but is rarely a serious problem in the UK. The larvae move into the sinuses where they develop over about 6 weeks, or much longer in winter, before the sheep sneeze them out onto the ground where they pupate and complete their life cycle. The adult flies cause a nuisance to the sheep and the larvae cause nasal discharge. Anthelmintics containing ivermectin, doramectin or moxidectin can be used to treat individual animals with clinical signs but preventative treatment is not usually warranted.

Enzootic nasal tumor

This is not a problem in the UK but may be seen in some other countries, for example in southern Europe. It is caused by a retrovirus (ENTV-1) similar to that causing OPA.

Helen Williams and Niall Connolly

16 Ticks and Tick-borne Diseases

JOHN GRAHAM-BROWN*

Department of Livestock and One Health, Institute of Infection, Veterinary and Ecological Sciences, University of Liverpool, UK

Abstract

This chapter covers problems and diseases caused by ticks. These are a world-wide problem but only diseases of importance in UK are covered here, particularly tickborne fever, tick pyaemia and louping-ill. Control is difficult because of the short time spent on hosts and the involvement of wildlife in their life cycle.

Sheep act as a host for many tick species and their associated tick-borne diseases (TBDs) throughout the world with wide-ranging diversity in terms of their epidemiology and significance. This is especially in tropical regions. The majority of these will not be discussed here. This chapter covers ticks of importance in the UK and the diseases they transmit.

UK Tick Rcology

There are presently two tick species notable for their role in primary parasitism and transmission of TBDs to and from sheep in the UK:

1. *Ixodes ricinus* (sheep tick or castor bean tick) is by far the most important and common with nation-wide distribution and a particularly high prevalence in the south of England, Wales and the Scottish Highlands. It is commonly found in areas of scrub, heath and woodlands, and the pastures adjoining these areas (Figs 16.1. and 16.2). Wildlife, particularly deer, birds and rodents play an important role in supporting and distributing tick populations. Outside the UK, *I. ricinus* has a wide geographical distribution from the Atlas Mountains in North Africa in the south, to Iceland, Sweden and Russia in the north, extending eastwards to Iran and westwards to Ireland. It is found extensively throughout central Europe including Austria, Switzerland, Poland and Slovenia.

2. *Haemaphysalis punctata* (red sheep tick) has a much more localized distribution in the UK, limited to south-east England and the western coastal area of Wales due to its predilection for grasslands, and in particular, chalk downs and marshland. Reports suggest populations of *H. punctata* are increasingly abundant in many of the regions in which it is present.

Both of these species are hard ticks (Ixodidae) and follow broadly similar life histories with three blood-feeding developmental stages (six-legged nymphs, eight-legged larvae and mature adults). Both species are 'three-host ticks', meaning over the course of their life cycle they will mount and feed off three separate hosts for a period of 3–5 days as larvae and nymphs, and 2–3 weeks as adults. After feeding, nymphs and larvae moult to the next life stage in the environment. Adult ticks (males and females) reproduce during their final feed, with the female subsequently producing clutches of several thousand eggs into the environment before dying. Despite their common names, neither tick species is host-specific. Nymphs and larvae are more usually found parasitizing small mammals (rodents) and birds, whilst adult ticks tend to parasitize larger mammals, including sheep, cattle, deer, companion animals (dogs, cats, horses) and humans.

Tick activity in the UK is highly dependent upon climate, particularly temperature and humidity. The majority of questing (seeking out a host) and feeding activity occurs between March and November once temperatures are consistently elevated above

*Email: J.Graham-Brown@liverpool.ac.uk

© CAB International 2025. *A Handbook for the Sheep Clinician, 8th Edition* (A.C. Winter and D. Grove-White eds)
DOI: 10.1079/9781800626355.0016

151

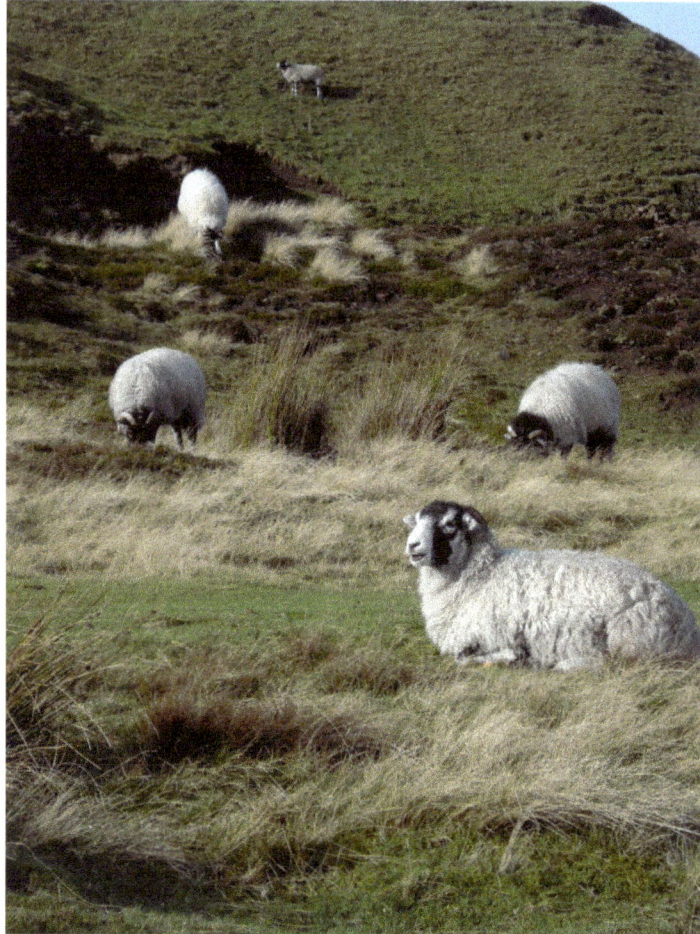

Fig. 16.1. Moorland with heather is a typical tick habitat (photo Agnes Winter).

7°C, with peaks of activity and pasture burdens observed in the spring due to re-emergence of over-wintered ticks following a period of diapause (arrested development), and autumn once new life stages emerge post-moult following a blood meal earlier in the season. These spring and autumn peaks may be further accentuated by hot, dry summers when ticks will reduce their questing behaviour to avoid desiccation. These various aspects of climate and tick biology lead to the classical view of *I. ricinus* (and *H. punctata*) requiring three years to complete their life cycle from larva to adult, with diapause over winter between consecutive moults and blood meals. There is, however, increasing evidence in the UK to show ticks can remain active throughout the winter months and, under optimal conditions, achieve up to two moults within the season. This is largely attributed to changing weather patterns and is of significance since it has the potential to fundamentally alter the generation interval and reproductive potential of these native tick species in a manner that is detrimental to animal health. Importantly, these changing weather patterns combined with the role of migratory birds and/or companion animals travelling abroad as competent hosts, also have implications for the introduction of new tick species (and their associated diseases) to the UK.

John Graham-Brown

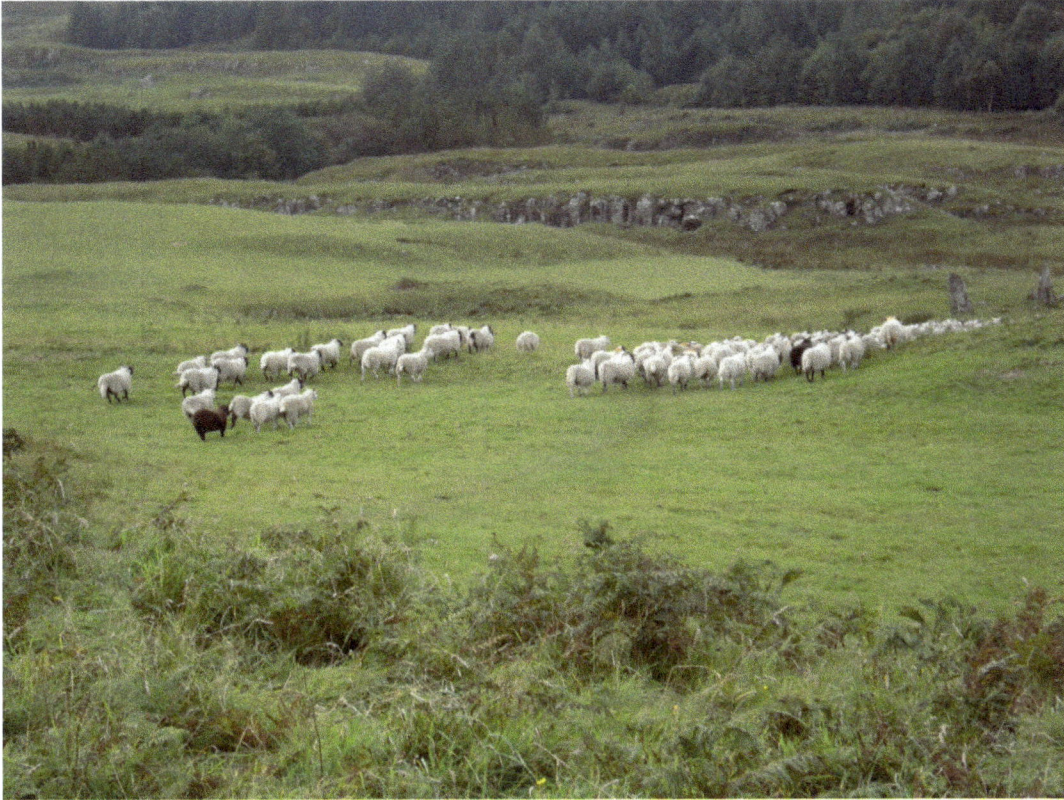

Fig. 16.2. The rough vegetation in the foreground could provide a habitat for ticks (photo Agnes Winter).

Clinical significance

Ticks are commonly found attached and feeding on sheep in areas of hairy or bare skin, particularly the axillae, inguinal and peri-anal regions, and less so in full fleece. Burdens can vary significantly between animals even when grazing the same pastures. Typically, older (bigger) animals have higher burdens, which is principally important from the perspective of onward transmission rather than clinical disease, since these animals are usually also more resilient.

As blood-feeding parasites, ticks are a cause of primary pathology and 'worry' in their own right, in particular causing anaemia and general malaise when young lambs are exposed to high-risk pastures soon after turnout. Bite wounds can become purulent and non-healing, allowing establishment of secondary infections (including with blowflies). More usually, however, primary effects form part of a wider impact on animal health that includes TBDs. In the UK, at present, tick-borne fever (TBF), tick-bite pyaemia and louping-ill are the most common and clinically significant TBDs of sheep. Additionally, a number of piroplasms (*Babesia* and *Theileria* species) have been detected in UK sheep and tick populations. It is also important to note that sheep and their tick populations are important from a wider One Health perspective, acting as a reservoir for various (anthropo-) zoonoses, most significantly Lyme disease, but also rickettsial diseases (e.g. Mediterranean spotted fever) and piroplasms (*Babesia venatorium* and *B. motase*), all of which have been identified in UK sheep and/or their associated ticks. Whilst Q fever is sometimes discussed in the context of ticks and TBDs, there is no evidence to suggest this is a significant route of transmission in the UK.

Tick control

For the reasons discussed relating to changing climate, it is likely control of ticks (and TBDs) will become more challenging. It is important to be realistic when devising control programmes in tick-infested areas. The fact that ticks spend virtually none of their time on hosts (~30 days spent feeding over a 3-year lifespan) combined with the role of sylvatic host species (rodents, birds, deer etc.) makes their elimination from suitable habitats impossible. Disease-control measures should therefore be aimed principally at minimizing risk. Importantly, this must include balancing ongoing exposure to allow animals to become acclimatized to tick burdens and establish immunity to any TBDs present without precipitating clinical disease.

Improving pastures and environment practices

Historically, draining and re-seeding lower pastures bordering high hills in tick-infested areas to improve lambing percentage and live-weight gains in lambs has had a dramatic effect on their tick populations. Where they are still grazed alongside unimproved scrub and heathland, such pastures may become re-infested over time, particularly in those areas bordering wilder habitats. Whilst not performed specifically for tick control, controlled burning of heather on moorlands, where practised, can similarly have a significant impact in reducing tick populations, although this is clearly a highly contentious issue in the wider debate on land management and the environment. Relating to this, consideration should also be given to the implications of modern concepts such as regenerative farming where livestock are used as part of a wider strategy to restore biodiversity and ecological balance to the rural landscape; whilst these are laudable concepts, it is likely such changes will be favourable for ticks, TBDs and their sylvatic hosts, potentially necessitating more frequent acaricide treatments with their own environmental implications.

Acaricide treatments

Both organophosphate (OP) diazinon dip and synthetic pyrethroids (SP), namely deltamethrin and cypermethrin 'pour-on' or 'spot-on' products, are licensed and available in the UK for control of ticks in sheep. All of these products have persistent activity of several weeks against ticks.

Whilst used principally for the treatment and elimination of sheep scab in the UK, plunge-dipping with diazinon is highly effective against ticks. This option is logistically challenging, usually requiring specialist equipment and qualified, certified personnel

to conduct safely and effectively. Dipping of lambs can also lead to mismothering. Post-treatment dipped animals will be protected against re-infestation for up to 6 weeks.

The SPs represent a more convenient means of chemical control, although their use is generally considered more problematic in terms of their environmental implications when compared with OPs. To maximize efficacy and minimize environmental contamination it is important that these are applied as per the manufacturer's recommendations. These usually stipulate topical application directly onto the skin by parting the fleece down the midline from the shoulders towards the rump. It is also important that their application is not immediately prior to periods of rainfall that may wash off the product prematurely. After correct application the drug spreads over the skin surface in the sebum and will provide continuous control ticks for 3–12 weeks depending upon the product used (check the data sheet for claims of specific products). Pour-on SPs are particularly useful for treating lambs during peak risk periods of infestation, since they rapidly kill feeding tick (within hours) and protect lambs from further infestation and exposure for an extended period. Treating ewes in advance of lambing to reduce pasture infestations in successive years may also be indicated in high-risk areas, as is re-treatment of animals to coincide with the autumn peak.

Fortunately, the percentage of the tick population exposed to such treatments at any one time is very low, minimizing selection pressure for drug resistance. To date, there is no evidence of acaricide resistance in the UK. Whilst resistance in ticks has been reported in other parts of the world it is important to distinguish the species commonly implicated, as these can have very different epidemiologies in terms of the proportions of their populations *in refugia*. Nonetheless, it is important to consider the use of acaricide products and their application sparingly where possible from a sustainability perspective, in terms of their potential environmental impact and, in the case or diazinon, its critical importance in the control and elimination of sheep scab. Furthermore, overuse of tick treatments will also limit natural exposure, ultimately impacting flock resilience and immunity.

Tick-borne diseases

Tick-borne diseases of sheep are usually transmitted through tick bites and subsequent blood-feeding,

John Graham-Brown

whilst transmission within ticks can be transstadial and/or transovarial. TBDs are a major source of animal health and economic burden in areas of high prevalence. Some hill-farming regions of the UK have reported losses of up to 20% of lamb crops from tick-borne diseases.

Tick-borne fever (TBF)

Caused by *Anaplasma phagocytophilum* and transmitted by *I. ricinus* (in the UK), this disease is present in tick-infested regions throughout the world, including the USA. *Anaplasma phagocytophilum* can also infect and cause clinical disease in a wide range of hosts including humans, cattle, companion animals and wild ruminants. It is an intracellular pathogen, infecting the host's neutrophils and monocytes leading to neutropenia and subsequent immunosuppression, the predominant feature of disease. Transmission in ticks is transstadial, meaning only nymphs and adults are infective, although prevalence within these life stages is very high. In sheep, disease is most commonly seen in young lambs aged 3–6 weeks. Clinical signs are often mild and not noticed – lambs may be listless, fail to suck and have a transient pyrexia (up to 41 °C) lasting a few days. In more severe cases, due to their increased susceptibility, animals succumb to other pathogens. Commonly, these include tick pyaemia, louping-ill and pasteurellosis. In the case of the latter, this may occur even where animals have been vaccinated, such is the degree of immunosuppression. Immunity usually develops at an early age post-exposure but requires continual re-exposure throughout life. There is no colostral transfer of immunity from immune ewes to their lambs. Severe signs of disease are occasionally seen in adult sheep bought in from a tick-free area. The pyrexia accompanying exposure may result in abortion in pregnant ewes (although this is unusual due to the time of year) and temporary infertility (up to 3 months) in rams. This is of considerable importance since rams are usually purchased and become infected in the autumn at exactly the time they are expected to perform their reproductive duties. It is therefore not recommended to move non-immune rams and/or pregnant ewes into a tick-infested area, at least during the breeding season.

Diagnosis of TBF is achieved most effectively through PCR of whole blood, or spleen from tissue obtained post-mortem. Serology is also available and can be useful as a screening tool to determine whether exposure has occurred. However, it should be noted both tests can return positive results for extended periods of time even after clinical disease has resolved. Organisms can also be found by Giemsa staining of a thin blood film, although this lacks sensitivity by comparison to its modern counterparts. In terms of treatment, *A. phagocytophilum* is susceptible to tetracyclines, sulfonamides and other broad-spectrum antibiotics. However, it is more important to obtain satisfactory immunity in lambs and to produce acclimatized sheep.

Tick-bite pyaemia

The exact aetiology of tick pyaemia is not fully understood, but it is known to involve generalized infection with *Staphylococcus aureus* in association with tick bites (*I. ricinus* or *H. punctata*) in lambs typically aged 2–12 weeks. This disease is characterized by fatal septicaemia and sudden death or by localized multi-focal abscesses with a range of associated clinical signs dependent on their location; lameness with painful enlarged joints, hindlimb paralysis (in the spinal cord), meningitis (in the brain and meninges) and unthriftiness (in liver, lungs, kidneys, etc.). Diagnosis based on clinical signs and farm history is often sufficient, although culture and sensitivity of abscess material can be used for confirmation and to inform antibiotic choice should treatment be pursued. Whilst not always present, co-infection with TBF is an extremely common presentation, with neutropenic lambs shown to be highly susceptible to staphylococcal septicaemia. Consequently, lambs rarely show signs of tick pyaemia before 2 weeks of age. Colostral transfer of antibodies may also play a role in this early period of protection.

It has been shown that half the lamb losses and virtually all lameness cases seen in lambs on tick-infested farms are associated with tick-bite pyaemia. Up to 50% of affected lambs may die, whilst survivors recover only slowly. Antibiotics (e.g. penicillin) may be effective against *S. aureus* if treated early, but success is generally limited once abscessation has occurred. Consequently, prophylactic use of SPs from 7 days of age, prior to tick exposure habitats may be employed to limit exposure in very young animals and delay infection until they are older to reduce severity.

Louping-ill ('trembling')

Spread by *I. ricinus*, this viral disease (flavivirus) affects sheep as well as many other hosts, including cattle, deer, humans, dogs and red grouse. Grouse are an important species epidemiologically, acting as a reservoir of infection for ticks since they are a preferred host species for larvae and nymphs, and viral transmission within the tick population is only transstadial. It is, however, also important to appreciate in the wider context of animal health that red grouse are also very susceptible to disease, with high rates of mortality (up to 80%) reported. Whilst grouse can increase risk of disease in sheep by acting as a reservoir, the same is therefore true in reverse. It has been shown that effective control in sheep through vaccination and treatment for ticks reduces infection and mortality in co-habiting grouse on moors. Unlike TBF, louping-ill virus is far less prevalent in tick populations, with only about 1 in 1000 ticks carrying the disease even in areas of higher prevalence.

Disease is seen in all ages of sheep, with lambs considered at greatest risk around weaning, particularly where this coincides with a waning of maternally derived antibodies acquired through the colostrum of their immune mothers. Usually only a small proportion of the flock is affected in a given year, but explosive outbreaks with high levels of mortality are occasionally reported. Clinically, viraemia usually occurs 2–6 days after the initial infecting tick bite, accompanied by transient pyrexia (42°C) and a general non-descript malaise following which the majority of sheep become acclimatized and recover rapidly. In some cases, however, the virus invades the CNS and, after a longer 6–18-day incubation period, manifests as severe neurological disease characterized by (i) resting the head on the ground; (ii) head pressing; and (iii) abnormal jerky gait ('leaping'), staggering, circling, paralysis, fine tremors of the facial muscles and ears, nystagmus and twitching or nibbling of the lips. In such cases coma and death commonly occurs within 1–4 days of onset, with the latter often assisted by predators. Some animals may recover from this acute neurological form of disease, but this is protracted and animals often show some residual paresis. As mentioned in relation to tick pyaemia, co-infections with TBF are very common, and increase host susceptibility and the likelihood of severe disease.

Diagnosis

In a disease outbreak is usually made on clinical signs, flock and grazing history, but other neurological conditions such as CCN, listeriosis, swayback etc. should also be considered. A serological assay (haemagglutination inhibition test) is available to determine whether animals have had recent exposure to louping-ill virus based on the relative proportion of IgM to IgG, whilst definitive diagnosis can be made post-mortem via immunohistopathology of neurological tissue. It is important to note here the zoonotic threat louping-ill poses, since transmission may occur through the handling of viraemic tissues as well as via ticks. When handling animals and samples in suspected cases, necessary care and precaution is therefore required.

Treatment and control

There is no effective treatment for louping-ill, but housing and nursing may save some cases and improve recovery times in post-viraemic animals. The aim of control is to ensure that ewes are immune and that lambs are protected passively. An inactivated vaccine previously available was discontinued in 2017, meaning at present, immunity can only be achieved through natural exposure. At the time of writing, the Moredun Research Institute is in the process of developing and licensing its own louping-ill vaccine for sheep. This has been funded in part by grouse moor owners.

Piroplasmoses

There are a number of tick-borne piroplasms reported in UK sheep and ticks including *Babesia ovis* and *B. venatorum* (transmitted by *I. ricinus*), and *B. motasi*, *Theileria orientalis* and *T. iuwenshuni* (transmitted by *H. punctata*). Whilst generally these are not considered of major clinical significance, they are occasionally implicated in cases of clinical disease. For example, an outbreak of clincal disease and deaths in Kent in 2005 was linked to *T. iuwenshuni* infection. Furthermore, *B. motase* and *B. venatorum* are also of note from a public health perspective due to their anthropozoonotic potential. Where there is a suspicion or uncertainty, a pan-piroplasm PCR has been developed by APHA that can detect and distinguish between these various species. Whilst not presently listed on their routine test portfolio, this may be available through discussion with a Veterinary Investigation Officer.

Lyme disease

Lyme disease, caused by the spirochaete *Borrelia burgdorferi*, is transmitted in the UK by *I. ricinus*.

Serological studies in Scottish sheep show as many as 40% of hoggs have circulating antibody, with only small numbers of lambs and older ewes showing significant antibody titres. In sheep, this pathogen is generally not associated with clinical disease, although severe lameness associated with high titres of antibody and heavy tick infections has been described in 6-month-old lambs in Norway. The principal concern with Lyme disease in sheep is therefore the role they can play as a reservoir for infection, the anthropozoonotic potential of *B. burgdorferi* and its profound and long-lasting impact on humans (and their dogs). It is increasingly recognized as a disease of hill walkers as ticks will readily feed on humans. Whilst this could potentially be used to justify more robust tick-control measures in sheep from a One Health perspective, public education initiatives highlighting the risks and necessary precautions to take to mitigate these are likely to be a more realistic option.

17 Notifiable Diseases and Diseases Exotic to the UK and Northern Europe

EMMA FISHBOURNE*

Department of Livestock and One Health, Institute of Infection, Veterinary and Ecological Sciences, University of Liverpool, UK

Abstract

There are many diseases of sheep globally that, because of their severe economic or zoonotic potential, are controlled by government legislation and must be reported if suspected, i.e. are notifiable. Arthropod-borne diseases are of particular concern because of climate change – these include tick-borne and mosquito – and midge-borne diseases. In the UK, keeping the country free of foot and mouth disease, which devastated the ruminant population in 2001, is a particular concern.

Notifiable Diseases

All sheep-rearing countries take measures to avoid the introduction of serious diseases and to control them in the event that they do become introduced. These measures include the legal requirement for owners of animals to report sheep showing clinical signs associated with a list of notifiable diseases to government veterinary authorities. In addition, many countries require the reporting of other named diseases which do occur in the country but for which special measures are being taken to control or eradicate the disease or which are of particular importance, notably of zoonotic potential. Which animal diseases are considered notifiable is determined by the World Organisation for Animal Health (WOAH, founded as OIE) and their website (https://www.woah.org/en/?OIE - accessed 9/11/24) has useful information with details on clinical signs, routes of transmission and diagnosis on listed and emerging diseases. The World Animal Health Information System (WAHIS) is the global animal health reference database of the WOAH and currently has a subscription service which enables you to receive email animal health alerts on the current global situation of listed and emerging diseases. Promed (promed@isid.org) is a free internet-based emerging disease and outbreak detection reporting service for all human, animal and plant diseases. It is noteworthy that it played a key role in the identification of Schmallenberg virus in 2011.

Worldwide, one of the biggest threats to human and animal health is arthropod-borne diseases. Across Europe there is growing evidence that distribution of ticks and tick-borne disease transmission is increasing from the movement of people, pets and livestock, from migratory birds and changes in climate and habitat (Fig. 17.1). Mosquito- and midge-borne diseases can also be introduced via migratory birds, through the importation of infected animals and via the wind.

In the UK, both animal keepers and veterinary surgeons are legally obliged to report all suspect cases of notifiable diseases to the Animal and Plant Health Agency (APHA). Notifiable diseases of sheep in the UK include bluetongue, *Brucella melitensis*, contagious agalactia, contagious epididymitis, foot and mouth disease (FMD), sheep and goat pox, peste des petits ruminants (PPR), rabies, Rift Valley fever and scrapie. One of these, scrapie, is endemic in the UK and is discussed in Chapters 12 and 14. There are also two notifiable diseases of sheep which are not endemic but have been seen in recent years and which are of considerable significance – these are bluetongue and FMD, which

*Email: emma.fishbourne@liverpool.ac.uk

© CAB International 2025. *A Handbook for the Sheep Clinician, 8th Edition*
(A.C. Winter and D. Grove-White eds)
DOI: 10.1079/9781800626355.0017

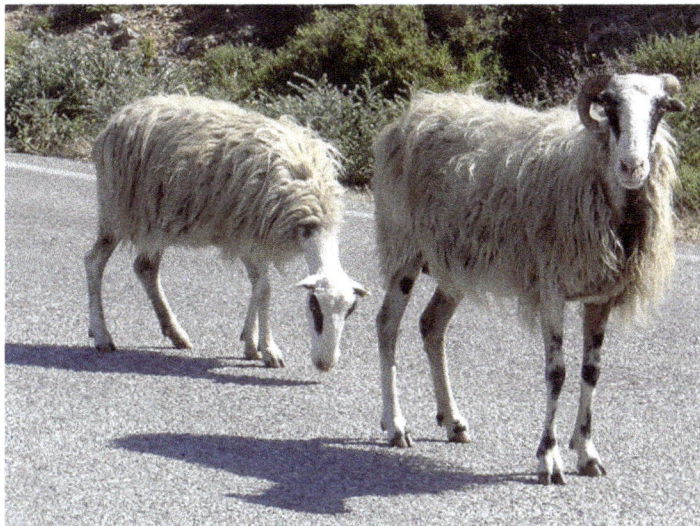

Fig. 17.1. Diseases affecting sheep in the Mediterranean area could spread further north as a result of climate change (photo Agnes Winter).

will be discussed here along with some of the more important notifiable diseases which occur in some parts of the world but not in the UK (Fig. 17.2).

One extremely important disease, known for thousands of years, that has in the past affected sheep as well as cattle, was rinderpest (cattle plague, murrain), which occurred as epidemics in Great Britain in the 18th and 19th centuries. The last epidemic in 1865–1867 led to the setting up of the State Veterinary Service. Rinderpest is only the second disease to be eradicated from the world (in 2011) after smallpox and there are plans to try to eradicate a third morbillivirus, namely peste des petits ruminants (PPR), which causes severe disease and high mortality in sheep and goats and has spread widely in recent years. It should also be noted that, whilst we may be aware of what disease may be close to our borders, new and emerging pathogens and diseases can arise, seemingly out of nowhere, as did Schmallenberg disease in 2011 (see Chapter 5). As vets we need to remain vigilant.

Foot and mouth disease

FMD is caused by a virus (FMDV) and affects all cloven-hoofed animals and is highly contagious, with rapid replication and a short incubation period. FMD is endemic in many countries bordering Europe. There are 7 serotypes and within each

serotype, genotypes can be geographically restricted (referred to as topotypes).

The massive outbreak in the UK in 2001 resulted in over 6 million animals being slaughtered, around 5 million of which were sheep (this number does not include young animals at foot, especially lambs which were not recorded. An estimate of their number resulted in the often quoted figure of 10 million animals being slaughtered and valued at around £4 billion). The primary outbreak was in pigs but large numbers of sheep farms were affected early in the outbreak, associated with the movement of sheep via a market in the affected area to many other areas of the UK, since there was a considerable delay in reporting disease on the pig farm.

Clinical signs

The disease is severe in young lambs with high mortality and in pregnant ewes, resulting in abortion but many sheep do not show obvious clinical signs. Where clinical signs occur, sudden, severe lameness, usually in more than one leg, is the most obvious feature but since lameness due to other causes is so common in sheep, it is easy to miss the significance of the lameness. Sheep lie down and are often unwilling to rise or stand in a crouching position.

Early lesions are blanching and separation of the interdigital skin at the coronary band; after

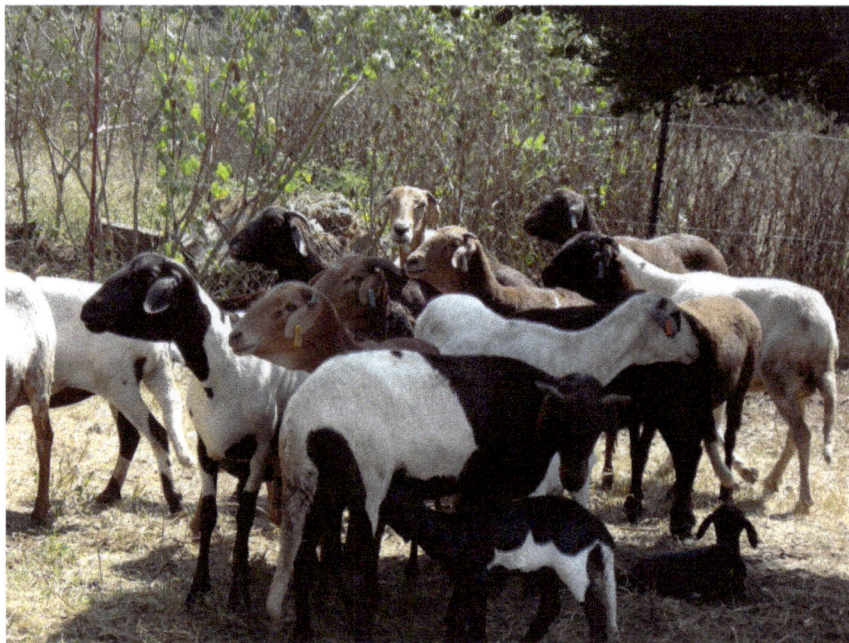

Fig. 17.2. Sheep specialists should have some knowledge of exotic diseases such as those that may affect these sheep in South Africa (photo Agnes Winter).

a day or two, the lesions become ulcerative and granulomatous and are easily confused with early FR. The severity of disease and lesions depends in part on the serotype involved, age of animal and infective dose.

Mouth lesions are less obvious than in cattle and affected sheep may eat normally with no excessive salivation as occurs in cattle. Blanching and separation of the mucous membrane occurs, particularly on the dental pad and, less often, on the tongue, and ulceration occurs within 1–2 days of the initial blister. The careful examination of the mouths of many sheep during the outbreak led to the recognition of mouth lesions that looked similar to FMD but were due to other causes, probably associated with mechanical damage. Initially called OMAGOD (ovine mouth and gum obscure disease) or idiopathic oral ulceration, they made diagnosis difficult. A retrospective study on stored samples showed that 23% of premises suspected of having FMD did not actually have the disease. Since the aim was to kill the animals on a suspect farm within 24 h, this was often before viral confirmation was possible, which has led to the ongoing development of 'pen-side' tests for on-farm use. If you as the vet have any

doubts about a possible case, you must speak to someone in APHA immediately.

Control

FMD is easily spread through fomites and animals can be infected via respiratory aerosols with the virus being carried over large distances, particularly over water. Animals can also be carriers and meat and by-products are also sources of infection. FMD virus has entered the UK in the past by: (i) swill-feeding in pigs which is now banned; (ii) imported carcasses from South America; (iii) wind from the continent of Europe with outbreaks in the Isle of Wight in the 1980s traced to outbreaks in France; and (iv) escape from a laboratory which worked on the disease. Careful surveillance of the FMD status of countries from which meat is imported helps to reduce the risk associated with the meat industry. All countries in the EU fall into the highest international FMD status of FMD-free and no country is allowed to use prophylactic vaccination. In addition, the movement of animals in the UK is now much more carefully regulated which would reduce

Emma Fishbourne

the risk of rapid spread which occurred in 2001 and swill-feeding in pigs has been banned.

The control strategy relies on the rapid reporting of suspect animals by farmers and veterinary surgeons followed by diagnosis and typing of any FMD virus isolated. All susceptible animals on the infected premises and on farms which are considered to be dangerous contacts are slaughtered. The EU directive allows emergency vaccination along with the implementation of the slaughter policy but a decision to vaccinate can only be made in the UK by the Secretary of State for the Environment, Food and Rural Affairs after a positive diagnosis has been made. It is believed that this vaccination policy, perhaps of a ring nature of susceptible animals on farms surrounding the infected premises, will limit the spread of the disease. Banks of vaccine and antigens from a range of FMD strains are held in EU countries.

Bluetongue

Bluetongue is a viral infection caused by bluetongue virus (BTV) of ruminant animals which occurs widely in tropical and subtropical countries throughout the world. There are more than 29 serotypes of BTV, each of which is immunologically distinct. Bluetongue does not affect or infect humans and so has no public health significance.

In recent years, there have been many outbreaks in several Mediterranean countries, and it has been suggested that global warming has encouraged the northern and western spread of the insect vector, the midge *Culicoides imicola*. It is believed that the virus spread into Europe from Turkey and North Africa and there are multiple strains circulating in Europe, with outbreaks due to BTV1, 3, 4 and 8 in 2023/2024.

In September 2023, BTV-3 infections were confirmed in The Netherlands. The route of incursion is currently unknown. Following this, there was a large outbreak in northern Europe, with high mortality in sheep. In November 2023, disease was detected in the south-east of England; by November 2024, over 150 farms were affected, mostly in eastern England. The spread to the UK is believed to be from infected midges blown across the North Sea. The previous 2006 outbreak in UK was associated with BTV-8, again following disease in The Netherlands. For the latest information visit https://www.gov.uk/government/collections/bluetongue-information-and-guidance-for-livestock-keepers (accessed 13/11/24).

Epidemiology

The virus is transmitted by species of biting midges of the genus *Culicoides*, some of which are widespread in the UK. Direct animal-to-animal transmission does not occur. In temperate climates the adult fly is not active during the winter and clinical disease is seen only from July to December so it was believed that the outbreaks on the continent would die out during the winter. However, this did not prove to be the case and outbreaks in northern Europe were more numerous and more virulent in summer 2007 than in 2006, and in 2008 there were over 30,000 outbreaks in the EU. It has been shown that the bluetongue virus overwinters in northern Europe more effectively than had been expected, probably due to a combination of: (i) animals maintaining a viraemia for a long time; (ii) the survival of some midge species; and (iii) the transplacental transmission of the virus.

Clinical signs

Usually, cattle remain as carriers with few signs, and the disease is more virulent in sheep, but in the 2007 Netherlands cases, cattle were also seriously affected. Mortality in sheep can be as high as 70% but the severity varies according to the breed of affected sheep.

In sheep, the disease is characterized by fever up to 42°C that may last for several days. Increased respiration rate and hyperaemia and swelling of the lips, mucous linings of the mouth and nose and eyelids are seen, accompanied by salivation and frothing at the mouth (Fig. 17.3). Nasal discharges are common. There is sometimes oedema of the head and neck. The tongue may be cyanotic, giving rise to the name bluetongue. Laminitis and inflammation of the coronary band may result in lameness and reluctance to stand. Animals lose condition rapidly, including muscle degeneration. Infection during pregnancy may result in abortions and congenital abnormalities. PME shows typical almost pathognomonic haemorrhages in the pulmonary artery.

Control

As a result of a successful vaccination campaign, the UK was granted bluetongue-free status in July 2011 which removed the restrictions on the export of cattle and sheep introduced in 2007. BTV cases were identified only in home-bred ruminants in

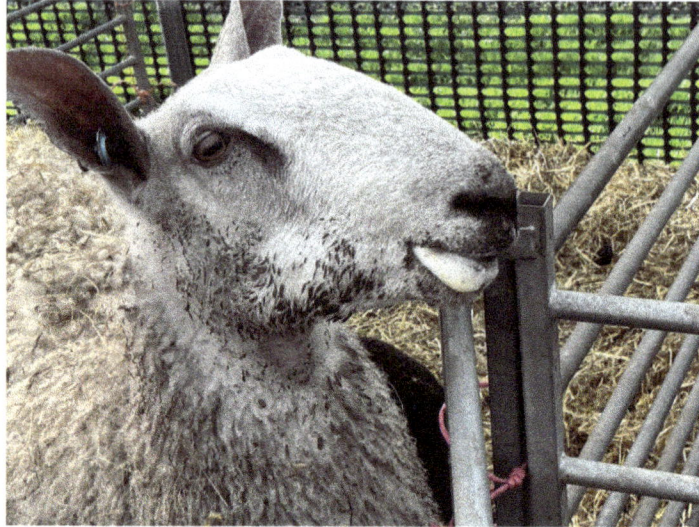

Fig. 17.3. This sheep is frothing at the mouth but otherwise appears healthy so is unlikely to be suffering from a systemic disease. Tooth problems are more likely (photo Agnes Winter).

England though a case in an imported cow from Germany was found in Scotland. No cases were seen in Wales.

Control was based on vaccination with new dead vaccines which became available from May 2008, a remarkably rapid development by several drug companies. The use of vaccine was voluntary in England, with the farmer bearing the full cost but the Scottish Parliament decided that vaccination would be compulsory with the farmer only paying half the cost. The vaccination campaign was so successful that a total of only 149 farms had infected animals. No cases had been seen since 2008, until disease caused by BTV-3 was introduced in September 2023, most likely by windborne spread. EU directives stated that prophylactic vaccination could not be used in a bluetongue-free country, but, to deal with the current situation, three vaccines became available for BTV-3 control, and use of these vaccines in England was permitted by Defra, subject to licence. These vaccines are not preventive but reduce the severity of disease. See https://www.gov.uk/government/collections/bluetongue-information-and-guidance-for-livestock-keepers (accessed 13/11/24). Control in countries where the disease is endemic is by vaccination but the high number of serotypes makes this difficult.

Diseases Exotic to the UK and Northern Europe

This book is based primarily on sheep diseases experienced in the UK, much of which also applies to sheep kept throughout northern Europe. Where appropriate, we have tried to indicate which of those diseases are also important in other major sheep-keeping countries such as Australia, New Zealand and South Africa, and, to a lesser extent, in North and South America. There are a number of serious diseases that do not occur in northern Europe that affect sheep in large areas such as the Mediterranean region, Africa, the Middle East and the Far East, of which it is important that the complete sheep vet has an appreciation. Some of these require vectors not present in temperate countries, but others could occur almost anywhere as a result of uncontrolled or illegal animal or animal product movements. This section briefly brings together some information on the most important of these.

Peste des petits ruminants

This is caused by a member of the genus *Morbillivirus*, closely related to that causing rinderpest. PPR is widespread in many parts of the world including most of Africa, the Middle East, the Indian subcontinent and China. Clinical signs include fever, catarrhal head discharges, necrotic stomatitis and diarrhoea, often with a high mortality rate (can be as high as 90%). It also causes immunosuppression. Transmission of PPR can occur directly from close contact with an infected animal or indirectly from contact with infected fomites. Control is by vaccination and there is currently a global programme to eradicate PPR, led by the WOAH.

Rift Valley fever (RVF)

This disease is caused by a member of the genus *Bunyavirus*, which is transmitted by mosquitoes. It occurs in sub-Saharan Africa and in 2000 the first cases of RVF were identified outside of Africa on the Arabian Peninsula. Infection in young lambs leads to a high mortality rate (70–100%) which can also occur in adult sheep (20–70%), though some may show a milder illness. Signs are mostly non-specific and include fever, listlessness, anorexia, and a reluctance to move, but in pregnant animals RVF causes nearly 100% abortion. Outbreaks of RVF typically present with numerous abortions and high mortality in young lambs with disease in humans. People become infected through contact with blood, body fluids or tissues of infected animals, or through bites from infected mosquitoes. Control is by vaccination.

Nairobi sheep disease (NSD)

This is also caused by a member of the genus *Bunyavirus*, transmitted by *Rhipicephalus* ticks in East and Central Africa. A variant of NSD (Ganjam virus) has been reported from parts of Asia including India and Sri Lanka. NSD causes similar signs to those seen in PPR with very high mortality rates. After infection, adult ticks can transmit this virus for more than two years. Control is by the use of acaricides to control the tick vector.

Akabane disease

This is caused by yet another member of the genus *Bunyavirus*, transmitted mainly by *Culicoides* spp. midges. Akabane virus is common in many tropical and subtropical areas including parts of Asia, Africa, the Middle East and Australia. Fetal infection has been the most common presentation, leading to congenital birth defects such as arthrogryposis and hydranencephaly. Diagnosis is by serology and vaccines have been developed but are not widely used

as most animals in endemic areas are exposed before sexual maturity and so control is achieved by moving animals into an endemic area and allowing immunity to develop before the most susceptible period of pregnancy.

Sheep and goat pox

These viral diseases occur in sheep and goats and are caused by members of the genus *Capripoxvirus*. Outbreaks have been reported in European countries including Spain. Animals can be infected by direct contact with infected animals or indirectly through contaminated fomites and the virus is present in respiratory aerosols. Clinical signs vary according to the breed of sheep and to the strain of virus and the mortality rate can be high with younger animals more severely affected. Affected animals develop fever with swollen lymph nodes and macules and ulcerating papules develop on the skin and mucous membranes. Internally there are lung haemorrhages and cases may present with breathing difficulties. Control in endemic areas is by the use of live, attenuated vaccines.

Rabies

This fatal disease, caused by a member of the genus *Lyssavirus*, occurs in areas such as North Africa and the Near East where stray dogs are a problem. Rabies presents similarly in our common farm species. In one study where 20 cattle and 5 sheep were challenged with rabies the average incubation period in sheep was 10.0 days, and the average morbidity period was 3.25 days. Major clinical signs in sheep included muzzle and/or head tremors (80%), aggressiveness, hyperexcitability, and/or hyperaesthesia (80%), trismus (60%), salivation (60%), vocalization (60%) and recumbency (40%) with the furious form of rabies manifested in 80% of the sheep.

Anthrax

This bacterial disease, caused by the spore-forming *Bacillus anthracis*, is found worldwide. In some countries such as parts of Africa it is endemic. In others, such as the UK, it occurs very occasionally, mostly in cattle, though sheep can be infected. It causes sudden death, the most characteristic signs being dark blood oozing from body orifices and an enlarged spleen. In endemic areas it is controlled by vaccination.

Contagious agalactia

Contagious agalactia is a mycoplasmal disease of sheep and goats and is present in many parts of the world including southern Europe. *Mycoplasma agalactiae* (Ma) is the main cause of the disease in sheep and goats, but *M. capricolum* subsp. *capricolum* (Mcc), *M. mycoides* subsp. *capri* (Mmc) and *M. putrefaciens* (Mp) produce a clinically similar disease. Clinical signs include mastitis, arthritis, keratoconjunctivitis and occasionally abortion. Transmission is through the milk from the dam to her offspring or via aerosols during milking.

Vaccines are available including ones inactivated with formalin which are widely used but are not considered to be very efficacious.

Brucella ovis

This causes epididymitis in rams. It does not occur in the UK but is common in many other countries. See Chapter 2.

Brucella melitensis

This is an important cause of abortion and human disease (Malta fever) in the Mediterranean region, Middle East, India and parts of Africa.

Emma Fishbourne

18 Health and Welfare Schemes

JENNIFER DUNCAN*

Department of Livestock and One Health, Institute of Infection, Veterinary and Ecological Sciences, University of Liverpool, UK

Abstract

This section describes the various types of health and welfare schemes for sheep flocks. These will vary from country to country and may be government-backed national or private individual farm schemes. The national schemes aim to produce a pool of sheep flocks of recognized health status regarding certain specified diseases but also encourage farmers to increase the welfare standards of flocks. Individual farm schemes are provided by practising veterinary surgeons for their clients and are 'tailor-made' for a particular flock.

National and Regional Health and Welfare Schemes

Most sheep-producing countries have a list of exotic notifiable diseases (see Chapter 17), designed to prevent their introduction into the country. Other notifiable diseases endemic to the country may be subject to special control measures if they are widespread and of considerable economic and welfare importance. In addition, certain other non-notifiable diseases may be of such significance that organized voluntary schemes are designed to improve their control. All these diseases may be included in national or regional health schemes.

UK Animal Health and Welfare Pathway

This government-backed scheme was introduced in England (with similar schemes in the devolved regions of UK) in 2023 as part of the Sustainable Farming Initiative. It aims to financially reward farmers to produce healthier higher-welfare animals and includes a fully funded veterinary visit which will address issues such as optimizing body condition of ewes, reducing lameness, improving pain management, tackling important endemic diseases and generally supporting good stockmanship through training. The effectiveness of the scheme will be reviewed after 3 years.

See https://www.gov.uk/government/publications/animal-health-and-welfare-pathway/animal-health-and-welfare-pathway (accessed 15/2/24). See also https://ahdb.org.uk/annual-health-and-welfare-review (accessed 15/2/24).

UK Sheep Welfare Strategy 2023–2028

This is an industry-based independent network of bodies involved in supporting sheep production in the UK in order to help farmers to build the health and welfare status of the national sheep flock. See Ruminant Health and Welfare at https://ruminanthw.org.uk/uk-welfare-strategies/sheep/ (accessed 15/2/24).

Premium Sheep and Goat Health Schemes

The Premium Sheep and Goat Health Schemes are administered by SRUC and are the official UK sheep health schemes for testing for various important endemic diseases. They are all voluntary and aimed at improving the health and welfare of sheep throughout the UK. Strategic animal testing is performed in addition to ensuring specific biosecurity practices are adhered to. Based on test results, certification as to disease status (monitored or accredited) is awarded, providing assurance to potential

*Email: jsduncan@liverpool.ac.uk

© CAB International 2025. *A Handbook for the Sheep Clinician, 8th Edition*   165
(A.C. Winter and D. Grove-White eds)
DOI: 10.1079/9781800626355.0018

buyers; thus these schemes are especially useful for farmers selling or exporting breeding stock.

The diseases covered are:

- maedi visna (MV)
- enzootic abortion of ewes (EAE)
- Johne's disease (paratuberculosis)
- scrapie

Full details are available on the website: https://www.sruc.ac.uk/business-services/veterinary-laboratory-services/sheep-goat-health-schemes/premium-sheep-goat-health-schemes/ (accessed 15/2/24).

SRUC Veterinary Services, Greycrook, St. Boswells, TD6 0EQ; Tel: 01835 822 456, Email: healthschemes@SRUC.ac.uk

Flock health clubs

Communication between sheep farmers and vets has traditionally operated on a 'fire brigade' basis, i.e. veterinary input in response to specific problems, e.g. lambings and caesarean sections in response to dystocia, with little communication or interaction regarding health and production in general. In part, this has been attributed to the perceived relatively low economic value and profitability inherent in sheep production. A recent development specifically aimed at addressing this communication and knowledge transfer gap has been the formation of Flock Health Clubs by veterinary practices (https://www.flockhealth.co.uk/#:~:text=FLOCK%20HEALTH%20CLUBS,meeting%20and%20deliver%20the%20; accessed 9/11/24). Whilst exact details vary between practices, the clubs are aimed at the more enthusiastic flock keepers and aim to deliver cost-effective advice on disease control via group meetings and strengthen the vet–client bond to the benefit of all. They are generally operated on a subscription basis and may offer subsidized services, e.g. regular faecal egg count reduction testing (FECRT) to identify anthelmintic resistance.

Individual farm health schemes

Veterinary surgeons with their special knowledge of epidemiology, control and the economic importance of disease have made a considerable contribution to the improved welfare and success of livestock health and production throughout the world. There are numerous studies on the adverse economic effects of conditions in dairy cows like lameness, mastitis and infertility which show that the distinctive knowledge and expertise of the veterinary profession can be applied to improve the finances of a farm as well as the health and welfare of the cows.

A great opportunity exists for UK veterinary surgeons to be involved in the formulation of health programmes with farmers as these are required as part of the many farm assurance schemes and government initiatives such as the Health and Welfare Strategy mentioned above. Successful on-farm schemes often start in a modest way with reaction to a particular disease event. If the control plan has a positive outcome, it may then lead to a more detailed discussion with the farmer and the production of a more comprehensive health plan (Fig. 18.1). However, experience has shown that it is usually best to concentrate on a limited number of diseases or issues at first, rather than going for a hugely complicated plan consisting of many pages of information and instructions. All farms have unique features and so an individual health plan is needed for each. The consultancy Flock Health Ltd (https://www.flockhealth.co.uk; accessed 19/2/24) works directly with all involved in sheep production from farm to abattoir and supports veterinary practices in setting up flock health clubs for their clients. Since the foundation of effective health planning is accurate data collection and analysis, there is increasing interest in the use of computer software for recording key information and events, ideally allowing the identification of areas of concern (Fig. 18.2).

The following is an account of the components of a health scheme which we and others have used on UK commercial sheep farms.

Objectives

To produce, monitor and maintain a unique health scheme for a particular farm, believing that this will decrease disease, increase production and improve the welfare of sheep in the flock.

The scheme

The scheme has three components:

1. a written health programme containing recommendations for the control of expected diseases and to improve production and welfare;

Jennifer Duncan

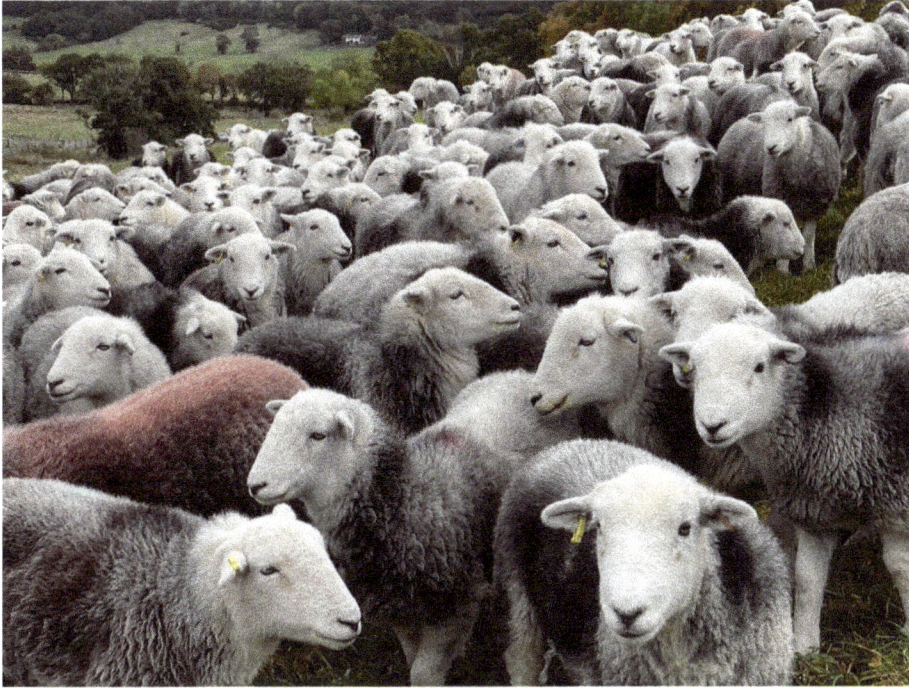

Fig. 18.1. Health programmes are aimed at minimizing losses from disease and achieving the aims of the flock owner (photo Agnes Winter).

2. planned visits to monitor health and production; and
3. reactions to events and advice on new advances during the year, to keep the programme up to date.

Its success hinges on the degree of co-operation between the farmer and the practising veterinary surgeon and other advisors and requires honest pooling of information.

Health programme

Prior to producing a health programme, information about some or all of the following aspects of the flock will need to be obtained:

- objectives of the flock;
- breeds, numbers, age structure;
- pasture and grazing management (including possible fluke habitats);
- feeding plans (types, quality and quantity);
- housing availability and management;
- lambing management including labour;
- clinical diseases experienced in the past;
- laboratory findings (including PME) if available; and
- production and financial data as available.

As a result of the first planned visit during which a full and open discussion should take place, a programme, in the form of a diary of important management events through the year, together with brief information on disease areas highlighted as being particularly important, is tailor-made to suit the needs of the farm. It is based around the fixed dates of the sheep-breeding cycle – the proposed dates for tupping, housing, lambing and weaning. It should address some or all the following major areas, depending on the commitment and interest of the farmer involved and on them having identified the areas of most concern to their flock. The document may range from its most basic form of a simple calendar of important events to a sophisticated computerized web-based system.

- Rams – examination and preparation for tupping time; use of teaser rams or other control of breeding.
- Ewes – condition scoring and culling if not done previously.
- Breeding schedule – date rams go in with ewes and date removed (to produce a compact lambing period).

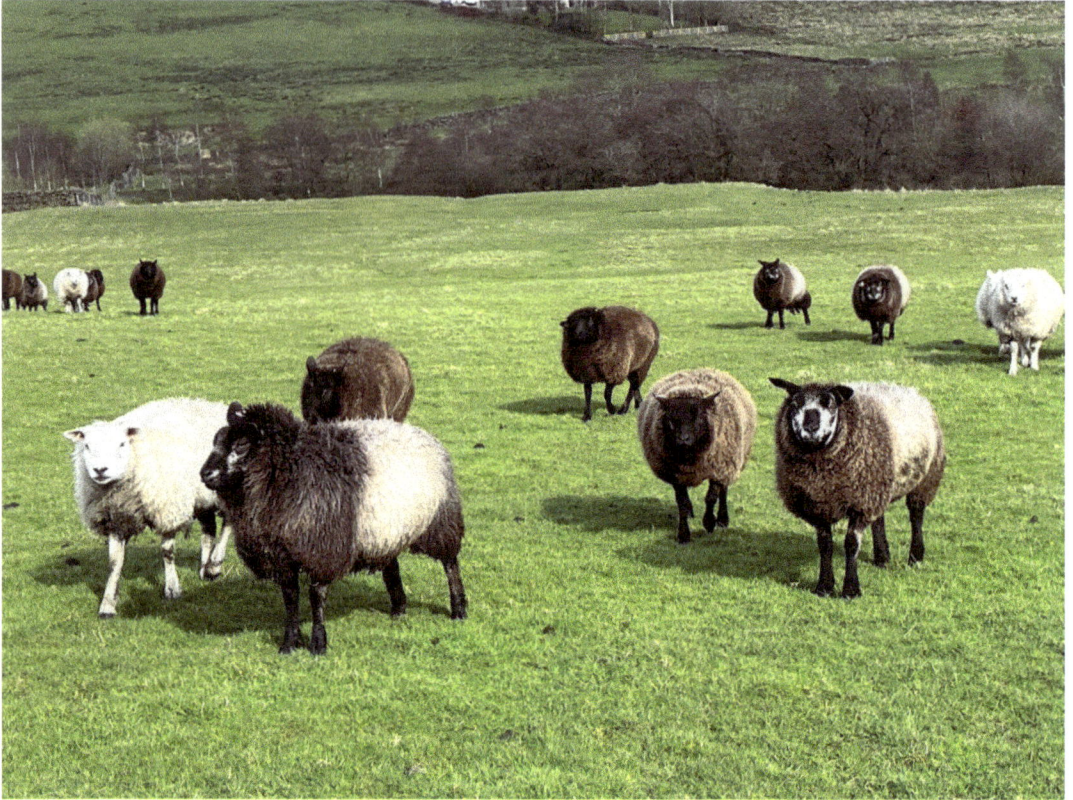

Fig. 18.2. Owners of small hobby flocks are often very keen to follow health plans and economics are usually not very important (photo Agnes Winter).

- Vaccination schedule – essential and optional disease cover.
- Lameness – identification of major cause(s) and control.
- Ectoparasites – status and control.
- Endoparasite – control including anthelmintic use and detection of possible anthelmintic resistance.
- Nutrition – BCS and LWG targets and nutrition planning
- Trace elements – known deficiencies including tests if necessary.
- Lamb morbidity and mortality – main causes and control.
- Farm Biosecurity Plan.
- Assessment of any welfare issues.

Planned visits

Several visits will be needed in order to assess the application and usefulness of the health programme. In the first year, three or four visits are recommended though in subsequent years fewer visits and samples will be required.

Reactions to events

It will be necessary to modify the original health programme from time to time during the year, because of unexpected events or following information obtained during and in-between the planned visits. The programme will need amendment at the end of each year to incorporate new research, drugs and vaccines in the light of the experience of the past year and any alteration in the aims of the farmer.

Jennifer Duncan

Appendix 1
Clinical Examination

Systematic Examination of a Sick Sheep

Carry out the examination in the order shown, examining in more detail where necessary. If signs indicate a neurological problem, a full neurological examination should be carried out. Use of an ultrasound scanner may be helpful particularly for the thorax and abdomen.

From a distance

Parameter	Some possible findings
Grade of illness	Mild, severe, dying
Duration of illness	Acute, chronic
General appearance	Normal, excited, depressed
Facial expression	May indicate pain
Mobility	Recumbent, unwilling to move, lame, ataxic, circling
Feeding	Poor appetite, off food, difficulty eating, quidding, ruminating, regularity of jaw movements if eating or cudding
Condition	Thin, fat (beware of fleece masking)
Fleece	Broken, patchy, rubbing
Faeces	Loose, scour, absent
Respirations (count)	Distressed, very fast, deep, coughing, nasal discharge
Head	High, low, turn, tilt, ear(s) drooping, dribbling
Eyes	Blinking, blepharospasm, discharge

On handling standing

Parameter	Some possible findings
Condition score (CS)	1–5 (emaciated, thin, fit, fat)
Temperature	Normal is 39–40°C
Pulse (femoral) and/or heart rate	Strong, weak, rapid (may be fear, recheck later)
Fleece and skin	Wool break, itchy (rub test), ectoparasites, scabs, sores
Age and teeth	
Incisors	Number of temporary/permanent, broken mouth, periodontal disease, apposition
Mandibles and molars (feel through cheeks)	Thickening of mandibles, lumps, discharging sinuses, pain, sharp edges, irregularities, food impaction
Lips and gums	Sores, scabs, smell breath, gum colour (may be pigmented), ulcers, dribbling, capillary refill time
Cheeks	Impacted food, paralysis
Nostrils	Movement, discharge

Continued

© CAB International 2025. *A Handbook for the Sheep Clinician, 8th Edition* (A.C. Winter and D. Grove-White eds) DOI: 10.1079/9781800626355.appx

Continued.

Parameter	Some possible findings
Eyes	Discharge
Menace and palpebral reflexes	Presence/absence
Eyelids	Entropion
Conjunctiva	Anaemia, toxaemia
Sclera	Vessels injected, jaundice
Cornea and anterior chamber	Keratitis, uveitis
Pupils and lens	Size, symmetry, cataract
Ears	Position, paralysis, discharge, haematoma, mites
Lymph nodes	Enlargement, abscesses
Larynx	Obstruction causing stridor
Chest	
Auscultate heart	Rate and sounds
Auscultate lungs	Abnormal sounds, absence of sounds
Wheelbarrow test	Excess fluid from lungs
Ultrasound chest	Abscesses, tumours
Abdomen (size, consistency, ballot, ultrasound). Right kidney may be palpable behind last rib	Distended, tucked up, gas, fluid, solid
Rumen (palpate, feel contractions, listen)	Irregular or absent contractions, abnormal resonance, gas, abnormal consistency
Abomasum and intestines (listen, ballot)	Abnormal sounds, no sounds, gas, solid
Faeces	Pellets, soft, scour, blood, smell
Vulva and vagina (F)	Discharge, fetal membranes, smell, injury, bruising, haemorrhage
Prepuce, penis, testes (M)	Urethral obstruction/rupture, orchitis, epididymitis
Legs and joints	Stiff, pain, swelling, abrasion, muscle wasting

Tipped up, sitting comfortably with back against legs of examiner

Parameter	Some possible findings
Abdomen (palpate, ballot)	Fluid, solid, fetus
Udder (palpate udder and teat canal)	Swelling, mastitis, fibrosis, abscess, gangrene, milk, colostrum, serum, blind teat, sores, scabs
Feet (locate painful digit by manipulation and pressure if not obvious)	Overgrown/loose horn, interdigital lesions/growths/foreign body, smell, under-running (wall or sole), swelling, cracks, coronary band lesions
Joints (knees, elbows, hips, stifles, hocks)	Pain, stiffness, swelling (fluid/firm)

Samples

Blood	From jugular vein (tube type depends on tests needed)

Appendix 2
Neurological Examination of Sheep

By working through the following sequence, noting down any abnormalities, it should be possible to localize any lesion(s) to assist in making a diagnosis.

Indicator	Some possible abnormalities
Behaviour	Wandering, circling, head pressing, fits
Mental state	Hyperexcited, depressed, stuporous, comatose
Head position	Turn, tilt, high/low carriage, star gazing
Head coordination	Jerkiness, intention tremors
Cranial nerves	
Menace test	Visual deficit
Pupil size	Dilated/constricted
Pupil symmetry	Asymmetry
Pupillary light response	Absent
Eye position	Strabismus
Eye movement	Nystagmus
Palpebral reflex	Absent
Facial sensation	Absent
Jaw tone	Slack
Facial symmetry	Facial paralysis
Balance	Loss of balance, rolling
Prehension	Difficulty
Swallowing	Drooling saliva
Stance	Wide-based
Gait	Ataxia, hypo/hypermetria
Neck sensation and movement	Stiffness, opisthotonus
Forelimbs	
Skin sensation	Absent (where?)
Muscle tone	Flaccid, spastic
Proprioception	Placing reflex absent
Wheelbarrow test	Difficulty right/left/both
Hemiwalking test	Difficulty right/left/both
Triceps reflex	Reduced/increased/absent
Pedal reflex	Reduced/increased/absent
Deep pain sensation	Absent
Trunk	
Panniculus reflex	Absent (side? level?)
Hind limbs	
Skin sensation	Absent (where?)
Muscle tone	Flaccid, spastic
Proprioception	Placing reflex absent
Hemiwalking test	Difficulty right/left/both
Sway response	Can push over (side?)
Patellar reflex	Reduced/increased/absent

Continued

Continued.

Indicator	Some possible abnormalities
Pedal reflex	Reduced/increased/absent
Deep pain sensation	Absent
Tail/anus	
Anal reflex	Absent, rectum distended
Tail tone	Flaccid
Bladder control	Incontinence

Blindfold (each eye in turn, then both) then reassess balance and gait, repeat wheelbarrow and hemiwalking tests.

Appendix 3
Checklist for Examination of a Sick Lamb

Indicator	Select applicable description
Age	Minutes/hours/days
Birth	Normal/assisted/difficult/caesarean
Litter size	1/2/3/4/5
Lamb size	Normal/small/large (? kg)
Ewe condition score	1/2/3/4/5
Ewe age	? years
Colostrum intake	Sucked unaided/sucked with help/not fed/not known/ tube-fed (volume ? ml)
Temperature	Normal/hypothermic/pyrexic (?°C)
Respiration	Normal/slow/rapid/laboured (?/min?)
Heart rate	Normal/slow/rapid/murmur (?/min?)
Demeanour	Normal/depressed/comatose/fits
Posture and gait	Normal/standing but weak/sitting/lateral recumbency/ ataxic/shaking/lame
Birthcoat	Normal/poor/hairy/pigmented
Head	
Jaw	Normal/abnormal
Salivation	Excessive
Eyes	Normal/entropion/discharge/other abnormality
Chest	Fractured ribs
Abdomen	Normal/empty/distended (gas/fluid?)
Navel	Wet/dry shrivelled/swollen/pus
Anal area	Atresia/meconium/scour/blood
Legs	Normal/swollen joints/fracture/contracted tendons
Castration	No/yes (When? How?)
Tailing	No/yes (When? How?)

© CAB International 2025. *A Handbook for the Sheep Clinician, 8th Edition*
(A.C. Winter and D. Grove-White eds)
DOI: 10.1079/9781800626355.appx

Appendix 4
Assessing a Feed Ration for Adequacy – a Practical Problem

One of the simple nutritional problems which the practising veterinary surgeon can carry out is to decide if a group of sheep is thin because of inadequate feed or if some specific disease is involved. The following steps illustrate how to investigate the problem by an examination of what is being fed to the thin ewes. It should be emphasized that it is a simplification but will indicate if there is a gross imbalance in the requirements and the intake of the ewes. It has been used by student groups over many years and usually works.

Is thinness in a group of ewes due to feeding or is something else responsible?

The most common problem is when a group of pregnant ewes are housed and a significant number of them are in poor condition.

Work on metabolizable energy (ME) only

STEP 1. Assume the following approximate ME requirements of a 70 kg ewe, which is around the average weight of a lowland ewe:

Maintenance	10 MJ
At lambing with two/three lambs	20 MJ
Full lactation	30 MJ

These figures are easy to remember and any stage of gestation can be obtained by linear extrapolation between maintenance at 80 days and lambing at 145 days (e.g. day 115 is approximately 15 MJ).

If the ewes are significantly different in weight from this, maintenance ME can be obtained by the formula:

$$ME = 0.4(body\ weight)^{0.75}$$

For example for a 70 kg ewe ME = $0.4 \times 24.2 = 9.7$ MJ (rounded off above to 10 MJ).

Does the ration supply these requirements?

STEP 2. Examine the concentrate consumption. The farmer may know how many kilograms are fed daily or may state, for example, that 'six bucketsful are given to the group'. Weigh a bucketful and calculate how many kilograms are fed to the group. Count the number of ewes and let the quantity fed per ewe be 'c'.

1. Check the ME of the concentrate.
This may be: (i) obtained by asking the manufacturer; (ii) calculated from formulae; or (iii) assumed to be about 12.4 MJ/kg DM. This assumption is risky since some feeds (usually the cheaper ones) may be as low as 11.0 MJ/kg DM. Take great care to distinguish between values given by manufacturers for air-dry or oven-dry material. It is assumed that the value obtained is for oven-dry material (i.e. true DM).
2. Remember that the megajoule in (1) will be per kilogram DM. Since concentrates have a DM of about 85%, the DM intake will be 0.85c.
3. Calculate the mean intake of each ewe from the concentrate:

$$ME\ intake\ concentrate = 0.85c \times MJ$$
$$(e.g.\ \ 0.85c \times 12.4 = 10.5c)$$

STEP 3. Examine the forage consumption: The farmer may state that this is given *ad libitum* which should mean that there is always some available for the ewes (i.e. hay in the rack all day or self-feed silage). If this is not true when you visit the farm, the quantity fed must be measured by weighing a bale and asking how many bales are fed per day. If the forage is truly available *ad libitum*, work on

© CAB International 2025. *A Handbook for the Sheep Clinician, 8th Edition* (A.C. Winter and D. Grove-White eds)
DOI: 10.1079/9781800626355.appx

forage being consumed to appetite. (This is a problem in the calculation since so many factors influence food intake but a check is included later – see STEP 5).

(In the example given below it is assumed that the ewes are being given hay, but the calculation for other forages such as silage is identical. It is probably even more important to have the forage analysed as there are greater variations than for hay. The DM content of hay is around 85–90% whereas that for silage is 25–30% so a much greater weight of silage must be eaten to provide the same energy. It should be remembered that care must be taken with silage production to reduce the risk of listeriosis.)

1. Calculate forage consumed.
Assume a 70 kg ewe has an intake of approximately 2% of bodyweight equating to 1.5 kg DM, which is reasonable if they are fed medium or good quality hay. If the hay is poor, with a ME of 8, the intake will be less, around 1.25 kg DM.

> DM forage consumed
> $= 1.5 - $ concentrate consumed
> $= 1.5 - 0.85c$

2. Calculate the ME of the forage.
This can be obtained by: (i) analysis; (ii) calculation; or (iii) by estimating the quality and assuming that poor, medium and good quality hay will have values of approximately 8, 9 and 10 MJ/kg DM, respectively. The values for silage are higher than for hay and the corresponding values are 9.5, 10.6 and 11.7, respectively.

> ME intake forage $= (1.5 - 0.85c)$
> $\times$ ME forage
> For example with medium quality hay
> $= (1.5 - 0.85c) \times 9$

STEP 4. Calculate the total ME intake:

> Total ME intake $=$ ME from concentrate
> plus ME from forage
> $= 0.85c \times$ ME concentrate
> $+ (1.5 - 0.85c)$
> $\times$ ME forage

For example:

> Total ME intake $= 0.85c \times 12.4$
> $+ (1.5 - 0.85c) \times 9$

STEP 5. Look at modifying factors on the farm: These calculations have made a number of assumptions, some of which can be checked on the farm.

1. Check that your calculation of forage agrees roughly with what is fed (i.e. weigh and count bales).

2. Allow for wastage of forage if this is not fed *ad libitum*, which will depend on its quality. Look at the bedding and see how much hay can be seen and observe the ewes eating and see how much they reject. As an estimate, wastage of good hay will be about 5% and can be ignored but poor hay may have wastage of 20%. Make an allowance for this in your calculations unless the hay is truly *ad libitum*.

3. Look at the trough space which should be at least 45 cm for each ewe in the group. Watch the ewes when they are given concentrates and see if many are forced to snatch small quantities and keep moving. Each ewe should be able to stand fairly quietly and eat its share. Watch for bullying which may give rise to a small number of thin (bullied) ewes with the rest normal or overfat.

4. Ask if there are any ewes with particular requirements. We have assumed that the ewes are uniform but different lamb numbers, initial condition, etc. may need to be taken into consideration.

A calculated example

A 70 kg Mule ewe at 115 days of gestation given hay *ad libitum* with an analysis of 9.0 MJ/kg DM and 0.25 kg of a concentrate with ME of 12.4 MJ/kg DM. Is this diet adequate to maintain body condition?

> Requirement $=$ approximately 15 MJ
> Intake $= 0.85 \times 0.25 \times 12.4 + (1.5 - 0.85$
> $\times 0.25) \times 9$ (from STEP 4 above)

Intake $=$ 14.2 MJ ME, which is just less than requirement, so some loss in condition will result and it would be preferable to increase the concentrate fed slightly.

Appendix 5
Professional Development – Specialist Societies

Most countries with a significant sheep population have an organization with a specialist interest in sheep, small ruminants or perhaps one combined with beef cattle, for which details will be available from country or state veterinary organizations.

Sheep Veterinary Society (SVS)

This is a specialist division of the British Veterinary Association (BVA) and membership is open to all members of the veterinary profession (whether BVA members or not) and others interested in sheep. The Society holds two meetings a year – in spring (now often on Zoom) and in autumn – which usually include farm visits as well as lectures and discussion in a friendly atmosphere. Membership is a must for all who wish to keep up with developments in sheep veterinary work. Sometimes the Society holds a meeting in another country (for example, meetings have been held in Denmark, Holland, Germany, Spain and Canada). Contact the Secretariat at:

Sheep Veterinary Society (www.sheepvetsoc.org.uk)
Moredun Research Institute
Pentlands Science Park
Bush Loan
Penicuik
Midlothian
EH26 OPZ
UK

International Sheep Veterinary Congresses and the International Sheep Veterinary Association

International meetings for veterinarians interested in sheep have been held every fourth (moving to every third) year for over 35 years, initiated by the SVS in the UK. Meetings have been held in the UK, New Zealand, Australia, South Africa, Greece, Norway and Spain. The International Sheep Veterinary Association has been set up to foster relationships between sheep veterinarians worldwide and to oversee decisions regarding the sites for future international congresses (www.intsheepvetassoc.org).

SPECIALIST QUALIFICATIONS FOR SHEEP VETERINARIANS

The Royal College of Veterinary Surgeons (RCVS)

The RCVS offers the Certificate in Advanced Veterinary Practice (CertAVP) which has a flexible modular approach that enables vets to design their own post-graduate certificate according to their particular interests. This includes sheep. See https://www.rcvs.org.uk/lifelong-learning/postgraduate-qualifications/certificate-in-advanced-veterinary-practice-certavp/ (accessed 9/11/24) for full details. The RCVS Diploma in Sheep Health and Production (DSHP) is no longer offered.

European College of Small Ruminant Health Management

This college is a member of the European Board of Veterinary Specialities and is responsible for approving residents and training establishments and for awarding the DipECSRHM. The diploma is only achievable by examination. Although this is a European college, several notable *de facto* diplomates are from countries outside Europe, for example New Zealand, South Africa and Canada. Details are on their website https://ecsrhm.org.

Many other countries have schemes for achieving specialist sheep veterinary qualifications and information about these will be available from country or state veterinary authorities or other local veterinary organizations.

DOI: 10.1079/9781800626355.appx

Index

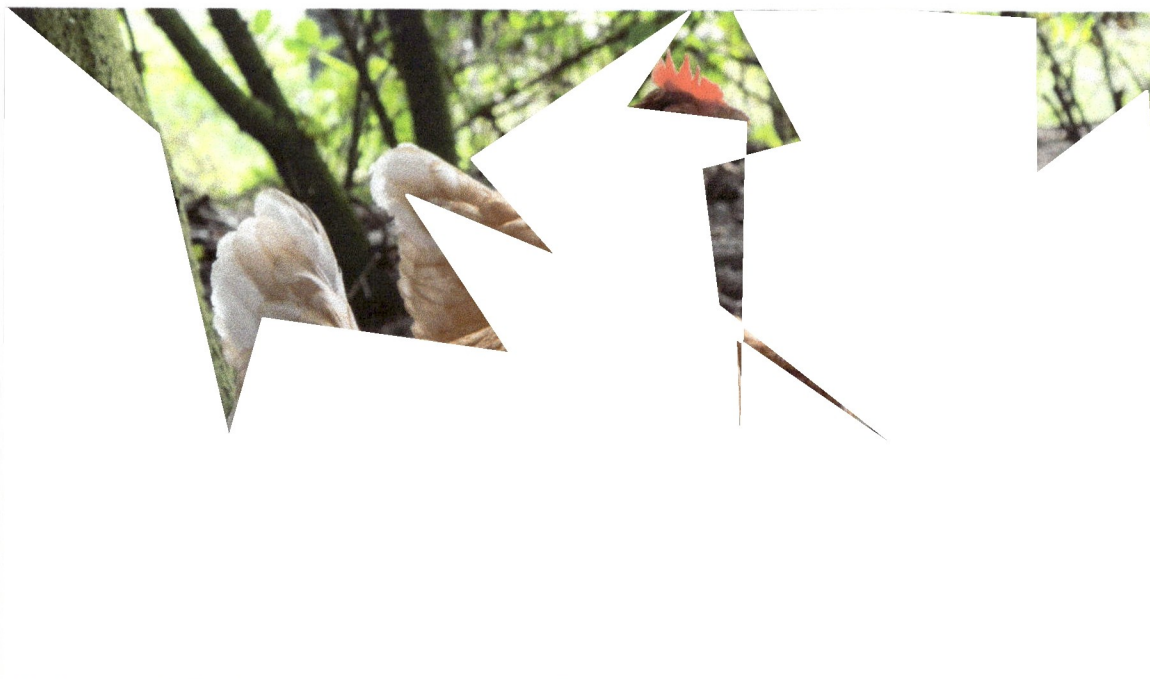

This book is published by **CABI**, an international not-for-profit organisation that improves people's lives worldwide by providing information and applying scientific expertise to solve problems in agriculture and the environment.

CABI is also a global publisher producing key scientific publications, including world renowned databases, as well as compendia, books, ebooks and full text electronic resources. We publish content in a wide range of subject areas including: agriculture and crop science / animal and veterinary sciences / ecology and conservation / environmental science / horticulture and plant sciences / human health, food science and nutrition / international development / leisure and tourism.

The profits from CABI's publishing activities enable us to work with farming communities around the world, supporting them as they battle with poor soil, invasive species and pests and diseases, to improve their livelihoods and help provide food for an ever growing population.

CABI is an international intergovernmental organisation, and we gratefully acknowledge the core financial support from our member countries (and lead agencies) including:

UKaid
from the British people

Ministry of Agriculture
People's Republic of China

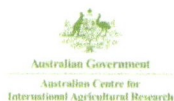

Australian Government
Australian Centre for
International Agricultural Research

Agriculture and
Agri-Food Canada

Ministry of Foreign Affairs of the
Netherlands

Schweizerische Eidgenossenschaft
Confédération suisse
Confederazione Svizzera
Confederaziun svizra

Swiss Agency for Development
and Cooperation SDC

Discover more

To read more about CABI's work, please visit: **www.cabi.org**

Browse our books or explore our online products at **https://www.cabidigitallibrary.org**

Interested in writing for CABI? Find information for authors here: **https://www.cabidigitallibrary.org/books/authors**